A Handbook for Dental Hygienists

CW00793246

A Handbook for Dental Hygienists

FOURTH EDITION

W. J. N. Collins MSc, BDS, FDSRCPS (Glas)
Chief Dental Officer, Northern Ireland
Formerly Director, Schools of Dental Hygiene
Glasgow Dental Hospital and Royal Army Dental Corps

T. F. Walsh DDS, BDS, MSc, FDSRCS (Eng)
Professor of Restorative Dentistry, University of Sheffield
Honorary Consultant, Central Sheffield University Hospitals NHS Trust

K. H. Figures MDS, BDS, FDSRCS (Edin)
Director, School of Dental Hygiene and Dental Therapy,
School of Clinical Dentistry, University of Sheffield

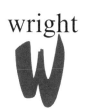

wright

EDINBURGH LONDON NEW YORK OXFORD PHILADELPHIA ST LOUIS SYDNEY
TORONTO 1999

Wright
An imprint of Elsevier Limited

First published 1978
Second edition 1986
Third edition 1992
Fourth edition 1999
    Reprinted 2000, 2001, 2002, 2003, 2004, 2005

ISBN 0 7236 1740 6

British Library Cataloguing in Publication Data
A catalogue record for this book is available from the British Library

Library of Congress Cataloguing in Publication Data
A catalogue record for this book is available from the Library of
Congress

your source for books,
journals and multimedia
in the health sciences

www.elsevierhealth.com

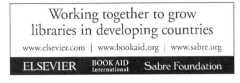

Working together to grow
libraries in developing countries

www.elsevier.com | www.bookaid.org | www.sabre.org

ELSEVIER   BOOK AID International   Sabre Foundation

The
publisher's
policy is to use
**paper manufactured
from sustainable forests**

Typeset by Bath Typesetting
Printed and bound in China

Contents

Foreword to the Fourth Edition		*vii*
Foreword to the Third Edition		*viii*
Foreword to the First Edition		*ix*
Preface		*xi*
1	The training and employment of dental hygienists	1
2	General histology	11
3	Systems of the body	21
4	Regional anatomy	38
5	Tooth morphology	59
6	Oral histology and physiology	68
7	Microbiology, cross-infection and immunity	90
8	General pathology	106
9	Plaque, calculus and stains	111
10	Dental caries	119
11	Inflammatory periodontal diseases	129
12	Epidemiology of dental diseases	150
13	Oral medicine	158
14	Abnormalities of the teeth	167
15	Dentine sensitivity	173
16	Emergencies in the dental surgery	178
17	Patients with special needs	185
18	Instrument care and use	199
19	Rubber dam application	210
20	Prevention of dental diseases	215
21	Dental radiography	239
22	Local analgesia and pharmacology	252
23	Oral health education	262
Index		275

Foreword to the fourth edition

By Dr Margaret Seward CBE
MDS, FDS, MCCD, DDSc, DDS, Hon FDSRCS (Edin)
President of the General Dental Council
Former Vice-President of the British Dental Hygienists' Association

When a book appears in its fourth edition you can be assured that it is a winner. This is the case for the Handbook for Dental Hygienists which has indeed become a winner with student hygienists, not only in the schools of dental hygiene and other training establishments in this country, but also around the world. This is not surprising as the three eminent authors have brought their lifetimes' experiences of training dental hygienists to the task. Now, in this edition they have not only redesigned the format so that it is more reader-friendly but have also incorporated the important and exciting advances that have recently occurred in the practice of dentistry, particularly in the field of dental hygiene.

The developing role of the oral health team in the delivery of dental health care and the increasing realization that maintenance of oral health is essential for general well being, brings new significance to the role of the hygienist as a member of a profession complementary to dentistry.

Changes currently proposed by the General Dental Council, supporting the philosophy of skill mix working in primary dental care, could increase the opportunities for hygienists to use their unique skills and knowledge for the benefit of patients. If and when these changes occur, it will be essential to possess the firm basis of theoretical knowledge which is provided comprehensively by the authors in this Handbook.

Today learning is a continuum, and a hygienist in company with all members of the dental team, is obliged as a health professional to keep up to date. This Handbook also provides an excellent refresher course for those returning to practice after a career break, as well as giving suggestions for further reading on selected topics. I welcome this fourth edition, confident that it will become even more popular than its predecessors, with a new generation of readers.

Foreword to the third edition

By Professor David K. Mason
BDS, MD, FDS, FRCPath
President of the General Dental Council

As Dr G. H. Leatherman predicted in his Foreword to the first edition, this Handbook for Dental Hygienists has become a standard textbook for dental hygienists and training establishments throughout the world. Another new edition, the third, so soon after the second, is testimony both to the continuing usefulness and attractive format of this text and also the many changes that have occurred in the practice of dentistry.

The book incorporates much new information and still maintains its objective of being comprehensive and covering the whole dental hygienists' course. The format of this new edition has changed somewhat in that in some sections the information is updated and yet presented even more concisely. As a consequence of the recent changes which have allowed hygienists to give local analgesia under supervision in the United Kingdom this subject is given particular emphasis and a new section on cross-infection is included.

The authors are to be congratulated on maintaining the high standard of the first two editions whilst encompassing new developments and further broadening the scope of this book. These days when the role of all members of the dental team is under consideration it is invaluable to have the present educational course for hygienists so clearly defined.

Foreword to the first edition

By Gerald H. Leatherman
DMD, FDS, RCS (Eng & Edin), FFD, RCS (Ire), DSc, DOdont
Executive Director Emeritus of Fédération Dentaire Internationale,
Honorary President of the British Dental Hygienists' Association

The whole of my professional life as a practising dentist was based on the necessity for a clean mouth as a sound foundation for oral health.

Socio-economic and manpower developments in the delivery of dental services to the world's populations have influenced not only the dental profession, but governments, to plan for an ever-increasing use of auxiliary services, including the dental hygienist.

As an 'operating auxiliary' the dental hygienist can be described as a 'person who is permitted to carry out to the prescription of a supervising dentist certain specific preventive and treatment measures, including some operative procedures in the treatment of periodontal disease. The dental hygienist is not permitted to carry out any operative procedures for the treatment of dental caries' (Slack G. L. (1974) *Dental Public Health: An Introduction to Community Dentistry*. Bristol, Wright, p. 205).

The authors of this book are to be commended for producing a textbook which not only provides a comprehensive theoretical course for student hygienists, but will have great, continuing, educational value for all members of the dental team and those concerned with its maintenance and function.

I can visualize this publication becoming a standard textbook in many of the training establishments for dental hygienists throughout the world.

The authors are to be congratulated on their efforts to assist in the training of personnel who are able to play a major part in improving the dental health of the peoples of the world.

Preface

Since the publication of the third edition of this book in 1993, a number of important changes have taken place in relation to the training and the scope of work of dental hygienists in the United Kingdom. Not least of these is the extension of the minimum length of training from one to two years. This improvement has allowed for some easing of what had become an excessively crowded course content; for more time to allow assimilation of the facts being taught and for the inclusion of new topics such as practical dental radiography.

Recently, the General Dental Council has ruled that the application of rubber dam is a legitimate role of the dental hygienist. It has also recommended that the regulations be altered to permit the dental hygienist to place a temporary restoration in a situation where a filling is dislodged during treatment. Naturally these changes have been reflected in the content of this edition.

The publication of the important Nuffield Report *The Education and Training of Personnel Auxiliary to Dentistry* in 1993 gave impetus to a great deal of activity in this field. Possible future outcomes are the registration of all dental professionals, including dental nurses and technicians, with the General Dental Council, the extension of the clinical duties of existing groups such as dental hygienists and therapists and the development of new professions complementary to dentistry such as orthodontic auxiliaries and clinical dental technicians. It has also stimulated a significant increase in the training of dental therapists and of joint hygienist/therapist courses. These are exciting changes that will undoubtedly affect the content and format of future editions of this book, but it is too early in their development for them to influence this edition.

We have also taken account of the numerous requests received to increase the information given in relation to the cause and management of dentine sensitivity. A new chapter has been added in which the various references to this subject in previous editions have been incorporated and extended.

As would be expected, there has been a great deal of updating of the information contained within this book, but we have also extensively changed and modernized the format in the hope of making it more readable and more easily assimilated. In order to accommodate the increased information contained in many important areas without significantly increasing the size and cost of the book, we have taken the opportunity to prune some of the peripheral topics.

Our aim in producing this book is to provide the student dental hygienist with a general text covering all aspects of the theoretical content of the training course. Clearly reference must be made by the student to other more detailed texts where appropriate and for this reason we have attempted to provide guidance on further reading at the end of each chapter. As with previous editions, we make no attempt to describe in detail the practical skills required by the dental hygienist. These can only be learned whilst treating patients in the clinic.

We would like to acknowledge the help received from many sources in producing this fourth edition. In particular we would like to thank Paul Nixon for his advice on the dental radiography sections and our wives for their understanding and support.

W. J. N. Collins
T. F. Walsh
K. H. Figures

1

The training and employment of dental hygienists

Historical background

The first training programme for dental hygienists was organized in the USA in 1913. Since then the role of the hygienist has changed only in scope. Originally, their main task was that of 'dental prophylaxis' (that is the prevention of dental disease), a term which has now become synonymous with routine cleansing of the surfaces of the teeth by the dentist or dental hygienist.

At its inception, the dental hygienist programme met with considerable opposition in the USA, principally from dentists, and it would be foolish to deny that there are still opponents within the profession; happily in ever diminishing numbers. The opposition was inspired initially by fear of the lesser qualified intruder, with what was seen as 'dilution of the profession', and by a lack of appreciation of the true role of the hygienist in the field of dentistry. Gradually there has been, and continues to be a better appreciation amongst dentists and their patients of the true value of a team approach to dental care. Dr Leatherman, who wrote the foreword to the first edition of this book, once stated that the relationship between the dentist and the hygienist could be compared to gin and tonic. When tonic is added to gin, it is seen to enhance it rather than dilute it.

Currently in the UK, following the publication of the 1993 Nuffield Inquiry into the 'Education and Training of Personnel Auxiliary to Dentistry', there has been much interest in the possible expansion of the types, roles and usage of dental auxiliaries. No doubt there will be many exciting developments in this area in the future, but it is to be expected that dental hygienists will remain centrally important to the prevention of dental diseases. All indications suggest that their numbers and their contribution to improving dental health will continue to increase.

It can be argued that, in the past, there has been a misapprehension within the dental profession of the correct approach to the dental problems of mankind. For years the dentist was taught and applied a mechanistic attitude to dental breakdown and was content to repair as well as possible, with the tools and materials available, the ravages of disease. The more complicated and intricate the repair procedures, the higher the dentist's status in the profession.

There have always been dentists who were dissatisfied with this approach and who felt that dental disease could and should be prevented. As early as 1844, Dr D. D. Smith of Philadelphia was advocating preventive treatment for 'the reduction of decay and general betterment of mouth health'. Early observations showed that the cleaner the mouth was kept, the healthier the gums around the teeth became, but even had the early 20th century dentists not been able to demonstrate this to their entire satisfaction, they were advancing into an age where cleanliness was synonymous with health in all aspects.

Since 1913, when the first dental hygiene school was opened in Bridgeport, Connecticut by Dr Alfred C. Fones, the training and employment of dental hygienists has spread throughout much of the world. In the UK the hygienists' history is just over fifty years long. Whereas there were dentists contemporary with Smith in the 19th century who believed in prevention, no organized hygienist programme came into existence until World War II. The Royal Air Force Dental Branch commenced training young women in 1943 in a 16-week intensive course, and by the end of the war much excellent work had been carried out by these women, especially in the field of gingival health. The importance today of the success of the RAF dental hygienist service during the war is not only that this was used as a basis on which all later training methods were built, but that hundreds of young dentists, many of whom had gone straight into the service from dental school, were able to work with and observe the excellent results obtained by these trained 'technicians'. There was also the beginning of a team approach to dental problems and so, at a later date, the introduction of the dental hygienist to the profession as a whole was made much easier by the more favourable attitude of the same dentists, many of whom were in practice or other positions of importance by this time.

Much of the credit for the development of the dental hygienist profession within the UK must be given to the vision of Sir William Kelsey Fry whose drive initiated the programme in the RAF and later inspired the civilian training plans.

In 1948, an experimental government-sponsored training scheme was set up in the Eastman Dental Hospital, London, for a period of 5 years. By the time it ended in 1953 about 150 hygienists had been trained. Government regulations were finally formulated in 1957 and the first definitive training of hygienists started in Manchester Dental Hospital in 1959; other schools soon followed. Currently there are 17 UK dental hygiene schools. Two schools have also been established in the Republic of Ireland (Table 1.1).

A number of the UK dental hygiene schools run programmes designed in such a way that the student can qualify simultaneously as both dental hygienist and dental therapist. Others run shortened training courses to allow hygienists to gain the additional therapist qualification or vice versa.

Since the formal training programmes came

Table 1.1 The location of dental hygiene schools in the UK and Ireland

Dental hygiene schools are located at the following places.

In the UK
- The dental hospitals of Belfast, Birmingham, Bristol, Cardiff, Dundee, Edinburgh, Glasgow, Leeds, Liverpool, Manchester, Newcastle and Sheffield.
- In London, at the Eastman, Guy's, Kings and St Bartholomew's & Royal London dental hospitals.
- At the Defence Dental Agency's Training Establishment in Aldershot.

In the Republic of Ireland
- In Dublin and Cork dental hospitals.

into existence there has been a steady increase of interest in the employment of hygienists within the profession, and the present situation in the UK is that the demand for hygienists by all sections of the profession exceeds the supply. The number of dental hygienists enrolled with the General Dental Council on 31st December 1990 was 2648. This number has shown a steady increase each year and on 31st December 1997 it was 3903.

Scope of work

The rules governing all aspects of the training and practice of dental hygienists are laid down in the Dental Auxiliary Regulations, 1986, but paragraph 23, relating to the scope of work permitted, was modified by the Dental Auxiliary (Amendment) Regulations of 1991 (Table 1.2).

In summary, these regulations allow the dental hygienist to carry out the full range of treatment listed, provided there is an outline of treatment written by the dentist. It need hardly be added that such written instructions should be retained as part of the patients' notes. Only when local analgesia is being administered by the hygienist, is the dentist required to be on the premises.

Just how detailed the written prescription must be cannot be fully set down in regulations. Such general phrases such as '*Scale and polish – three visits*', '*Maintenance visit every three months*' or '*Use local analgesia as necessary*'

Table 1.2 Dental hygienists' scope of work

Paragraph 23 of the Dental Auxiliary (Amendment) Regulations of 1991, which relates to a dental hygienist's scope of work states the following.

1. Subject to the provision of this regulation, a dental hygienist shall be permitted to carry out dental work (amounting to the practice of dentistry) of the following kinds.
    (a) Cleaning and polishing teeth.
    (b) Scaling teeth (that is to say, removal of deposits, accretions and stains from those parts of the surfaces of the teeth which are exposed or which are directly beneath the free margins of the gums, including the application of medicaments appropriate thereto);
    (c) The application to the teeth of such prophylactic materials as the Council may from time to time determine;
    A dental hygienist shall not be permitted to carry out dental work amounting to the practice of dentistry of any other kind except that the scaling of teeth under sub-paragraph (b) above may be carried out by a dental hygienist under local infiltration analgesia administered by the dental hygienist or any regional or block analgesia administered by a registered dentist.
2. A dental hygienist shall not be permitted to carry out such dental work authorized as aforesaid except under the direction of a registered dentist and after the registered dentist has examined the patient and has indicated in writing to the dental hygienist the course of treatment to be provided for the patient.
3. A dental hygienist shall administer local infiltration analgesia authorized as aforesaid only under the direct personal supervision of a registered dentist who is on the premises at which the hygienist is carrying out such work at the time at which it is being carried out.

would seem to be adequate, but specific mention should be made of anything beyond normal routine, such as the use of specific topical anti-microbial agents. No instructions exist with regard to the length of time a dental hygienist can care for a patient under a programme of maintenance without the dentist seeing the patient and renewing the prescription. It would be reasonable to expect this period to vary depending on the needs of individual patients, but it would seem prudent to avoid the time stretching much beyond a year.

The UK General Dental Council has from time to time given guidance on the interpretation of the regulations with regard to individual aspects of treatment. For example, fissure sealants, topical fluorides and desensitizing agents are all included in 23(1)(c) and sub-gingival slow release anti-microbial agents are included in 23(1)(b). It has also ruled that dental hygienists may place rubber dam in the course of procedures such as fissure sealing teeth. Some areas are quite complicated and new procedures are constantly being introduced. Consequently, should a dental hygienist be in any doubt about the legality of carrying out a certain form of treatment, either the GDC or a professional defence organization should be contacted for guidance.

Training

Guidelines for the running of UK dental hygienist training courses are set out in the 'Curriculum for Dental Hygienists', published by the GDC. This document points out that a course of training 'should extend over a period of two academic years' and should involve at least 50% of the training time being 'devoted to clinical dental practice'. It also identifies the entry requirements (Table 1.3).

Table 1.3 Requirements for entry into UK dental hygiene schools

To gain entry to a UK dental hygiene school, applicants must have the following educational qualifications

Without dental nurse experience:
*   Five GCSE passes at grade C or above or five Scottish Standard Grades at grade 3 or above; plus
*   Two A level passes at grade E or above or three Scottish Higher Grades at grade C or above; or
*   other equivalent qualifications.

With dental nurse experience:
*   Five GCSE passes at grade C or above or five Scottish Standard Grades at grade 3 or above, or some other equivalent qualification; plus
*   a nationally recognized dental nursing certificate.

The 'Curriculum for Dental Hygienists' lists the following details with regard to the training course content.

Course theoretical content

Outline guidance in relation to courses is given below. Educational establishments and other organizations requiring further detail of the course should refer to the Dental Hygiene Course Syllabus and Training Objectives produced by the Directors and Tutors of Schools of Dental Hygiene Group.

Foundation course

A Foundation Course outlining the work to be undertaken by the dental hygienist and including their professional, legal and ethical obligations, Health and Safety issues and first aid. The precise content of this course will depend on the previous educational background and experience of students.

An introduction to Teamwork in Health Care, dental auxiliaries and current national and international trends in the delivery of dental care.

An introduction to patient care and management including the need to follow a written treatment plan and the need to keep adequate records.

Cell biology and general histology

An understanding of cell biology including the cellular structure and function of human tissues and organs.

General anatomy and physiology

A general understanding of all the systems of the body, with a more detailed knowledge of the structure and function of the following systems: circulatory system, respiratory system, digestive system, nervous system, skeletal system, lymphatic system, endocrine system.

Regional anatomy

An overall understanding of the regional anatomy of the head and neck, with increasing content in relation to the para-oral structures and fine detail of the oral cavity structure.

Dental anatomy

An understanding of:
- the anatomy and development of the human deciduous and permanent dentitions;
- the anatomy and development of oral tissues and related structures;
- the processes of eruption and resorption.

The identification of teeth and the use of current terminology and methods for nomenclature and charting.

A knowledge of the morphology of the permanent and deciduous teeth.

Oral and dental histology and embryology

An understanding of the histology and embryology of human teeth, their supporting structures and other oral tissues.

An understanding of the functions of these various tissues.

Oral physiology

An understanding of:
- the composition and functions of saliva;
- the processes of mastication and deglutition;
- the physiology of taste.

Diet and nutrition

A knowledge of the principles of the diet and nutrition and an understanding of their scientific basis with particular reference to:
- the composition of diet;
- the relationship of diet to general health, dental and oral health;
- the role of diet in the aetiology of dental caries;
- the dietary requirement of groups with special needs and the influence on diet of age, culture and occupation.

An ability to carry out diet analysis and provide advice and counselling for the prevention of dental disease.

General pathology

An ability to define the common terms and methods used in pathology.

An understanding of:
- acute and chronic inflammation;
- wound healing;
- routes of spread of infection;
- immunology;
- neoplasia.

A knowledge of the common pathological conditions relevant to patients' medical histories.

A knowledge of the relevant diseases of childhood and their dental implications.

Microbiology and infection control

An understanding of:
- the classifications and characteristics of micro-organisms;
- the relationship between micro-organisms and disease.

A precise knowledge of the modes of transmission of disease.

A detailed knowledge of the principles of infection control and an ability to implement them.

Pharmacology

A knowledge of:
- the legal control of drugs and the principles of pharmacokinetics;
- the therapeutic agents commonly used in medicine and dentistry with particular reference to those of significance to the dental hygienist.

Local analgesia

A detailed knowledge of the related oral anatomy and nerve supply.

A basic understanding of the physiology of nerve conduction.

A knowledge of the pharmacokinetics and use of local analgesic agents available in dentistry.

An ability to carry out the safe practice of local infiltration techniques.

Medical emergencies and their management

An ability to recognize potential and actual medical emergencies and to understand their causes.

The ability to follow the necessary procedures to deal effectively with an emergency and to carry out the technique of cardiopulmonary resuscitation (CPR).

Tooth deposits and stains

A comprehensive knowledge of 'dental plaque' and its formation and development from a clean tooth surface until its maturity with special reference to the micro-organisms involved.

A detailed knowledge of the role of plaque in the aetiology of caries and periodontal diseases.

The ability to recognize supragingival and subgingival calculus together with a knowledge of formation and the various means of detection.

The ability to recognize the common types of intrinsic and extrinsic staining and a knowledge of their origins and methods of removal.

Theory of periodontal instrumentation

An ability to describe:
- the principles of scaling, root planing/debridement;
- the design of scaling instruments and their use;
- the action of mechanical scalers, their advantages and disadvantages;
- the uses of polishing instruments and the different prophylactic pastes available.

Dental caries

A detailed knowledge of the aetiology of dental caries.

A general knowledge of the clinical and histopathological changes that occur in dental caries.

A good understanding of the epidemiology of dental caries relating this to the relevant studies.

Periodontal disease

A full understanding of the causes of all forms of periodontal diseases, including the initiating, predisposing and systemic factors.

An ability to:
- classify the different types of periodontal diseases;

- recognize a healthy periodontium and the clinical changes which occur in the presence of periodontal diseases;
- record and monitor various parameters associated with disease activity and its aetiology, e.g. pocket charting and indices;
- recognize and distinguish between acute and chronic periodontal disease;
- recognize those periodontal conditions which necessitate the immediate attention of a registered dentist.

A thorough understanding of the role of the immune system and other systemic factors in the aetiology of periodontal disease.

An understanding of:
- those factors which adversely affect the prognosis in periodontal disease;
- the features and aetiologies of lateral periodontal abscesses, apical abscesses (both acute and chronic) and perio-endo lesions.

Epidemiology

An understanding of the basis for epidemiological studies in the provision of oral health care.

A knowledge of the indices used in oral epidemiological studies and an ability to use common plaque, gingival and periodontal indices.

An understanding of the basic statistical methodology used in the planning and interpretation of epidemiological studies.

A knowledge of the major epidemiological studies of oral disease, the changing pattern of oral and dental diseases, and the cause and effect of the changes.

An ability to interpret the findings of epidemiological studies.

Dental public health

An understanding of:
- public health measures in the control of disease and the promotion of health;
- the principles of health promotion, including oral health promotion.

A knowledge of:
- the structures of public health services;
- community based oral health initiatives.

Oral pathology and oral medicine

A basic knowledge of the aetiology and features of tooth anomalies.

The ability to recognize and ascribe causes for tooth wear (tooth surface loss).

A knowledge of the features and aetiology of oral lesions e.g. ulcers, white lesions etc. and their implications.

The ability to recognize the common oral infections.

An awareness of the differing features of benign and malignant lesions and their significance.

A knowledge of the causes, significance and local management of xerostomia.

A basic knowledge of the common causes of facial pain and the relevance of temporomandibular joint (TMJ) disorders to patient care.

An ability to recognize changes from normal in the oral tissues and seek appropriate advice.

General dentistry

A general understanding of restorative dentistry including prosthetics, orthodontics, paediatric dentistry and oral and maxillo-facial surgery.

A thorough understanding of the role of the dental hygienist in these areas and in the holistic care of the patient.

A knowledge of the dental management of patients with special needs (mental, physical, medical, social) and their care in different environments.

A knowledge of the physiology of ageing and the management problems associated with the dental care of the elderly.

A knowledge of the principles and problems involved in providing domiciliary dental care.

Dental radiography

A knowledge of legislation and regulations relating to dental radiography and ionizing radiation.

A basic knowledge of ionizing radiation and its effect on tissues.

A full understanding of the hazards involved in dental radiography and the measures to be taken to protect patient and operator during the taking of dental radiographs.

A knowledge of the different types of radiographs and their uses in dentistry.

The ability to identify the anatomical features and common pathology visible on dental radiographs.

The ability to interpret dental radiographs, as relevant to dental hygienists.

A knowledge of:
- the techniques for taking dental radiographs;
- the principles of processing dental radiographs and the faults which may occur;
- the importance of quality assurance in dental radiography.

Preventive dentistry

A thorough understanding of the principles of prevention of dental disease with an appreciation of the dynamics involved including therapeutic, educational, social and environmental factors.

A comprehensive knowledge of:
- mechanical and chemical plaque control methods, including modified methods for patients with special needs;
- the role of fluoride in preventive dentistry; topical and systemic delivery;
- the principles and methods of dietary control of dental caries;
- the composition, properties, techniques and uses of fissure sealants and other preventive materials currently available.

Behavioural sciences

An understanding of human development with specific reference to:

- child growth;
- physical, mental and emotional development.

A sufficient knowledge of psychology and sociology to better understand human behaviour and in particular health behaviour.

An awareness in general of the influence of social, psychological, cultural and environmental factors on human behaviour and in particular the impact of these factors on oral health and the delivery of dental care.

A knowledge and understanding of the theories and methodology relating to communication and of the importance of developing inter-personal skills. An appreciation of the relevance of listening, and of verbal and non-verbal communication.

The ability to recognize potential barriers to effective communication and behaviour modification, the ability to develop skills to minimize such barriers.

An understanding of techniques for management of the anxious patient.

An appreciation of the relationship between behavioural science and patient education, patient management and successful teamwork including inter-professional collaboration and communication.

Oral health education

A detailed knowledge of the principles of education and of the methodology of oral health education with particular reference to planning, delivery and evaluation.

An appreciation of the fundamental role of communication skills.

A comprehensive knowledge of the scientific basis of oral health education.

An understanding of the relationship of oral health education to general health education.

Medical conditions of oral significance

A thorough knowledge of the following:

- the recording of a patient's medical history;
- patients' medical conditions which might affect the treatment given by a dental hygienist or the health of members of the dental team.

An understanding of the oral manifestation of systemic disease.

Practical training

Approximately half the time spent in training should be devoted to practical clinical procedures.

Pre-clinical training

Facilities should be available for students to develop their practical skills using phantom head and other appropriate laboratory aids, before working on patients.

The students should be able to identify and select the appropriate equipment, instruments and materials for the task to be carried out, use instruments safely and effectively, and maintain them to the required standard.

Students should be able to organize their working environment.

Clinical training

Scope

Adequate experience should be provided in the full range of practical procedures as permitted by the Council's Regulations including:

- preventive procedures such as topical fluoride applications and fissure sealant placement (including the fitting of rubber dam where appropriate);
- periodontal therapies such as the polishing of the teeth (including teeth previously filled or crowned), supra- and sub-gingival scaling, root surface debridement, pocket irrigation, the placement of sub-gingival anti-microbial agents and the care of dental implants;
- local infiltration analgesia;
- radiographic techniques of oral relevance including the taking of periapical, bite-wing, occlusal and panoramic radiographs and the processing of films;
- measurements and assessments, including periodontal charting and the use of oral hygiene, gingival and periodontal indices.

Types of patients

The Council considers that, during their training, student dental hygienists should, in association with other members of the dental team, treat the full range of adult and child patients, including medically compromised children and adults and those with physical or mental disabilities.

Locations

The Council also considers that the opportunity should be given for students to work or observe in a variety of working conditions, such as community dental clinics, in-patient hospital facilities, general dental practice and the domiciliary setting.

Practical oral health education

Practical participation in the planning, provision and evaluation of oral health education programmes and the practical demonstration of communication skills with individuals and diversity of target groups.

Preparation for employment

A knowledge of the organization of dentistry in the UK and the structure of the NHS.

An understanding of the legal position of enrolled dental hygienists, including the type of work they are allowed to carry out and the areas they are permitted to work in, under the direction and written prescription of a registered dentist.

An understanding of the standard of conduct expected of an enrolled dental hygienist and the kind of behaviour which may be regarded as misconduct.

An understanding of, and the need to comply with, the legal requirement for annual enrolment for dental hygienists in employment.

An understanding of the importance for dental hygienists in employment to have membership with a relevant medical/dental protection agency.

An understanding of the importance of a contract of employment.

An understanding of the role of the British Dental Hygienists' Association.

A full appreciation of the importance of continuing education, clinical audit and quality assurance programmes throughout a dental hygienist's professional working life.

A thorough knowledge of the Health and Safety regulations pertaining to dental practice.

An understanding of the role of the dental hygienist within the framework of a dental team.

Final examination

At the end of the course the students sit an examination which is set and controlled by the Central Examining Board for Dental Hygienists (Table 1.4).

Table 1.4 Student dental hygienists' final examination

The Central Examining Board's final examination has the following parts.

Two written papers
- Paper 1: the candidate must answer two essay-type questions from a selection of three.
- Paper 2: the candidate must answer one of two essay-type questions and fifty objective questions.

Practical test
The candidate must carry out the necessary scaling, root planing and polishing to an agreed part of the dentition of a patient who has received previous treatment by the candidate and be prepared to discuss the case history, previous treatment and advice given to the patient. Local analgesia should be used where appropriate. Other practical tasks can be set on a previously unseen patient should there be any difficulty with the patient originally chosen.

Oral examination
This lasts for ten minutes and is used to confirm the examiner's opinion of the candidate's competence.

After the examination, the successful candidates are awarded the General Dental Council Diploma in Dental Hygiene, which entitles them to enrolment on the General Dental Council's Roll of Dental Hygienists.

Employment

On qualification and before taking up employment as a dental hygienist, there are certain things which either must or should be done (Table 1.5).

Table 1.5 Tasks to be completed before starting employment

After qualifying and before starting to work as a hygienist in the UK, a hygienist should consider the following requirements.

- **Legal obligation:** enrol with the General Dental Council.
- **Important precaution:** join a professional defence organization.
- **Desirable professionalism:** join the British Dental Hygienists' Association.

Enrolment

It is against the law for a dental hygienist to practise without having enrolled with the GDC. Each year, on 1st December, the Registrar of the GDC sends out an application form for retention of a name on the roll to every hygienist currently on it. This must be returned immediately, with the required fee. If it is not received by the Registrar by 31st December, that name will be removed from the roll and it costs an additional fee to have it restored. Any hygienist continuing to practise, having allowed the enrolment to expire, whether wilfully or accidentally, will become liable to disciplinary action (Table 1.6).

Table 1.6 The General Dental Council

The address of the General Dental Council is:

The Registrar
General Dental Council
37 Wimpole Street
London W1M 8DQ
UK

Professional indemnity

There are compelling reasons for taking advantage of the inexpensive security offered by being a member of one of the defence organizations. Although hygienists work under the direction of dentists, that does not exempt them from professional responsibility nor from being faced with a lawsuit for malpractice or professional negligence. Furthermore, in any legal dispute, it is possible that the interests of the dentist may be at odds with those of the hygienist. In addition there is the possibility of contractual problems arising with an employer or the risk of being summoned to a GDC disciplinary hearing. Many employers will insist on such membership (Table 1.7).

Table 1.7 Professional defence organizations

The two professional defence organizations which accept dental hygienist members are:

- Dental Protection Limited, 80 Great Portland Street, London W1N 5PA, UK
- Dental Defence, Medical Defence Union, 3 Devonshire Place, London WIN 2EA, UK

British Dental Hygienists' Association

Although membership of the BDHA is not mandatory, the Association is the hygienists' own professional organization and has done a vast amount of good for its members and all hygienists in the UK. It publishes the journal Dental Health, containing professional articles, news, letters, job vacancies and new product details, which all its members receive. It is also the main source of continuing professional education and the need for such training is stressed by the GDC. The authors strongly recommend that all hygienists should join the BDHA (Table 1.8).

Table 1.8 British Dental Hygienists' Association

The address of the British Dental Hygienists' Association is:

> British Dental Hygienists' Association
> 64 Wimpole Street
> London W1M 8AL
> UK

Further reading

Curriculum for Dental Hygienists (1997) General Dental Council, London.

Department of Health (1986). *Statutory Instrument No 887. Dental Auxiliaries Regulations.* HMSO.

Department of Health (1991). *Statutory Instrument No 1706. Dental Auxiliaries (Amendment) Regulations.* HMSO.

The Education and Training of Personnel Auxiliary to Dentistry. (1993) The Nuffield Foundation.

2

General histology

The microscope

Structures which are easily distinguishable by the unaided eye may be described macroscopically, and this holds true even if the usual type of hand lens is used to assist in the examination of the object. The almost-invisible object may be examined by the microscope, which is a combination of lenses so arranged that a minute object will appear greatly enlarged and in great detail when illuminated and viewed through the system. A comparison may be made with another combination of lenses - the telescope - which will apparently bring closer the distant object upon which it is focused.

There are maximum limitations in the ability of both systems, so that the telescope is unable to show up very distant stars; the radio telescope is then employed. Similarly the light microscope has a limit of magnification of about 2000 times. Beyond this the image loses its clarity and detail. The electron microscope, however, will enlarge the object from 100 000 to 250 000 times. It uses an 'electron gun' in place of the light source, and the objective lenses and eyepieces are replaced by magnetic lenses. The resultant image is usually seen on a fluorescent screen similar to a television or radar screen. The introduction of the electron microscope has enabled us to increase our knowledge of the basic structures and cellular organization of our tissues, indeed to the level of the larger molecules.

The scanning electron microscope is one in which the object is examined from a number of different angles and a three-dimensional effect is obtained. An example of its usefulness is the enormous amount of new knowledge which has been obtained of the surface structure of dental enamel.

- **Macroscopic**: visible with unaided eye.
- **Microscopic**: requires use of lenses in a microscope to magnify object up to 2000 times.
- **Electron microscope**: uses a beam of electrons to magnify object up to times 250 000.

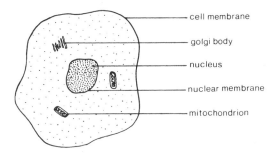

Fig. 2.1 Diagram of a cell.

The cell

All living organisms, whether vegetable or animal, are made up of microscopic units called cells. These are the smallest structures capable

Table 2.1 Cellular activity

The range of cellular activity includes the following behaviours

- **Irritability:** the ability to respond to various stimuli, such as heat and touch.
- **Motility:** independent movement. There are various forms of movement, such as contraction, expansion and rotation. Cells of the body are normally only described as motile if they are able to wander freely through the body tissues.
- **Nutrition:** the intake of foodstuffs which are converted to the energy required for all other functions.
- **Respiration:** taking in oxygen which is essential for metabolism. In this process the oxygen is converted to carbon dioxide which is then given off.
- **Excretion:** the removal of the waste products of metabolism.
- **Growth:** the increase in size of the cell, brought about by converting foodstuffs into cell components.
- **Reproduction:** the process by which cells multiply. Simple cells reproduce by dividing in half: each half forms a complete new cell. This is termed mitosis.

of independent life. Cells are composed of a jelly-like substance called protoplasm. They have a more or less centrally placed nucleus which is surrounded by cytoplasm. The whole cell is contained within the cell membrane (Fig. 2.1).

The nucleus is the control centre of the cell and is responsible for its development and the nature of its activity. It contains the genetic material of the cell in the form of deoxyribonucleic acid (DNA). The DNA molecules are called genes and these are strung together in long thin chains called chromosomes.

Cellular chemistry is dominated by carbon compounds which are capable of forming large complex molecules. Four basic types of carbon compound are utilized by cells. These are amino acids, fatty acids, sugars and nucleotides. These compounds can then be polymerized into larger macromolecules important for cell function. These macromolecules are nucleic acids (from nucleotides), lipids (from fatty acids), proteins (from amino acids) and polysaccharides (from sugars).

Most of the biochemical activity of the cell takes place in the cytoplasm. Various tiny structures called organelles are found there, each with a specific function. One such organelle is the Golgi apparatus, which is involved in the production of material to be secreted by the cell. It is prominent in cells which produce secretions and this includes cells such as odontoblasts, the cells which form dentine, and ameloblasts, which form enamel. Other organelles, termed mitochondria, act as the powerhouse of the cell, converting nutrients into energy.

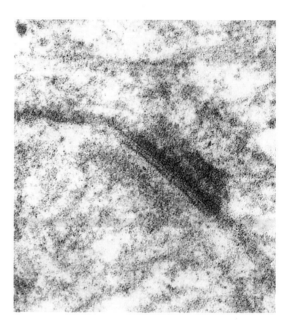

Fig. 2.2 A photomicrograph of the boundary between two cells with a desmosome clearly visible.

The cell membrane plays an important part in regulating the cell function. It controls the substances taken into and released by the cell. In some types of cell the presence of tiny structures associated with the cell membrane known as hemidesmosomes are seen. These are responsible for attaching the cell to neighbouring cells or structures. When the hemidesmosome of one cell sticks to that of another cell, the entire structure is termed a desmosome (Fig. 2.2 and see Fig. 6.14). Hemidesmosomes are commonly seen on epithelial cells. Most un-

Table 2.2 Cell function

Some specialized functions provided by cells include

- **Nerves** are long cells capable of transmitting electric impulses.
- **Endocrine glands** contain specialized cells capable of elaborating highly complex compounds (hormones) which have general control of the body's function.
- **Phagocytic cells**. The blood contains white cells that, like the amoeba, are capable of ingesting and then digesting or isolating foreign particles. Particles which remain free in the body could cause it harm. This activity is shown in Figure 2.3

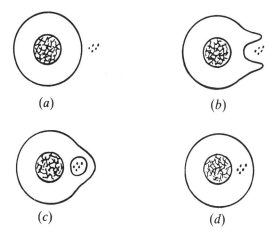

(a)   **(b)**   **(c)**   **(d)**

Fig. 2.3 The four stages of phagocytosis: (a) phagocyte attracted by foreign particles, (b) pseudopodia pushed out to surround material, (c) foreign material ingested into cell, (d) lysed material broken down inside phagocyte by enzymes.

specialized cells are capable of the range of activities shown in Table 2.1

The specialized activities of human cells are numerous. Indeed many of them have not yet been fully understood or described. A few examples of specialized cell functions are shown in Table 2.2

- Cell contents are known as protoplasm and this consists of the nucleus and cytoplasm.
- Four basic compounds are utilized by cells: amino acids, fatty acids, sugars and nucleotides.
- Mitochondria are the power houses of the cell.
- The cell membrane regulates substances leaving and entering the cell.

Cell renewal

The integrity of the body and its constituent tissues can only be maintained if the growth and division of each cell is programmed and co-ordinated with neighbouring cells. Many epithelial cells divide continuously throughout life whereas voluntary muscle and nerve cells, which are both very specialized cells, lose their mitotic ability once they have matured.

The process of cell division in the body is by mitosis or meiosis (when sperm or ova are produced). When a cell is not in division it is said to be *interphase*. However, when it divides it passes through the following phases.

- Prophase.
- Metaphase.
- Anaphase.
- Telophase where the cell finally divides to produce two daughter cells.

Growth factors act on cells to control mitosis and hence regulate cell growth. The rapid cell growth seen in some cancers reflects mitotic cell division that is out of control.

In meiosis similar stages of cell division are completed but an extra stage is included in this type of cell division to give a sperm cell or ovum exactly half of the normal number of chromosomes for that individual. Therefore, when the sperm cell and the ovum unite a new cell is produced with half its genetic make up from the male and half from the female.

The phases of mitosis are
- Prophase.
- Metaphase.
- Anaphase.
- Telophase.
- Interphase is the state of the cell when it is not dividing.

Tissues of the body

The tissues of the body are made up of groups of similar cells designed to carry out specific functions. They include muscles, nerves and those of most interest to the dental hygienist – epithelium and connective tissue.

Epithelium

Epithelium is embryologically (in the fetus) derived from ectoderm. It is the layer of tissue that covers all the surfaces of the body, both external and internal. Its functions are:

- To protect the underlying tissues from injury.
- To prevent bacterial invasion of the tissues.
- To prevent loss of fluid from the underlying tissues.

There are several types of epithelium, which are well suited to the different requirements of the various parts of the body (Fig. 2.4).

Simple squamous or pavement epithelium

This is composed of a single layer of flattened cells with varying shapes and sizes, resulting in an appearance resembling crazy paving (hence the name). This type of epithelium occurs where a thin smooth lining is required and where mechanical strength is not the main criterion, for example, the inner lining of blood vessels and the lining of the body cavities, such as the abdominal cavity.

Simple columnar epithelium

This is composed of a single layer of elongated cylindrical cells. Most of the alimentary canal is lined with this type of epithelium as are the ducts of most glands, including the ducts of the salivary glands.

Ciliated columnar epithelium

This is similar to columnar epithelium but is distinguished by the multitude of tiny hair-like processes, called cilia, which project from the free surface of the cells. Cilia are capable of a beating action – usually in one direction only. Since the cavity of the nose and most of the

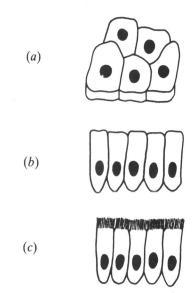

Fig. 2.4 Types of epithelium: (a) squamous or pavement epithelium, (b) columnar epithelium, (c) ciliated columnar epithelium.

respiratory passages are lined by ciliated epithelium it is often referred to as respiratory epithelium. Mucus, produced by cells called goblet cells, covers ciliated epithelium, and minute particles of dust which become trapped in the mucus are swept towards the opening of the cavity by the action of the cilia.

Stratified or compound squamous epithelium

Unlike the previous types of epithelium which are all composed of a single layer of cells, this is made up of several layers of cells (Fig. 2.5). The cells of the deepest layer continually multiply while those on the surface are continually being shed. This type of epithelium is found in areas which are exposed to mechanical damage and friction and it is therefore not surprising that the skin is composed of stratified squamous epithelium. It is this type of epithelium which is of most interest to the dental hygienist, since it also lines the whole of the oral cavity, where it is referred to as mucous membrane.

Stratified squamous epithelium may be keratinized or non-keratinized, i.e. it may or may not be covered by a layer of material called keratin. It is made up of several distinct zones. The zones of the keratinized epithelium are:

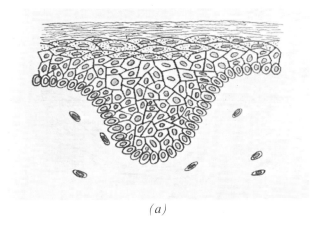

(a)

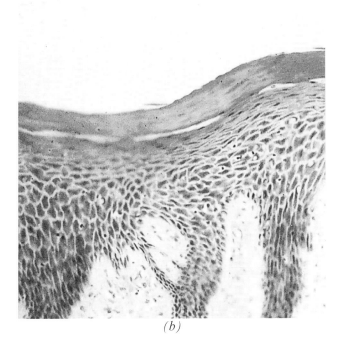

(b)

Fig. 2.5 (a) Diagram and (b) photomicrograph of keratinized stratified squamous epithelium showing the stratum germinativum, spinosum, granulosum, corneum and a layer of keratin at the surface.

Stratum germinativum

This is the single layer of cells at the base of the epithelium. The cells of the layer repeatedly divide to produce more cells, pushing those above them towards the surface. For this reason, this is also called the germinal layer. In areas which have to withstand a greater turnover of cells, the basal layer is increased in area by a series of folds, the rete ridges, similar to those of an egg box, leaving finger-like projections of connective tissue extending into the epithelium. These are called dermal papillae.

Stratum spinosum

This is composed of several layers of polyhedral cells. Because of their appearance this is also called the prickle cell layer. The prickles are the microscopic attachment mechanisms, by which adjacent cells stick to each other (desmosomes).

Stratum granulosum

This comprises several layers of flattened cells which contain keratohyaline granules in their cytoplasm. This is also referred to as the granular layer.

Stratum corneum

The outer layers of flattened cell remnants, which have lost their nuclei, are termed squames. Since they contain keratin, this layer is generally called the keratinous layer.

In non-keratinized stratified squamous epithelium, the last two zones are not found. The cells of the stratum spinosum simply become more and more flattened, with the outer layer of flattened cells being continually shed.

Epithelium is derived embryologically from ectoderm. Stratified squamous epithelium is the most common epithelial tissue and is made up of:
- stratum germinativum: the basal or germinal layer,
- stratum spinosum: the prickle cell layer,
- stratum granulosum: the granular cell layer,
- stratum corneum: the keratinous layer.

Connective tissue

This is derived embryologically from meso-derm. It serves as a supporting framework for the more specialized structures of the body. There are several different types, but they all consist of cells and fibres embedded in soft ground substance. In contrast to epithelium, the cells are always widely spaced from each other.

Cells

The main cells of connective tissue are fibro-blasts, histiocytes, plasma cells and mast cells.

Fibroblasts

Fibroblasts are the most numerous. They are flattened cells which are spindle-shaped when viewed from one aspect and more irregular with branching processes when viewed from the other aspect. Their function is closely linked with the formation of the fibres of connective tissue and some of the constituents of the ground substance.

Histiocytes

Histiocytes are wandering phagocytic cells, which means they can move freely through the tissues ingesting any foreign particles they find. These amoebic and phagocytic properties make histiocytes important defence cells. They are irregular in outline, with rounded branching processes, a small kidney-shaped nucleus and coarse granules within their cytoplasm. They may also be termed *macrophages* and, when circulating in the blood, are referred to as *monocytes* (see Chapter 3).

Plasma cells

Plasma cells are oval-shaped with an eccentrically placed nucleus, which when stained resembles a cartwheel. They are thought to be concerned with the formation of substances called antibodies, which are very important in the defence of the tissues against infection. It is not surprising, therefore, that they are much more numerous in areas where inflammation is present.

Mast cells

Mast cells are round cells that have a centrally situated round nucleus. They are most commonly found around blood vessels and, although the function is not definitely known, they are thought to be concerned with the response of the tissues to allergic conditions.

In addition to these cells, the connective tissue contains less of the blood cells which are described in Chapter 3.

Fibres

The three principal types of fibres found in connective tissue are collagen, reticular and elastic.

Collagen

Collagen fibres are the most common and widely distributed fibres. They are generally arranged in bundles that often have a wavy

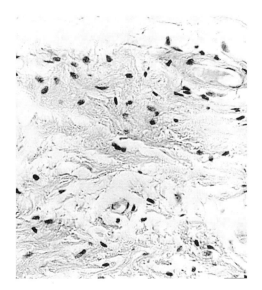

Fig. 2.6 Microscopic appearance of the dental pulp, which is a loose connective tissue. Numerous fibroblasts are seen, surrounded by collagen fibres and ground substance. A sectioned blood vessel can also be seen at the top right.

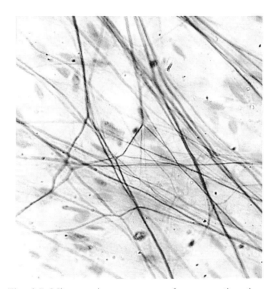

Fig. 2.7 Microscopic appearance of a connective tissue containing elastic fibres.

course. They cannot be stretched and are white in colour when viewed macroscopically when grouped together, for example in a tendon. Electron microscopy has shown that the fibres are transversely striated with alternating light and dark bands. Collagen fibres are illustrated in Figure 2.6.

Reticular

Reticular fibres are often closely associated with collagen and it is thought that they may be an immature form of collagen. They readily stain with silver dyes and, for this reason, are termed argyrophilic.

Elastic

Elastic fibres are yellow in colour and, as their name implies, are readily stretched. They are less common than collagen fibres and, unlike collagen, the fibres are branched. Elastic fibres are illustrated in Figure 2.7.

The several distinct types of connective tissue differ from each other mainly in the proportions of cells, fibres and ground substance to each other.

Embryologically connective tissue is derived from mesoderm. The main cells of connective tissue are the following.
- Fibroblasts
- Histiocytes (macrophages).
- Plasma cells.
- Mast cells.

The main fibres in connective tissue are as follows
- Collagen fibres.
- Reticular fibres.
- Elastic fibres.

Areolar tissue

Areolar tissue is often referred to as loose connective tissue, which aptly describes its histological appearance (Fig. 2.6). It is made up of a loose matrix of collagen and elastic fibres with connective tissue cells present in the abundant ground substance. This type of connective tissue occurs widely throughout the body. It is found immediately below the skin and mucous membrane and it will be seen in Chapter 6 that the dental pulp is composed of arcolar tissue.

Adipose tissue

Adipose tissue is similar to areolar tissue, but it contains large numbers of fat cells within the fibrous network. Each of these cells contains a large globule of fat within its cytoplasm. Adipose or fatty tissue is widely distributed throughout the body and, besides being a reserve supply of food, it acts as a protective cushion for some of the more delicate body structures. A layer of adipose tissue lies below the skin and helps to reduce heat loss from the body.

White fibrous tissue

This type of connective tissue is made up of densely packed collagen bundles with little ground substance and few elastic fibres. Each type of connective tissue cell is present. All the strong fibrous structures of the body, such as ligaments, tendons and the various protecting sheaths, are composed of white fibrous tissue, including the periodontal ligament which holds each tooth in its socket (see Chapter 6).

Yellow elastic tissue

As the name suggests, elastic fibres are the main constituents of this tissue. It is found wherever it is necessary for a tissue to be able to stretch, such as in the walls of blood vessels and in the lungs.

- Areolar tissue is a loose connective tissue found throughout the body.
- Adipose tissue is connective tissue composed of many fat cells.
- White fibrous tissue is the connective tissue found in ligaments and tendons.
- Yellow elastic tissue is a connective tissue found in the lungs and walls of blood vessels.

Cartilage

Cartilage consists of cells embedded in a resilient extracellular matrix that is usually uncalcified. There are three distinct types of cartilage found in the body:

- **Hyaline cartilage** covers the articular surface of most joints.

- **Elastic cartilage** is similar to hyaline cartilage but has a high content of elastin fibres. It is found in the external ear and epiglottis.
- **Fibrocartilage** which is found in intervertebral discs and the jaw joint.

Bone

Bone is a specialized connective tissue in which the ground substance has become impregnated with calcium salts. Being a rigid tissue, it is particularly well suited to supporting and protecting the more delicate body structures. Most bones have a dense outer layer called compact bone and an inner spongy layer called cancellous bone. The spaces in the meshwork of cancellous bone are filled with marrow, which is the tissue mainly responsible for blood cell formation in the adult.

Histologically, bone is composed of large numbers of haversian systems (Fig. 2.8). Each of these is a series of concentric layers of bone called lamellae that contain the mature bone cells called osteocytes. These lie around a central canal called the haversian canal, which contains blood vessels, nerves and lymphatics. The outer surface of bone is covered by a tough white fibrous tissue capsule called the periosteum. Between this and the bone is a thin layer of cells called osteoblasts, the cells responsible for bone formation. The cells that cause resorption of bone are large multinuclear cells called osteoclasts.

Bone is particularly significant to hygienists

- Bone is a connective tissue impregnated with calcium salts.
- It consists of compact bone (surface bone) and cancellous bone (the bone marrow).
- It is composed of haversian systems which contain osteocytes (mature bone cells).
- It is covered by periosteum (a white fibrous tissue) immediately beneath which lie osteoblasts (bone forming cells).

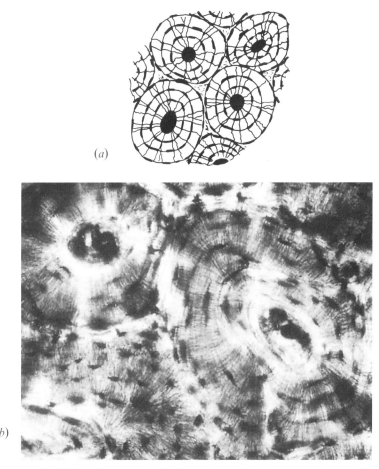

(a)

(b)

Fig. 2.8 (a) Diagram and (b) photomicrograph of haversian systems with their central canals and concentric lamellae.

Muscle tissue

Muscle tissue is composed of bundles of reddish fibres; each consisting of elongated specialized cells with the ability to contract. There are three distinct types: voluntary, involuntary and cardiac muscle.

Voluntary muscle

As the name implies, voluntary muscles are under the control of the will. In general these muscles are attached to the skeleton by fibrous tendons and are principally concerned with movement. Most muscles are attached at one end to a fixed bone, termed the origin, and at the other to a movable bone, termed the insertion. Histologically the muscle fibres are striped in appearance and, for this reason,

voluntary muscle is also termed striped or striated. The muscles of the tongue, of mastication and of facial expression are all of this type (see Chapter 4).

Involuntary muscle

Involuntary muscle has cells with no microscopic striations and therefore may be called smooth muscle. It cannot be controlled by the will. The muscles of the stomach, intestines, bladder, arteries and various glands are all of this type.

Cardiac muscle

Cardiac muscle is so called because it is found only in the wall of the heart. It is involuntary muscle, but its cells are striated and, unlike both previous types, they are branched. This enables the contraction of the cardiac muscle cells to spread to adjacent cells and the heart to function as a co-ordinated unit.

> Muscle tissue consists of three different types
> - Voluntary or skeletal or striped muscle.
> - Involuntary or smooth muscle.
> - Cardiac muscle is unique to the heart.

Nervous tissue

Nervous tissue is designed to carry messages from one part of the body to another. For example, nerves transmit information about temperature and touch from the skin to the brain and other nerves carry instructions from the brain to the muscles of the body.

The functional unit of nerve tissue is the nerve cell or neurone, which is made up of the cell body and its processes (Fig. 2.9). The nerve cell bodies mainly lie in the brain and spinal cord in the grey matter. The white matter of the brain and nerves is made up of the nerve cell processes, of which there are two types.

The process, which conducts signals or impulses away from the cell body, is called the axon and this process is often very long. For example, the axons of some neurones, which have their cell bodies in the spinal cord, run to the muscles of the arms and legs. Nerve cells also have a variable number of dendrites, the processes which conduct impulses towards the cell body. Where the axon of one neurone contacts the dendrite of another is termed a synapse and it is via synapses that impulses are transmitted from one neurone to another. Because nerves are very specialized, when they are damaged as in a patient who has suffered a head injury, they take a very long time to recover even partially, so the patient often remains in a coma for a long time. In addition in people who have strokes they may lose the function of part of the body permanently as damaged nerve cells never recover sufficiently for normal function to return.

Neural transmission

The passage of nerve impulses down the axons of any nerves occurs by the exchange of sodium

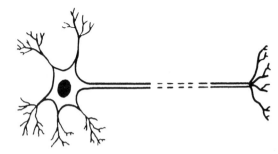

Fig. 2.9 Diagram of a neurone showing the long axon and five dendrites.

and potassium ions across the cell membrane as shown in Chapter 22 in Figure 22.1. The nerve message or electrical impulse is actually referred to as the *action potential* and is best visualized as similar to the wave that travels down a whip when it is cracked. When the action potential has passed, the sodium and potassium ions resume their previous relationship inside and outside the cell membrane, and they are helped to achieve this by means of the *sodium pump*.

It is thought that local analgesics such as lignocaine act by blocking the movement of the sodium and potassium ions and prevent the movement of the action potential down the axon.

> - Nerves convey sensation messages to the brain and action messages from the brain.
> - The functional unit of nerve tissue is the neurone.
> - Nerve cell bodies lie mainly in the grey matter of the brain and spinal cord.
> - Nerves communicate with other nerves via synapses which are similar to an electrical plug and socket.
> - Nerve cells are highly specialized cells which are fragile and easily damaged and show poor recovery after damage.

Further reading

Leeson T. S., Leeson C. R. (1988) *Atlas of Histology*. London: Saunders.

Rogers A. W. (1983) *Cells and Tissues*. London: Academic Press.

Ross J., Wilson K. J. W. (1995) *Anatomy and Physiology in Health and Illness*. 7th edition. Edinburgh: Churchill Livingstone.

3

Systems of the body

Introduction

The body is composed of a number of closely integrated specialized systems, which involve most of the tissue types described in Chapter 2. The tissues are grouped together into organs, which form the specialized systems. Thus the heart, blood vessels and blood form the circulatory system, whilst the lungs, air passages and respiratory muscles form the respiratory system.

Food taken into the body via the mouth is ingested by the alimentary canal and these organs form part of the digestive system. Control of these various organs is by the nervous and endocrine systems. The nervous system carries information between organs and tissues along nerves to and from the brain and spinal cord. The endocrine system acts by glands, which release hormones or chemical messengers. These circulate in the blood to act on distant organs.

In view of all the chemical interactions which take place in the body systems it is not surprising that a large number of waste products are formed. Some of these, for example carbon dioxide, are excreted via the lungs. The residue of food intake and the breakdown of digestive enzymes is excreted via the faeces. The urinary system is a most important means of ridding the body of toxic substances carried in the blood stream, and this is done via the kidneys.

The activity of these systems is very closely integrated, and variation in one system will directly affect all the others, which then attempt to compensate for the change. This compensatory mechanism is termed homeostasis. In young individuals, the capacity for compensation of the body systems is large. This capacity is reduced by injury, accident and the changes associated with age. A young person's circulatory system, for example, will compensate for a sudden bout of sustained physical exercise such as running for a bus. The older person is less able to cope with such activity.

For clarity this chapter describes the body systems separately, but the reader should remember the inter-relationship.

The cardiovascular system

The cardiovascular system has several components.

- The blood, which is a red viscous fluid.
- The heart, which acts as a pump.
- The blood vessels, which carry the blood from the heart throughout the body tissues and back to the heart.

The function of the cardiovascular system is principally to transport these substances to and from the tissues.

- Oxygen from the lungs to the tissues.
- Carbon dioxide from the tissues to the lungs.
- Foodstuffs from the alimentary canal to the tissues.
- Waste products from the tissues to the liver, kidney and intestine.
- Hormones from the glands in which they are produced to the tissues on which they act.
- Antibody substances to the site of any infection.

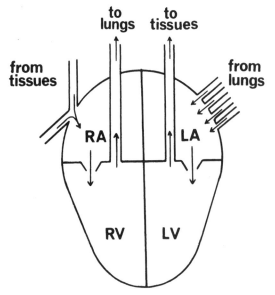

Fig. 3.1 Diagram of the heart: RA = right atrium, RV = right ventricle, LA = left atrium, LV = left ventricle. The direction of flow of the blood through the heart is indicated. It returns from the tissues through the two venae cavae, enters the right atrium and passes through the tricuspid valve into the right ventricle. It is carried from the right ventricle to the lungs by the pulmonary artery and returns to the left atrium through the pulmonary veins. It then passes through the mitral or bicuspid valve to the left ventricle, from where it is pumped through the aorta to the tissues.

The heart

The heart is situated in the chest between the lungs, behind and slightly to the left of the breast bone. It is a muscular organ which, by repeated contraction and relaxation, pumps the blood through the blood vessels.

It is divided into right and left sides, which are separated by a wall or septum (Fig. 3.1). Each side is subdivided into two chambers: the upper is called the atrium and the lower the ventricle. These two chambers are connected by an opening which has a valve designed to ensure the blood flows in one direction only, from atrium to ventricle. Between the right atrium and ventricle is the tricuspid valve and between the left atrium and ventricle is the bicuspid or mitral valve.

The blood returning from the tissues enters the right atrium through two large vessels named the superior and inferior vena cava. It passes through the tricuspid valve into the right ventricle and from this chamber, it is pumped

to the lungs through the pulmonary arteries. The blood returns from the lungs to the left atrium through the pulmonary veins. It then passes through the mitral valve into the left ventricle, from where it is pumped to the body tissues.

Each contraction begins in the upper part of the heart and, as the contraction spreads downwards, the blood in each atrium is forced down into the corresponding ventricle. Then, as the ventricles contract, the blood is pumped out of the heart. With relaxation of the two atria these chambers fill with blood, ready to refill the ventricles at the start of the next contraction. These heart contractions occur roughly at the rate of 72 per minute and it is these which can be heard or felt as heart beats. The rate at which the heart beats is controlled by the sinu-atrial node, situated in the right atrium near the opening of the superior vena cava. This structure is called the pacemaker of the heart.

When the heart contracts this is referred to as systole and when it relaxes it is called diastole. When it has stopped beating (as may occur after a heart attack) this is referred to as asystole.

Details of the heart

- Four chambers: two atria and two ventricles.
- The tricuspid valve between right atrium and ventricle.
- The mitral valve between left atrium and ventricle.
- The right side of the heart carries deoxygenated blood and the left side oxygenated blood.
- Systole is the term for a heart contraction and diastole for heart relaxation.
- The term asystole means the heart has stopped beating.

Blood vessels

There are three types of blood vessels.

- **Arteries**: which carry blood from the heart to the tissues.
- **Veins**: which return blood from the tissues to the heart.
- **Capillaries**: which form a network of small vessels in the tissues joining arteries to veins.

Arteries

Arteries vary greatly in size; the largest is the aorta, through which blood leaves the left ventricle. It divides and repeatedly subdivides into progressively smaller arteries; the smallest being termed arterioles (Table 3.1).

Table 3.1 Artery walls

The wall of an artery is made up of three layers

- **Tunica intima:** the innermost layer which is a thin layer of smooth endothelial cells forming the lining of the vessel.
- **Tunica intermedia:** a muscular layer which is controlled by the autonomic nerves described later in this chapter and which, when contracted, narrows or closes the vessel.
- **Tunica adventitia:** an outer fibrous layer of collagen and elastic fibres which supports the vessel and gives its wall a degree of elasticity.

With each heart contraction, blood is pumped into the arteries, which initially distend due to the pressure and then recoil to their original size as the blood is pushed further on towards the tissues. This gives rise to the pulse, which may be felt by placing the fingers over the skin covering an artery.

Capillaries

Capillaries are microscopic thin-walled vessels, which form a network called the capillary plexus in the tissues. Blood is pumped into the plexus by the arterioles and is drained from it by the smallest of the veins, termed venules. It is while the blood is in the capillaries that the oxygen and nutrient substances pass out into the tissues and carbon dioxide and waste products are removed from the tissues.

Veins

Veins also vary greatly in size. The microscopic venules merge to form small veins and these merge to form larger veins. Eventually all the blood from the tissues drains through two large veins, the superior and inferior vena cava, into the right atrium.

The walls of veins are thinner than those of

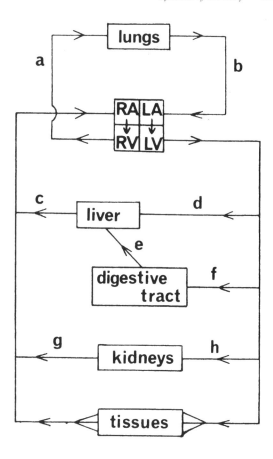

Fig. 3.2 Diagram of the blood circulation: RA = right atrium, LA = left atrium, RV = right ventricle, LV = left ventricle, a = pulmonary arteries, b = pulmonary veins, c = hepatic vein, d = hepatic artery, e = hepatic portal vein f = arteries to digestive tract, g = renal veins, h = renal arteries.

arteries and, although they are made up of the same three layers, the muscular middle layer is poorly developed. Since blood is not pumped into the veins but drains steadily from the capillaries, no pulse can be felt over them. They have numerous valves, which permit the flow of blood in one direction only and when the vein is compressed by the surrounding tissues, the blood is pushed onwards towards the heart.

The circulation

There are two distinct circulatory systems in the body: the systemic circulation and the pulmonary circulation (Fig. 3.2).

The systemic circulation has been described above, that is, the circulation of blood to the tissues of the body. The blood is pumped from the left ventricle, through the arteries and arterioles to the capillaries in the tissues and returns via the veins to the right atrium. By means of the systemic circulation oxygen is carried to the tissues, carbon dioxide is removed from the tissues and two other essential processes take place.

- Blood picks up nutrient substances.
- Blood is cleared of waste products.

The nutrients, which are absorbed in the stomach and intestines, are picked up by the blood circulating in their walls and carried by the hepatic portal vein to the liver, where those substances not required for immediate use are removed and stored. The kidneys and liver are the organs which remove waste products from the blood.

The kidneys are supplied with blood through the renal arteries. The blood is filtered in the kidneys and waste products including urea and uric acid are removed. Blood is returned to the heart via the renal veins.

The pulmonary circulation is the circulation of blood through the lungs. The blood vessels in this system are similar to those of the systemic circulation. The blood is pumped from the right ventricle through two large arteries (the right and left pulmonary arteries) to the lungs. These arteries divide and subdivide into smaller arteries, which eventually open into the capillary plexus in the lungs. In the capillaries the blood gives off carbon dioxide and takes up oxygen and then returns to the heart via progressively larger veins. It eventually drains into the left atrium through four large pulmonary veins.

The principal difference between the two circulations is that, in the systemic circulation, arteries carry oxygenated blood and veins carry deoxygenated blood whereas in the pulmonary circulation this is reversed: arteries carry deoxygenated blood and veins carry oxygenated blood.

Secondly, as the pulmonary system is small and the blood has therefore less distance to travel, the blood pressure supplied by the right side of the heart is lower than that on the left, and the blood vessel walls are consequently smaller. This pressure difference accounts for the variation in structure of the pulmonary and systemic blood vessels.

There are two circulatory systems in the body, the systemic circulation and the pulmonary circulation

- The pulmonary circulation takes blood through the lungs to allow gaseous exchange.
- The systemic circulation nourishes the tissues and removes waste products.

Blood

There are approximately 6 litres of blood in the average human adult body. Blood is a red viscous fluid, made of a liquid portion (plasma) and various cellular elements.

Plasma

This is a straw-coloured liquid, composed of 90% water and 10% dissolved substances. The dissolved substances include plasma proteins, hormones, nutrient and waste products and dissolved salts and gases (Tables 3.2 and 3.3.)

Table 3.2 Plasma proteins

Plasma proteins in blood include

- **Albumin**: responsible for the viscosity of blood and for maintaining the blood pressure.
- **Globulin**: a group of proteins, each identified by a letter of the Greek alphabet; alpha α, beta β or gamma γ. The gamma globulins are antibodies, or immunoglobulins – a major factor in the body's defensive system and of great significance in relation to, for example, periodontal disease.
- **Fibrinogen**: important in the process of blood clotting. It changes from a soluble substance into insoluble fibrin, which forms the meshwork of the clot.
- **Prothrombin**: another protein involved in clotting and discussed more fully later in this section.

Cells

There are three different cellular elements in blood: red blood corpuscles, white cells and platelets.

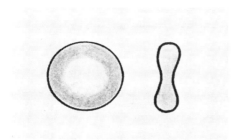

Fig. 3.3 Diagram of red blood corpuscles.

Table 3.3 Substances transported in blood

Substances transported in blood include

- **Hormones**: described in this chapter.
- **Nutrients**: principally glucose, fatty acids and amino acids.
- **Waste products**: principally urea and uric acid being transported to the kidneys for excretion.
- **Dissolved inorganic salts**: mainly sodium, potassium, calcium, chloride and bicarbonate.
- **Dissolved gases**: oxygen, carbon dioxide and nitrogen.

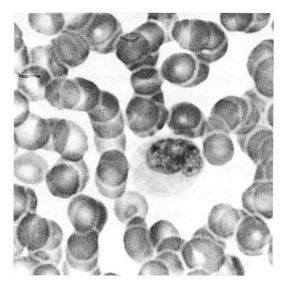

Fig. 3.4 Microscopic appearance of a blood film, showing large numbers of red blood corpuscles and a single leukocyte (monocyte).

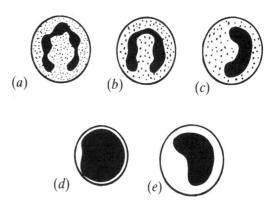

Fig. 3.5 The white blood cells of blood: (a) neutrophil polymorphonuclear leukocyte, (b) eosinophil polymorphonuclear leukocyte, (c) basophil polymorphonuclear leukocyte, (d) lymphocyte, (e) monocyte. (a), (b) and (c) are essentially the same but have different staining characteristics.

Red cells

These are biconcave discs which have no nucleus, these having been lost during cell growth (Figs 3.3 and 3.4). They contain the red, iron-containing protein haemoglobin and these corpuscles give blood its red colour. Haemoglobin is primarily concerned with the transportation of oxygen from the lungs to the tissues. In the lungs it picks up oxygen to form bright red oxyhaemoglobin and when the blood reaches the tissues the oxygen is given up and the haemoglobin becomes darker in colour. There are approximately 5 million red blood corpuscles in each cubic millimetre of blood.

White cells

White blood cells are termed leukocytes (Fig. 3.5). They have a nucleus, are larger than the red blood corpuscles and are far fewer in number than red blood corpuscles: approximately 8000 per cubic millimetre. Two different types of leukocyte exist: those which contain granules and their cytoplasm (granulocytes) and those which do not (agranulocytes) (Tables 3.4 and 3.5).

Platelets

Platelets, or thrombocytes, are not cells. They are merely small, irregularly shaped fragments which become detached from large bone marrow cells and as such have no nucleus. There are roughly 250 000 platelets in each cubic millimetre of blood and they are important in the process of blood clotting.

Table 3.4 Granular leukocytes

Granulocytes are often referred to as polymorphonuclear leukocytes, since their nuclei are irregularly shaped and have two or more distinct lobes. They are further subdivided according to the reactions of the granules to various dyes into neutrophils, eosinophils and basophils.

- **Neutrophils.** These have granules which stain purple with neutral dyes and nuclei which are divided into several lobes. They make up 65% of all the white cells and are important in the body's defence against infection. They are capable of moving freely through the tissues and of phagocytosis.
- **Eosinophils.** The granules of these cells stain red with acidic dyes and the nucleus of each cell is divided into distinct lobes. They make up approximately 3% of the white cells and, although their exact function is obscure, they are known to increase in the presence of allergic reactions.
- **Basophils.** These have granules which stain dark blue with basic dyes. They have kidney-shaped nuclei and make up roughly 1% of white cells. Their function is not known.

Table 3.5 Agranular leukocytes

Agranular leukocytes are divided into three types

- **Lymphocytes** are small round cells with darkly staining round nuclei which almost fill the cell. The nucleus normally has an indentation on one aspect. They make up roughly 25% of total white cells and play a major role in the process of immunity. They occur in large numbers in chronic infections. Lymphocytes can be divided into T and B types, which are discussed more fully later in the section on the immune response in Chapter 7.
- **Monocytes** are the largest of the blood cells and have large kidney-shaped nuclei. They make up 6% of the white cells. They are also capable of phagocytosis and are important in the body's defence against infection. They have already been discussed in Chapter 2.
- **Plasma cells** have also been described in Chapter 2 and will be discussed again in greater detail in the section on immunity in Chapter 7. They are developed from lymphocytes.

Blood

- Consists of plasma, red and white blood cells and platelets.
- The average human body contains about 6 litres of blood.
- Red blood cells have no nucleus but contain haemoglobin.
- Both agranular and granular white cells contain nuclei.
- There are roughly 250 000 platelets per cubic millimetre of blood.

Blood clotting

When the skin or mucosa is cut the torn blood vessels bleed freely which is nature's way of washing the wound clean of debris that may be present. After a minute or two the bleeding reduces due to the blood vessels in the area of damage starting to constrict. This slows the rate of blood loss down and allows the blood to begin to clot. The basic process involved in clotting is the formation of a fibrin meshwork by the conversion of the soluble plasma protein fibrinogen into insoluble fibrin. This reaction is brought about by the enzyme thrombin.

Thrombin is also derived from a plasma protein – prothrombin. The conversion of prothrombin to thrombin is caused by an enzyme which is not usually present in plasma. This enzyme is called thromboplastin and it is derived from either of two sources: damaged tissue cells or platelets. Several other factors are involved in the production of thromboplastin and a deficiency of any such factor can result in prolonged bleeding. For example, haemophilia is caused by a lack of factor VIII (antihaemophilic globulin) and Christmas disease is a deficiency of factor IX (Christmas factor). A diagrammatic representation of the process of clotting is shown in Figure 3.6.

Haemostasis is the term used to describe the

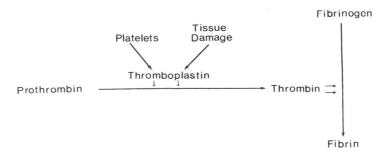

Fig. 3.6 The process of blood clotting.

halting of blood flow from a cut blood vessel. When a vessel is cut, its end constricts as a result of constriction of the smooth muscles in the wall. This slows down the flow of blood from the cut end. A plug of platelets then collects in the constriction, further reducing the blood flow, thus allowing the blood in that area to clot.

Haemostasis is achieved by the following mechanisms

- Thrombin converts fibrinogen into fibrin to start the formation of a blood clot.
- Thrombin comes from damaged tissues and platelets.
- There are also 12 blood clotting factors involved in blood clotting.
- In inflamed tissues it takes longer for the initial bleeding to stop.

Respiratory system

Oxygen is essential to the life of all cells of the body. It is needed for the conversion of nutrient substances into energy and as a by-product of this process carbon dioxide is given off. We have already seen that the blood carries oxygen from the lungs to the cells and returns carbon dioxide from the cells to the lungs. Respiration is the process whereby oxygen is taken up by the blood in the lungs and carbon dioxide is given off. The respiratory system consists of the air passages and the lungs (Fig. 3.7).

The air passages

The air passages connect the lungs with the air outside the body through the openings of the nose and mouth (Table 3.6). The nasal and oral cavities open backwards into the pharynx (Fig. 3.8). At its lower limits the pharynx divides into two tubes: the anterior one is the larynx or voice box and the posterior is the oesophagus, which is part of the alimentary canal and is described later. The larynx is continuous with the trachea, which passes downwards from the neck into the chest or thorax, where it divides into right and left bronchi. Each bronchus leads to one lung and, within the substance of the lung, it divides and repeatedly subdivides into progressively smaller bronchioles. The smallest of these terminate in blind-end sacs, called alveoli.

The respiratory passages are rigid tubes which are held open by cartilage within their walls. They are lined throughout by epithelium for the most part by respiratory epithelium.

Table 3.6 Respiratory passages

Functions of the respiratory passages are

- Conduct air to and from the lungs.
- Moisten and warm the air.
- Cleanse the air, by catching dust particles, etc. in the mucous membrane lining.
- Produce voice sounds by the action of the vocal chords within the larynx.

The lungs

The two lungs occupy most of the thorax and are situated one each side of the midline. They are separated by the heart, oesophagus, trachea and the large arteries and veins. Microscopically they consist of large numbers of alveoli, which have very thin walls containing the blood capillaries. In their walls, blood comes into close proximity to the air contained by the

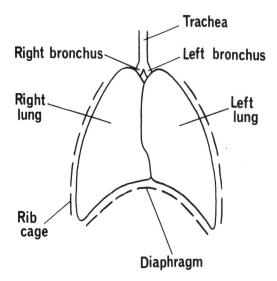

Fig. 3.7 Diagram of the respiratory system.

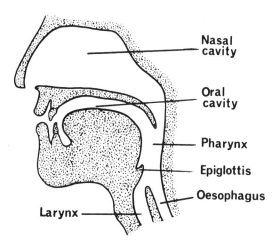

Fig. 3.8 Diagram of a vertical section through the nasal cavity, oral cavity and pharynx.

alveoli, allowing the exchange of gases to take place.

The lungs are elastic and are covered by a thin membrane called the visceral pleura. This is in close contact with the lining of the thoracic cavity, the parietal pleura: only a thin layer of lubricating fluid separates the two.

Respiration

The wall of the thorax contains the ribcage which, by muscular action, can expand and contract. Separating the thorax from the abdominal cavity is the dome-shaped diaphragm which, by muscular action, can flatten out, reducing the height of the dome. When the ribs expand and the dome of the diaphragm is depressed, the lungs are stretched and air is sucked into them. Then, when the muscles relax, the elasticity of the lungs makes them recoil to their original shape and size and air is expelled from them.

In this way a breath is taken and the build-up of carbon dioxide within the lungs is prevented. This happens at a rate which varies considerably with circumstances (such as physical exertion), but is roughly 16 breaths per minute at rest. Inspiration, or breathing in, is therefore an active muscular process, whereas expiration or breathing out is a passive process. This is the principle employed in the administration of exhaled air artificial respiration.

> The main features of the respiratory system are
> * The respiratory passages are rigid tubes lined by respiratory epithelium.
> * Gaseous exchange takes place in the alveoli.
> * The lungs are covered with a thin membrane called the visceral pleura which is in close contact with the lining of the thoracic cavity, the parietal pleura.
> * At rest there are about 16 breaths per minute.

Digestive system

The digestive system consists of a long, complicated tube called the alimentary canal. Food is inserted into one end of the tube (the mouth) and, as it passes through the tube, it is broken down mechanically and chemically by a process termed digestion. The nutrients of use to the body are absorbed into the blood stream while substances which are of no use are ejected from the other end of the tube (the anus).

Food

Before attempting to study the digestive system it is essential to have a basic understanding of what constitutes the food that humans eat. The enormous variety of foodstuffs may be broken down into the following substances.

Water

Since water makes up 70% of body weight, it is not surprising that it is the main constituent of the diet. A human being can last up to a month without food, but will die of thirst in only a few days. A total of 3 litres of water is needed each day by the average adult. Of this, some 2 litres are drunk as water in one form or other and the remaining litre is a component of other food-stuffs. Even the driest biscuit contains some water.

Vitamins

These are complicated substances which, in small amounts, are essential to life. They cannot be synthesized (i.e. made up) within the body and therefore must be absorbed unchanged from the foodstuffs of the diet. The different vitamins are identified by letters and some examples are described below.

Vitamin A
Vitamin A is a fat soluble vitamin which is found in fish-liver oils, such as cod-liver oil and halibut-liver oil. It also occurs in eggs, milk, green vegetables and carrots. A lack of this vitamin leads to changes in the body's epithelium and produces a condition termed night-blindness. This is the basis of the advice that children should eat carrots if they want to be able to see in the dark!

Vitamin B
Vitamin B complex are water soluble vitamins once thought to be a single vitamin but now known to be a complex of several. They are each identified by adding a number after the letter: e.g. vitamin B6, vitamin B12, etc. The B-complex vitamins are found in seeds, such as nuts, wholemeal, peas and lentils, but they are lost when wheat is excessively milled, as it is in the production of white bread. Deficiency of the B vitamins produces a variety of disorders, including digestive complaints, anaemia and skin lesions. The mouth may be affected with bleeding from the gums, and inflammation of the tongue (glossitis).

Vitamin C
Vitamin C is water soluble and its chemical name is ascorbic acid. It is important in the formation of collagen. It is found in citrus fruits, such as oranges and lemons, and in certain vegetables, including potatoes. A deficiency of ascorbic acid results in scurvy in which there is a generalized muscle weakness and a tendency for the bones to fracture easily. Multiple skin lesions occur and the gums and periodontal ligament supporting the teeth become badly infected.

Vitamin D
Vitamin D is fat soluble and is involved in the formation of healthy bones and teeth. Deficiency of this vitamin in childhood causes rickets, resulting in soft bones with typically bent legs and deformed chests. Vitamin D is found in milk, eggs and fish-liver oils and is also formed within the body by the action of sunlight on the skin.

Vitamin E
Vitamin E is fat soluble and its function is uncertain although it is known to be a powerful anti-oxidant.

Vitamin K
Vitamin K is fat soluble and is important in blood clotting. It can be stored in the liver.

Minerals

Some mineral salts are absorbed directly from the diet. One of the most important minerals is calcium needed for the healthy development of bone and teeth. The absorption of calcium is also dependent on vitamin D. Other necessary minerals include sodium, phosphorus, potassium, magnesium, iron, chloride and iodine. Fluoride is classified by the World Health Organization as an essential trace element and because of its value in the prevention of dental caries: the UK government recommends fluoridation of public water supplies.

Most of the other ingredients of the diet are too complicated to be absorbed unchanged into the blood stream and first need to be broken down into smaller units by digestion. Such ingredients may be divided into three groups: carbohydrates, proteins and fats.

Carbohydrates

As their name suggests, these are made up of carbon, hydrogen and oxygen. Carbohydrates are present in bread, potatoes and all sweetened foodstuffs. The simplest, called monosaccharides, are simple sugars such as glucose. Other sugars are composed of two monosaccharide molecules joined together and are called disaccharides, an example being sucrose or cane sugar. Some complex carbohydrates are made up of many monosaccharide molecules joined together: these are called polysaccharides. The most common polysaccharide in the average diet is starch. Since polysaccharides are too complex to be absorbed into the blood stream, they are digested into smaller units, most commonly the monosaccharide glucose.

Proteins

Proteins consist of highly complex molecules which contain nitrogen as well as carbon, hydrogen and oxygen. Their basic components are called amino acids and each protein molecule is a very long chain of numerous different amino acids. There is a multitude of different proteins which are present in all animal and vegetable tissue, and meat, fish, eggs and vegetables are particularly rich sources of dietary proteins. During digestion the proteins are broken down to their constituent amino acids, which are then absorbed.

Fats

Fats are also complex substances, which are made up of a combination of fatty acids and glycerol. They are present in both animal fats and vegetable oils. When digested they break down to fatty acids and glycerol, which are then absorbed.

Dietary fibre

Dietary fibre is the term used for the portion of the foodstuffs which cannot be digested and absorbed by the body. Although it has no nutritional importance, its significance in relation to the healthy functioning of the alimentary canal is definitely now recognized.

Essential dietary components are
- Proteins which provide amino acids.
- Fats which provide fatty acids and glycerol.
- Carbohydrates broken down to glucose to provide energy for metabolism.
- Vitamins: the fat soluble vitamins are A, D, E, K. The water soluble ones are the B complex and C.
- Minerals including iron, sodium, potassium.
- Fluoride is also an important mineral which is essential for life.
- Water: up to 3 litres per day are required by the average 70 kg adult.
- Dietary fibre: the undigested component of food necessary for good functioning of the alimentary canal.

Alimentary canal

This is divided into the following constituent parts (Fig. 3.9).

- Oral cavity: stops at the palatoglossal fold.
- Pharynx: otherwise known as the throat.
- Oesophagus: the food pipe.
- Stomach: where digestion begins and the food is gradually released into the intestines.
- Small intestine: where the majority of digestion takes place.
- Large intestine: where mineral salts and water are mainly absorbed.

Oral cavity

Food is placed into the oral cavity through the mouth. There it is prepared for its journey through the alimentary canal in the following ways.

- **Mechanical breakdown**. The food is chewed between the teeth and pulped by the action of the tongue on the roof of the mouth. This process is called mastication.
- **Lubrication**. The food is mixed with the saliva of the mouth, which moistens and lubricates it. In this way a softened, slippery ball of food, called a bolus, is made suitable for swallowing.

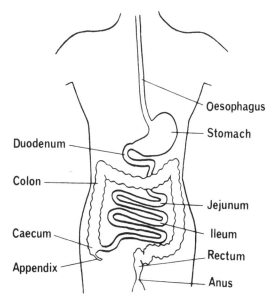

Fig. 3.9 Diagram of the alimentary canal.

- **Chemical breakdown**. Saliva contains the enzyme amylase which begins the breakdown of cooked carbohydrates such as starch. In view of the relatively short period of time the food is in the mouth, this is not an important function. It may be of significance in the aetiology of caries, by releasing sugars from starchy food particles lodged between the teeth. The composition and function of saliva is described in much more detail in Chapter 6 and the structure of the oral cavity is described in Chapter 4.

Pharynx and oesophagus

Once suitably masticated, the bolus of food is swallowed. It passes backwards into the pharynx and then down through the oesophagus into the stomach. This whole process from mouth to stomach is termed deglutition. Deglutition is the act of swallowing, in which food is carried from the mouth to the stomach. For descriptive purposes, it is normally divided into three stages: the first is voluntary and the other two are involuntary.

- **Stage 1.** When the food has been converted, by mastication, into a mucous bolus, it is ready to be swallowed. The teeth are first clenched together and the tip

of the tongue is pressed against the hard palate, behind the upper incisors. The bolus is pushed backwards into the pharynx by the action of the body of the tongue, which is pressed upwards against the hard palate, like squeezing toothpaste from a tube. At the same time the soft palate is raised upwards and backwards to close off the nasopharynx and prevent food passing up into the nasal cavity. The food bolus has now reached the pharynx and the voluntary phase of mastication is over.
- **Stage 2.** The bolus touching the walls of the pharynx triggers off a reflex contraction of the muscles in the pharyngeal wall, which pushes the food downwards into the upper part of the oesophagus. At the same time, the opening of the larynx is raised up under the cover of the epiglottis, to prevent food entering the lungs.
- **Stage 3.** The bolus is then pushed down the whole length of the oesophagus by a series of rhythmic contractions known as peristalsis. At the lower end of the oesophagus is a muscular sphincter, called the cardiac sphincter, which relaxes to allow the food to enter the stomach and then closes to keep it there. It takes roughly 6 s for a food bolus to travel the length of the oesophagus. It can be seen that deglutition is a muscular process and is little affected by gravity.

Stomach

The stomach is a strong muscular distensible bag. Its functions are as follows.

- **Storage of food**. The stomach can hold and store food from a large meal and, over a period of some hours, permit small quantities to pass on through the alimentary canal. This means that humans, in common with other animals, need not eat continuously, but can rely on periodic large meals. Both ends of the stomach are closed by muscular valves called sphincters: the cardiac sphincter above and the pyloric sphincter below.
- **Mechanical mixing of food**. While in the stomach the food is churned over by the action of the muscular stomach wall, so that it is broken down further and

becomes thoroughly mixed with the stomach secretions (gastric juices).

- **Digestion of food.** This is not a principal
  function of the stomach since most digestion takes place in the intestines.
- **Absorption of food**. Most absorption takes
  place in the intestines, but water, alcohol
  and glucose can be absorbed in the
  stomach. Alcohol is absorbed quite
  quickly and this is the reason why it is
  not advisable to consume alcohol when
  the stomach is empty.

Small intestine

It is principally in the small intestine that
digestion and absorption of food take place:
digestion in the short first part (the duodenum)
and absorption in the much longer distal parts
(the jejunum and ileum).

Table 3.7 Gastric juices

Gastric juices contain the following

- **Hydrochloric acid**, which has an antibacterial
  action and which aids the digestion of certain
  materials.
- **Rennin**, which coagulates milk.
- **Lipase**, an enzyme which begins the breakdown of fats.
- **Pepsinogen,** which is converted in the
  presence of hydrochloric acid to pepsin: this in
  turn starts the breakdown of protein.
- **Mucin,** which protects the lining of the
  stomach from the hydrochloric acid.

Digestion

In the duodenum, the food is mixed with
digestive juices from various sources: those
secreted by the walls of the duodenum itself,
termed succus entericus; the pancreatic juice
produced by the pancreas and carried to the
duodenum by the pancreatic duct; and bile
produced by the liver and carried to the
duodenum by the bile duct (Fig. 3.10). In the
duodenum, proteins are broken down by the
enzymes trypsin and chymotrypsin. Carbohydrates are digested by the enzymes amylase,
maltase, lactase and sucrase which convert
polysaccharide and disaccharide sugars into
monosaccharides. Fats are initially emulsified

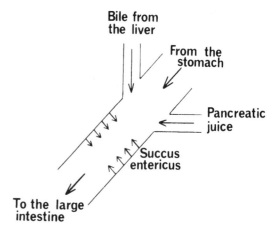

Fig. 3.10 Diagram of the duodenum.

(i.e. made soluble in water) by the bile salts and
are then broken down by lipase into glycerol
and fatty acids.

Absorption

Once suitably prepared, the foodstuffs are
passed on through the 6 metres of the jejunum
and ileum where absorption takes place. The
digested foodstuffs pass through the lining of
the intestine and are picked up by the blood
circulating through the intestinal wall. To
improve the uptake, the surface area of the
intestine is greatly increased in size by large
numbers of finger-like processes, called villi,
which project into the cavity.

Each of the cell surfaces of the villi are
covered with enormous numbers of tiny projections – microvilli – and thus the surface area of
absorption is vastly increased. The lining of the
gut wall has many specialized cells for the
intake of substances such as sodium salts,
amino acids and glucose. As these enter the
gut wall, the osmotic pressure of the contents of
the gut is lowered, and thus water follows the
solids into the blood stream via gut wall.

Large intestine

This is the last 2 metres of the alimentary canal
and is divided into the caecum, colon and
rectum. As the residues of the foodstuffs pass
through the caecum and colon, water and
mineral salts are absorbed, leaving the semi-
solid faeces. These are stored in the rectum and,
at intervals, are ejected through the anus.

Digestion of food
- Food is lubricated and initially broken down mechanically in the mouth.
- Chemical breakdown begins in the mouth with the enzyme salivary amylase.
- Further chemical breakdown occurs in the stomach with gastric juice.
- The main area for chemical breakdown is the small intestine.
- The large intestine only absorbs water and mineral salts.

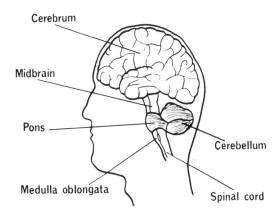

Fig. 3.11 The main parts of the brain.

Nervous system

The nervous system consists of two main parts: the central nervous system comprising the brain and spinal cord and the peripheral nervous system, which consists of a system of nerves carrying impulses to and from the central nervous system. The nervous system controls and co-ordinates body functions by transmitting messages from one part of the body to another. The basic cell of the nervous system is the neurone (see Chapter 2) with its cell body situated in the grey matter of the brain and spinal cord, and its processes running through the white matter of the brain, spinal cord and peripheral nerves. A nerve trunk contains the peripheral processes of many neurones.

Central nervous system

The brain and spinal cord make up the central nervous system. This is the controlling, co-ordinating part of the system and is also the site of more sophisticated mental activity, such as thought, understanding and memory. The brain lies in and is protected by the skull, whilst the spinal cord occupies the central canal of the vertebral column (Fig. 3.11).

The brain consists of three main parts – the forebrain, midbrain and hindbrain. Most of the forebrain is occupied by the cerebral hemispheres (cortex) which, amongst other functions, are concerned with sensory perception and motor control. The co-ordination part of the brain, the cerebellum, is in the hindbrain, as are the pons and medulla.

The cerebral cortex, unlike the spinal cord, has its grey matter (nerve cell bodies) situated

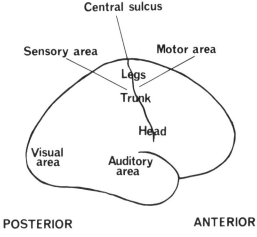

Fig. 3.12 Diagram to show the main areas of the cerebrum.

on the surface. The motor area is situated in front of the central sulcus of the cortex and the sensory area is situated behind this central sulcus (Fig. 3.12). The body areas are represented alongside this central sulcus in an upside-down fashion. The sensory impulses from the head, for example, arrive alongside the lower part of the sulcus whilst the impulses from the leg arrive in the upper part.

The spinal cord lies in the vertebral column and is protected by it. The spinal cord has a central H-shaped area of grey matter surrounded by white matter (Fig. 3.13).

From the central nervous system arise various nerves: 12 pairs of cranial nerves and 31 pairs of spinal nerves. Each of the spinal nerves arises from two roots, as illustrated in Figure 3.13, but these nerves are of much less

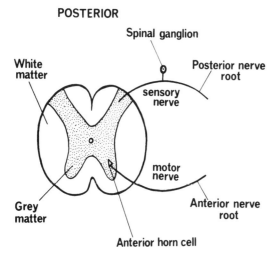

POSTERIOR

Spinal ganglion

White matter

Posterior nerve root

sensory nerve

motor nerve

Grey matter

Anterior nerve root

Anterior horn cell

Fig. 3.13 The spinal cord and nerve roots.

significance to the dental hygienist than the cranial nerves. Some of the latter are discussed in more detail in Chapter 4.

Peripheral nervous system

Nerves are of two types: those conducting impulses towards the central nervous system, afferent or sensory nerves, and those which conduct impulses away from the central nervous system, efferent or motor nerves. This is, however, a physiological classification rather than an anatomical one, since certain anatomical nerves contain both motor and sensory fibres. The mandibular nerve will be seen to be an example of one such nerve. Sensory nerves have specialized nerve endings or receptors which respond to differing stimuli (Table 3.8).

Table 3.8 Skin receptors
The four skin sensory receptors are
• Touch.
• Pain.
• Heat.
• Cold.

From deeper structures there are receptors which give information about the position of the body. These receptors are found, for example, in muscles, ligaments and joints, and are called proprioceptors. Proprioceptors in the temporomandibular joint capsule and muscles of mastication provide awareness of the position of the teeth and jaws and permit the high degree of control over jaw movements.

Table 3.9 Special senses
There are four special senses
• Sight.
• Hearing.
• Smell.
• Taste.

Autonomic nervous system

This is the part of the peripheral nervous system which is concerned with the regulation of essential body functions, such as respiration, blood circulation and digestion. The muscles concerned with these functions are influenced by the brain, but there is no conscious control, hence they are termed involuntary muscles. These muscles exhibit no striations and are called smooth muscles.

The autonomic nervous system is divided into two parts.
• The sympathetic nervous system.
• The parasympathetic nervous system.

The two systems tend to be mutually antagonistic. For example, when one type excites a muscle, the other inhibits the same muscle. In this respect the autonomic system differs from the nerve supply to striated muscles (Fig. 3.14 and Table 3.10).

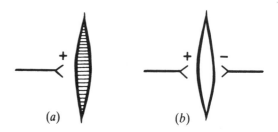

(a)   (b)

Fig. 3.14 Diagram to illustrate the difference between: (a) voluntary muscle innervation and (b) smooth muscle innervation.

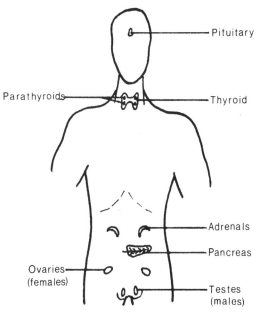

Fig. 3.15 The main organs of the endocrine system.

The sympathetic system provides the body with the 'fight or flight' reaction which prepares the body for action. Thus the heart rate is increased, the pupils and respiratory passages dilate, blood supply to striated muscles increases but digestion is inhibited. When the dental hygienist student is called on to undertake the first of the group teaching practices, she or he will recognize the increased heart rate and dry mouth!

The nervous system consists of the central and peripheral nervous systems

- The central nervous system is made up of the brain and spinal cord.
- Peripheral nerves can be afferent or sensory and efferent or motor.
- The autonomic nervous system regulates essential body functions.
- The autonomic system can be sympathetic or parasympathetic.

Endocrine system

Endocrines, or hormones, are produced by a series of glands situated in various parts of the body. The glands secrete the hormones into the bloodstream, which carries them to other tissues of the body where they have an effect. Whereas the nervous system regulates the immediate and short-term activities of the body, the endocrine system regulates the slower, more prolonged activities, such as growth and metabolism (Fig. 3.15 and Table 3.11).

Table 3.11 Principal endocrine glands

The principal endocrine glands are

- Pituitary.
- Thyroid.
- Parathyroids.
- Pancreas.
- Adrenals.
- Gonads.

Pituitary

This is a small gland which lies below the lower surface of the brain. It is especially important since it acts as an overall regulator of the other endocrine glands. It also produces hormones concerned with growth and water balance.

Thyroid

The thyroid gland lies in the front of the neck, its two lobes situated on either side of the trachea. It controls various functions, including growth and energy production in the cell.

Parathyroids

There are four parathyroid glands which are embedded in the thyroid gland, two in each of the lobes of the thyroid. They regulate the level of calcium in the blood.

Pancreas

Besides producing the pancreatic digestive juice which flows into the duodenum, the pancreas produces two hormones called glucagon and insulin. The endocrine-producing cells are different from those which produce the digestive juices and are collected together in patches referred to as the islets of Langerhans. Glucagon increases and insulin lowers the level of glucose in the blood and when inadequate amounts of insulin are produced, the condition is referred to as diabetes mellitus. This is of some importance to the dental hygienist since it will be seen later in this book that the health of the periodontal tissues is often undermined by diabetes.

Adrenals

There are two adrenal glands, one situated above each kidney. Each adrenal consists of an inner layer called the adrenal medulla and an outer layer called the adrenal cortex. The adrenal medulla secretes adrenaline, which produces an effect on the body similar to the action of the sympathetic nerves (i.e. it prepares the body for 'fight or flight'). The adrenal cortex produces three different hormones which control various processes including growth and sexual development. One of these hormones is cortisone and this is commonly used to treat chronic inflammatory conditions.

Steroid hormones come from the adrenal glands and help the body to cope with stress.

Gonads

The hormones secreted by the gonads – the ovaries in the female and the testes in the male – control sexual development and are largely responsible for the differing sexual characteristics in males and females. Those produced by the ovaries also control the female menstrual cycle and pregnancy. It is well recognized that, during pregnancy, gingival inflammation tends to be more severe.

Hormones are produced by the endocrine system

- The pancreas has both exocrine and endocrine functions.
- The adrenal cortex produces cortisone and the adrenal medulla adrenaline amongst other hormones. Cortisone helps the body to cope with stress.

Lymphatic system

All cells of the body are bathed in tissue fluid which passes into the tissue spaces from the capillaries. There is a continuous interchange of this fluid between the tissues and the capillaries, but not all the fluid that leaves the capillaries returns to them. Some of it is drained from the tissues by the lymphatic vessels. The lymphatic system is of great significance in relation to the control of infection, the spread of malignant tumours and the immune system.

Lymphatic vessels

The lymphatics are very thin-walled, blind-ended vessels which form a network within the tissues. When tissue fluid enters these vessels it is referred to as lymph and, because the vessels have thinner walls than capillaries, larger particles can escape from the tissues in the lymph than can enter the blood stream. This is an important factor in the clearing of the products of inflammation from the tissues.

The microscopic lymphatic vessels merge with each other to form progressively larger vessels, in the same way that venules merge to form veins. The larger lymphatics are similar in structure to veins, having thin walls and valves to ensure the flow of lymph in one direction only. The lymph flows through progressively larger vessels and eventually empties into the large veins of the neck through the thoracic duct on the left and the smaller right lymphatic duct on the right.

Although the lymphatics are not normally visible in the tissues, when severe inflammation is present, they may appear as red lines running away from the site of inflammation.

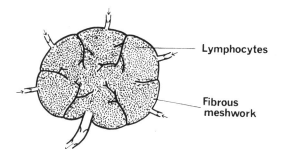

Fig. 3.16 Diagram of a lymph node with five vessels emptying into it (afferent vessels) and one large vessel draining from it (efferent vessel).

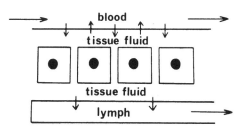

Fig. 3.17 Diagram of the interchange of fluid between the capillaries, intercellular tissues and the lymphatic vessels.

Lymph nodes

At periodic intervals the lymphatic vessels empty into lymph glands or nodes (Fig. 3.16). Several vessels empty into each node and a single larger vessel drains from it. The nodes consist of a fibrous meshwork containing large numbers of lymphocytes, mainly B lymphocytes and plasma cells, and they filter the lymph as it passes through the lymphatics to the blood (Fig. 3.17).

The lymphatic system of the body

- Returns tissue fluid to the blood stream.
- Lymph nodes filter this tissue fluid and remove foreign material before entering the blood stream.
- Lymph nodes also contain lots of plasma cells which can make antibodies to neutralize foreign material when necessary.

Further reading

Department of Health (1991) *Dietary Reference Values for Food Energy and Nutrients for the United Kingdom.* HMSO.

McNaught A. B., Callander R. (1983) *Illustrated Physiology.* 4th edition. Edinburgh: Churchill Livingstone.

Ross J., Wilson K. I. W. (1990) *Anatomy and Physiology in Health and Illness.* 7th edition. Edinburgh: Churchill Livingstone.

4

Regional anatomy

Introduction

The knowledge of anatomy which a dental hygienist requires becomes more detailed the nearer it is to the area of work: the oral cavity. There is a need for a general understanding of the anatomy and functions of the systems of the body discussed in Chapter 3, with a more detailed knowledge of the structures of the head and a thorough knowledge of the oral cavity and para-oral structures.

Osteology

When studying anatomy it makes sense first to examine the bony structure of the area, since the position of other anatomical features then can be related to this skeletal framework. The study of bones in general is osteology and the bones which are of most concern to the hygienist make up the bones of skull.

The skull

For simplicity the skull is considered as consisting of two parts, the cranium (or 'brain box') and the facial skeleton (Figs 4.1 and 4.2 and Tables 4.1 and 4.2). Between them they are made up of 22 bones which are joined together by immovable fibrous joints called sutures in a manner similar to that in which crazy paving is joined by cement. There is one exception: the mandible, which is attached by a movable joint, the temporomandibular joint.

Table 4.1 Posterior view of the skull

The skull mainly consists of the occipital bone, with the following features to be noted

- The external occipital protuberance.
- The foramen magnum through which the spinal cord exits from the cranial cavity.
- The nuchal lines for the attachment of neck muscles.
- The lambdoid and sagittal sutures.
- The occipital condyles.

Cranium

This is the hollowed-out upper part of the skull (Table 4.3). It contains and protects the brain. Therefore, on the whole, the bones forming it are very thick and solid and shaped for maximum resistance to injury.

The upper domed part of the cranium is the vault (Fig. 4.2). The lowest part is the base of the skull. On each side of the vault is a semicircular ridge; the temporal line, below which is the temporal fossa.

Numerous foramina are found in the base of the skull (Fig. 4.3). Through them pass the many nerves leaving the brain and the arteries that carry the brain's rich blood supply. Several of these nerves and blood vessels are described in more detail later. The largest structure leaving the cranial cavity is the spinal cord which exits via the foramen magnum. The maxillary nerve exits through the foramen rotundum and the

Table 4.2 Lateral view of the skull

A lateral view of the skull reveals the following of note

- The ascending ramus of the mandible, its condyle and coronoid process.
- The zygoma and zygomatic process which together form the zygomatic arch from which the masseter muscle originates.
- The styloid process: an unmistakable sharp spike which gives attachment to styloglossus, stylohyoid and stylopharyngeus muscles and the stylohyoid and stylomandibular ligaments.
- The mastoid process.
- The temporal fossa: a large concave area giving origin to the temporal muscle.
- The infratemporal fossa which communicates with the pterygopalatine fossa.

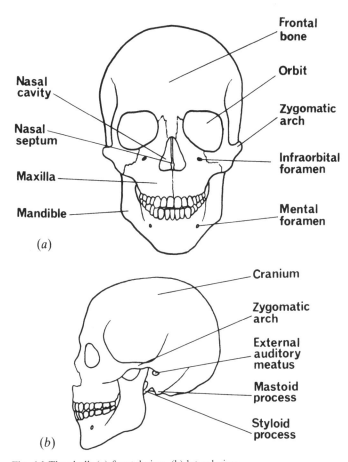

Fig. 4.1 The skull: (a) frontal view, (b) lateral view.

mandibular nerve through the foramen ovale.

Many of the blood vessels entering the cranium are large because the brain requires a high level of oxygen and nutrients to function effectively. The internal carotid artery enters via the carotid canal and the jugular vein leaves via the jugular foramen.

The external auditory meatus (outer opening of the ear) lies between the glenoid fossa, the hollow facet with which the mandible articulates, and the mastoid process.

When viewed from above, the upper teeth and hard palate lie in front of the base of the skull. The hard palate is made up of parts of

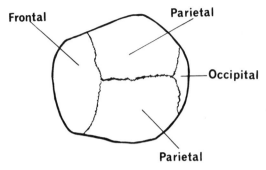

Fig. 4.2 The cranium viewed from above.

Table 4.3 The cranium
The following eight bones make up the cranium
Frontal bone

Parietal		Parietal
Temporal		Temporal
	Ethmoid	
	Sphenoid	
	Occiptal	

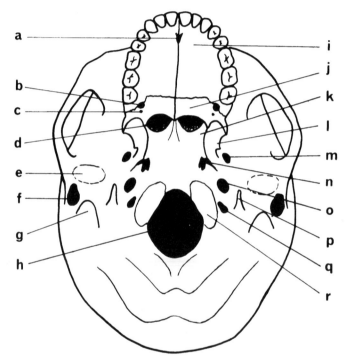

Fig. 4.3 The base of the skull: **a** incisive fossa, **b** greater palatine foramen, **c** lesser palatine foramen, **d** pharyngeal opening of the nasal cavity, **e** mandibular fossa, **f** external auditory meatus, **g** mastoid process, **h** foramen magnum, **i** palatine process of maxilla, **j** horizontal plate of palatine bone, **k** medial pterygoid plate, **l** lateral pterygoid plate, **m** foramen ovale, **n** foramen lacerum, **o** carotid canal, **p** styloid process, **q** jugular foramen, **r** occipital condyle.

four bones: the palatine processes of the right and left maxillae in front and the horizontal plates of the two palatine bones behind. Projecting backwards and outwards from the hard palate is a wing-shaped plate of bone called the lateral pterygoid plate from which arise the lateral and medial pterygoid muscles (two of the muscles which control movement of the mandible).

Facial skeleton

This is the lower anterior part of the skull and is the supporting structure for the face (Table 4.4). Clearly, a more detailed understanding of this area is required by the hygienist.

The functions of the facial skeleton are:

- to give protection to the delicate organs of sight and smell,

Table 4.4 The facial skeleton

The 14 bones of the facial skeleton which support the facial features are

Maxilla	Maxilla
Zygomatic	Zygomatic
Palatine	Palatine
Nasal	Nasal
Lacrimal	Lacrimal
Inferior turbinate	Inferior turbinate
Vomer	
Mandible	

- to hold the teeth, via the maxilla and mandible,
- to form part of the masticatory and respiratory system.

The facial skeleton is oval in shape and is wider above than below. The main features are the two orbital cavities, each of which also has a supraorbital and infraorbital foramen or notch, the nasal cavity and the large separate bone of the mandible whose teeth meet with those of the two maxillae.

Of the facial bones mentioned above, this text is interested mainly in those involved in the structure of the oral cavity. Therefore, the maxilla and the mandible will be described in some detail. The remaining bones of the facial skeleton should be known by name and the student should be able to identify each on the dried skull.

Table 4.5 The maxilla

The four processes of the maxilla are

- The zygomatic process, which projects laterally towards the zygomatic arch.
- The frontal process, which projects upwards to form the medial wall of the orbit.
- The palatine process, which projects horizontally to form part of the hard palate.
- The alveolar process which projects downwards and supports the upper teeth.

Maxilla

The maxillae are fixed to the other bones of the skull by sutures and are immovable. Each one

consists of a body and four processes (Figs. 4.4 and 4.5 and Table 4.5).

The body of the maxilla is roughly pyramidal in shape, the base of the pyramid being the lateral wall of the nasal cavity and the apex being the zygomatic process. The posterior surface forms the anterior wall of the pterygo-palatine fossa (mentioned later in connection with the maxillary nerve), the superior surface forms the floor of the orbit and the anterior surface forms part of the facial skeleton. In the superior (orbital) surface is a groove in which run the infraorbital nerve and blood vessels. Passing forwards, these enter the infraorbital canal and emerge onto the facial surface through the infraorbital foramen, which, as its name suggests, lies slightly below the lower border of the orbit.

The body of the maxilla is hollowed out by

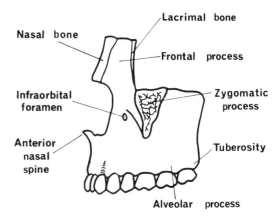

Fig. 4.4 The maxilla viewed from the lateral aspect.

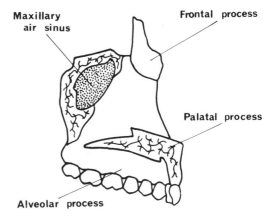

Fig. 4.5 The maxilla viewed from the medial aspect.

the maxillary air sinus which opens into the nasal cavity through an opening in the nasal wall. The sinus is one of a group referred to as the paranasal air sinuses, because they all open into the nasal cavity. The other sinuses are in the ethmoid, sphenoid and frontal bones. Their function is not known, but various suggestions have been made.

- They may serve to lighten the skull.
- They may add resonance to the voice.
- They may insulate the delicate tissues of the head against temperature changes.

The roots of the upper posterior teeth often project into the maxillary sinus, being covered by only a thin layer of bone. The sinus is plainly visible on intraoral radiographs taken of these teeth.

Mandible

The mandible is the lower jaw (Figs 4.6 and 4.7). It is a horseshoe-shaped bone formed by the midline union of right and left halves. Each half has a horizontal, tooth-bearing portion called the body, and a flattened, vertical portion called the ramus. The junction between the body and the ramus is the angle.

The body

The body is roughly pear-shaped in section, the narrower part being the alveolar ridge, which supports the lower teeth. After loss of the teeth this part of the mandible resorbs. In front, the thicker lower part of the body forms the prominence of the chin and is termed the symphysis.

On the outer surface of the body, a ridge of bone, called the external oblique line, runs downwards and forwards from behind the last molar tooth and is a part of the attachment area of the buccinator muscle. Above the external oblique line, at the level of the premolar teeth, is the mental foramen, from which emerge the mental nerve and vessels.

On the inner aspect of the body there is another ridge of bone similar to the external oblique line. It also runs downwards and forwards from behind the last molar and is called the mylohyoid line. This forms the attachment of the mylohyoid muscle and it separates the submandibular fossa below from the sublingual fossa above. These concave areas

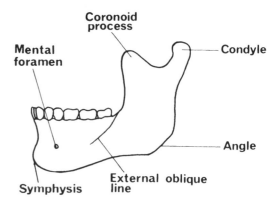

Fig. 4.6 The outer aspect of the mandible.

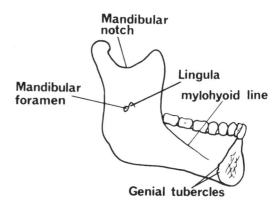

Fig. 4.7 The inner aspect of the mandible.

are respectively the sites of the submandibular and sublingual salivary glands. The inner aspect of the body has a third fossa situated anteriorly near the lower border. It is the digastric fossa and is the attachment area of the digastric muscle. On either side of the midline are two bony projections called the inferior and superior genial tubercles, the attachments of the geniohyoid and genioglossus muscles respectively.

The ramus

The ramus is roughly rectangular in shape. It has two large bony processes projecting upwards which are separated by the mandibular notch. The posterior process is called the condyle and is the part of the mandible which articulates with the base of the skull. Its rounded upper portion is called the head and the narrower lower portion the neck. The

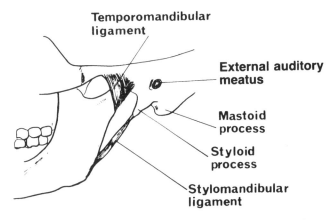

Fig. 4.8 Ligaments of the temporomandibular joint from the lateral aspect.

lateral pterygoid muscle is inserted into a shallow fossa on the anterior surface of the neck. The anterior process is the coronoid process. The temporal muscle is inserted into its tip and to the whole of the anterior edge of the ramus.

The masseter muscle is inserted into a roughened area covering most of the outer aspect of the ramus. In the centre of the inner aspect is the mandibular foramen through which the mandibular nerve and vessels enter the mandible. It is guarded anteriorly by an upward projection of bone called the lingula. Between the mandibular foramen and the angle of the mandible is a roughened area into which is inserted the medial pterygoid muscle.

The temporomandibular joint

The temporomandibular joint (Figs 4.8 and 4.9) is the hinge between the mandible and the base of the skull and is the only movable joint of the skull.

Structure
The temporomandibular joint consists of the head of the condyle articulating with the glenoid fossa of the temporal bone. In front of the glenoid fossa is the articular eminence. Between the head of the condyle and the temporal bone lies the articular disc, an oval pad of dense fibrous tissue, and the whole joint is enclosed in a fibrous capsule. The position and movements of the condyle are controlled by ligaments which act as strengtheners and limit excessive movements during muscle con-

tractions.

- **The articular capsule** envelopes the whole of the joint.
- **The temporomandibular ligament** is involved with the outer surface of the capsule and joins the zygomatic process of the temporal bone to the posterior and lateral border of the condyle. It supports the articular capsule by strengthening its outer surface and limiting excessive movements.
- **The sphenomandibular ligament** runs from the spine of the sphenoid bone to the lingula on the inner aspect of the ramus in the region of the entrance to the inferior dental canal.
- **The stylomandibular ligament** runs from the styloid process to the angle and posterior border of the ramus.

Movement
The joint has two basic movements which occur simultaneously. When the mouth is opened, the head of the condyle rotates through a horizontal axis and, at the same time, slides forward on to the bony prominence in front of the glenoid fossa. The articular disc consists of a lower layer of collagenous tissue attached to the condyle, so that it slides forwards with the condyle. Its upper layer is elastic fibrous tissue and is attached to the posterior edge of the mandibular fossa, which limits the forward slide of the condyle.

When right and left joints function together, the anterior part of the mandible is depressed, the teeth separate and the mouth opens. This is

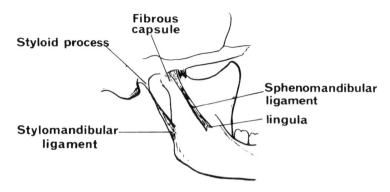

Fig. 4.9 Ligaments of the temporomandibular joint from the medial aspect.

the movement used, for example, when biting into an apple. If one joint operates alone, the mandible swings to the opposite side, grinding the upper and lower teeth. During chewing both these types of movement are used. This is discussed in more detail in the section below on the muscles of mastication.

Maxillae
- Pyramidal shaped body.
- The maxillary sinus: structure and functions.
- Four processes: zygomatic, frontal, palatine and alveolar.
- Four surfaces: nasal, facial, orbital and posterior.

Mandible:
- The body: symphysis, mental foramen and alveolar, mylohyoid and external oblique ridges.
- The ramus: mandibular foramen, mandibular notch, condyle, coronoid process.
- The angle.

Temporomandibular joint:
- Structure: condyle, glenoid fossa, articular disc.
- Ligaments: capsular, stylomandibular, sphenomandibular, temporomandibular.
- Movements.

Oral cavity

The oral cavity extends from the lips to the palatoglossal fold, a ridge of soft tissue running

from the soft palate to the base of the tongue, immediately in front of the tonsils. The roof of the cavity is formed by the hard palate in front and the soft palate behind. Its lateral walls are the cheeks and the tongue projects upwards from its floor. It contains the upper and lower alveolar ridges and teeth and the space between these structures and the lips is called the vestibule. The entire cavity is lined by stratified squamous epithelium, which is keratinized in some areas, such as the gingivae and hard palate, and is non-keratinized in others, including the inner aspect of the lips and the floor of the mouth. Because the epithelium is moistened by a layer of mucus, it is referred to as mucous membrane.

Lips

The lips are muscular structures designed to close off the entrance to the oral cavity. Where the upper and lower lips meet they form the angle of the mouth and the junction of upper and lower lips is the labial commissure. Their bulk is made up principally by the orbicularis oris muscle, a circular muscle which circumscribes the mouth and which, when contracted, closes and purses the lips. Several other muscles are inserted into parts of the orbicularis oris and contribute to various facial expressions (see the later section on the muscles of facial expression). Like all of the muscles of facial expression the orbicularis oris muscle is supplied by the facial nerve (the VIIth cranial nerve).

The lips are covered on the outer aspect by skin and on the inner aspect by non-keratinized mucous membrane. In the midline of the outer surface of the lips is a shallow vertical groove called the philtrum, which ends below in a slight prominence. On each side the upper lip is separated from the cheek by the nasolabial groove.

Between the muscle layer and the mucous membrane lie numerous salivary glands which are roughly the size of small peas and open into the vestibule. Each side of the lips receives its blood supply from branches of the facial artery of that side; the lower lip by the inferior labial arteries and the upper lip by the superior labial arteries. In both lips the right and left arteries anastomose across the midline. Drainage of blood is via the superior and inferior labial veins to the facial vein.

Cheeks

The cheeks are also muscular structures, covered on the outside by skin and on the inside by mucous membrane. The mucous membrane of their inner surface is non-keratinized, with the exception of an area of keratinization corresponding to the level of the occlusal surfaces of the teeth. The bulk of the cheeks is made up of the buccinator muscle, which is attached behind to the outer aspect of the upper alveolus in the region of the molar teeth, to the external oblique line of the mandible and to the pterygomandibular raphe between these two. It is inserted in front into the lateral part of the orbicularis oris and, like this muscle, is supplied by the facial nerve. The buccinator plays an important role in mastication by pushing food from the vestibule back into the oral cavity proper.

The cheeks also contain a large quantity of fat tissue and have numerous salivary glands situated between the buccinator and the oral mucous membrane.

Floor of the mouth

This is the area which is largely covered by the tongue and is bounded laterally and anteriorly by the teeth (Table 4.6).

The bulk of the floor of the mouth is made up by the mylohyoid muscles which anastomose (interweave) with each other in the median line. The muscles originate from the mylohyoid line of the mandible and are inserted into the body of the hyoid bone. The submandibular salivary gland lies both above and below the sheet of muscle, folding around its posterior free edge.

The genioglossus is a triangular-shaped muscle which originates at the superior genial tubercle on the inner side of the mandible. The muscle spreads out in a fan shape backwards and upwards and is inserted into the base of the tongue.

Table 4.6 The floor of the mouth

The floor of the mouth is made up of the following paired (i.e. right and left) structures

- Mylohyoid muscle.
- Genioglossus muscle.
- Geniohyoid muscle.
- Anterior belly of the digastric muscle.
- Sublingual salivary gland and ducts.
- Submandibular salivary gland and duct.

The geniohyoid is a narrow muscle originating from the inferior genial tubercle and running backwards and downwards is inserted into the hyoid bone.

The digastric muscle has two parts; an anterior and posterior belly. The anterior belly originates from the digastric fossa of the inferior border of the mandible. It is attached to the hyoid bone by a fibrous sling and then continues backward as the posterior belly which is inserted into the digastric notch in the mastoid process of the temporal bone. The digastric is an accessory muscle of mastication and assists in controlling and depressing the mandible.

Noteworthy features visible on the floor of the mouth are the following.

- The lingual frenum which connects the under surface of the tongue to the floor of the mouth.
- The sublingual papillae: one on either side of the fraenum. These are the openings of the ducts from the submandibular salivary gland.
- The sublingual fold extends backwards and laterally in the floor of the mouth from the papilla and has minute openings in the surface from the ducts of the sublingual salivary gland (Fig. 4.10).

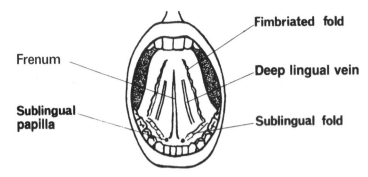

Fig. 4.10 The ventral surface of the tongue and floor of the mouth.

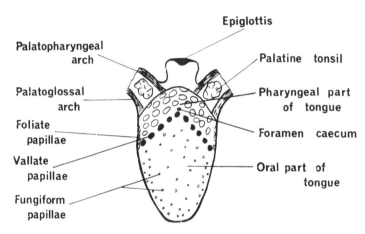

Fig. 4.11 The dorsum of the tongue.

The tongue

The tongue is a muscular organ projecting upwards from the floor of the oral cavity (Figs 4.10 and 4.11). It has a tip, a superior surface, called the dorsum, and an inferior, or ventral surface. A median fibrous septum runs backwards from the tip, dividing it into two halves.

The surfaces of the tongue

The dorsum is, for descriptive purposes, divided into the anterior two-thirds, which lie in the oral cavity, and the posterior one-third, which forms the anterior wall of the pharynx. The two parts are separated by a shallow V-shaped furrow; the sulcus terminalis, running outwards and forwards from a small midline pit called the foramen caecum.

The anterior two-thirds are covered with thick keratinized epithelium and have a median

furrow running from the foramen caecum to the tip. There are three types of papillae found on its surface: filiform, fungiform and vallate (Fig. 4.12 and Table 4.7).

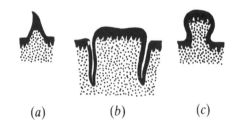

Fig. 4.12 The papillae of the tongue: (a) filiform, (b) vallate, (c) fungiform.

The posterior one-third of the dorsum extends from the sulcus terminalis to the epiglottis, which protects the entrance to the lungs. It is covered with thin non-keratinized

Table 4.7 The papillae of the tongue

The papillae of the tongue

- Filiform papillae are small and conical. They cover the whole surface and give this part of the dorsum its rough appearance and texture.
- Fungiform papillae are less numerous than the filiform type. They are roughly mushroom-shaped and are visible as small red dots.
- Vallate papillae are larger than the others and, being 1–2 mm in diameter, are clearly visible to the naked eye. There are between 10 and 12 of them, forming a V-shaped line immediately in front of the sulcus terminalis. They are cylindrical in shape and each one sits in a depression in the tongue, with part of the cylinder projecting above the surface. Numerous taste buds (the receptors for taste sensation) are present in the walls of the trench that surrounds the papilla and serous (or watery) saliva is secreted into the trench by glands at its base.

epithelium, with no papillae, but a nodular appearance produced by underlying lymphoid tissue.

The sensory nerve supply of the anterior two-thirds of the dorsum differs from that of the posterior third. The anterior part receives its sensory supply from the lingual nerve, a branch of the mandibular division of the trigeminal (Vth cranial) nerve. The nerve fibres which carry taste sensation travel initially in the lingual nerve, but then pass via the chorda tympani to the facial (VIIth cranial) nerve. Both touch and taste sensations are carried from the posterior third by the glossopharyngeal (IXth cranial) nerve.

The inferior surface of the tongue is smooth and purplish in colour. It is covered with thin non-keratinized epithelium which is continuous with the epithelium covering the floor of the mouth. On either side of the lingual fraenum lies a fold of mucous membrane, the fimbriated fold, and between the two the deep lingual vein can be seen showing through the epithelium.

The muscles of the tongue

The muscles of the tongue are divided into two groups of four on each side: the intrinsic muscles, which are contained entirely within the tongue, and the extrinsic muscles, which originate outside the tongue and are inserted into it (Table 4.8).

The function of the intrinsic muscles is to alter the shape of the tongue.

- The superior longitudinal muscles run backwards from the tip of the tongue, just below the dorsal mucous membrane.

- The inferior longitudinal muscles also runs backwards from the tip, but close to the under surface. Contraction of both longitudinal muscles shortens the tongue, while contraction of the superior muscles alone turns the tip upwards and contraction of the inferior muscles alone pulls the tip downwards.
- The vertical muscles extend from the dorsal surface to the inferior surface. These muscles flatten the tongue.
- The transverse muscles consist of fibres which originate in the median septum and pass laterally to be inserted into either side of the tongue. They narrow and lengthen it.

Table 4.8 The muscles of the tongue

The muscles of the tongue are

Intrinsic muscles.
- Superior longitudinal.
- Inferior longitudinal.
- Vertical.
- Transverse.

Extrinsic muscles.
- Genioglossus.
- Hyoglossus.
- Palatoglossus.
- Styloglossus.

The extrinsic muscles of each side of the tongue are primarily responsible for moving the bulk of the tongue around the oral cavity.

- The genioglossus is attached to the superior genial tubercle of the mandible and fans out backwards and upwards to be inserted into the whole of the under surface of the tongue. Its action is to pull the tongue forwards so that the tip pokes out of the mouth.

- The hyoglossus arises from the hyoid bone, a horseshoe-shaped bone in the neck, and passes upwards to be inserted into the side of the tongue. It depresses the tongue.
- The palatoglossus is a small, narrow muscle which arises from the aponeurosis of the soft palate and is inserted into the side of the tongue. It lies within the palatoglossal arch which marks the posterior limit of the oral cavity and its action is to lift up the tongue, closing off the mouth from the pharynx.
- The styloglossus is a short muscle, originating on the styloid process and passing downwards and forwards to be inserted into the side of the tongue. It draws the tongue upwards and backwards.

The motor nerve supply to all the muscles of the tongue, with the exception of the palatoglossus, is the hypoglossal (XIIth cranial) nerve. The palatoglossus is supplied by the accessory (XIth cranial) nerve. The blood supply reaches the tongue via the lingual artery, a branch of the external carotid, and drains principally through the lingual vein.

The functions of the tongue

The functions of the tongue are as follows.

- The mastication and deglutition of food.
- Speech. Although the basic voice sounds are produced in the larynx, they are modified by the action of the soft palate, lips and tongue.
- Taste. This is discussed in Chapter 6.
- Oral hygiene. The tongue is used to clean food debris from the surface of the teeth.
- Some gestures, not all of them polite.
- In the baby, the tongue has an important role as a sensory organ. It is used to explore and identify objects in its new surroundings.

Alveolar ridges and gingiva

The upper and lower alveolar ridges are horse-shoe-shaped projections of the maxilla and mandible respectively (Figs 4.13 and 4.14). They are covered by keratinized epithelium and support the teeth, which project through the epithelium into the oral cavity proper.

The epithelium covering the alveoli is termed gingiva and is firmly adherent to the underlying bone. It is pale pink in colour (often described as salmon or coral pink) and, in dark-skinned people, diffuse areas of pigmentation may be found. Its surface is not smooth but stippled, meaning that it is covered with numerous tiny pits, resembling the texture of orange peel.

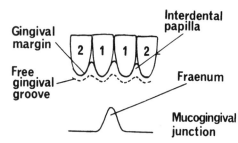

Fig. 4.13 The labial gingiva of the lower teeth.

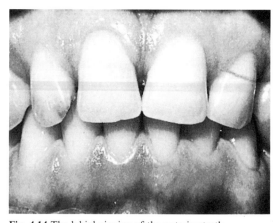

Fig. 4.14 The labial gingiva of the anterior teeth.

On the outer aspect of the alveoli, the gingiva is continuous with the non-keratinized epithelium covering the inner surface of the lips and cheeks, forming the vestibular sulcus. There is a clear line of demarcation between the pink gingiva and the much redder oral mucous membrane, which is termed the mucogingival junction. Several folds of soft tissue run from the lips and cheeks to the alveoli and reduce the depth of the vestibular sulcus. Each of these folds is called a fraenum and the largest are generally found in the midline. The lingual gingiva of the lower alveolus is continuous with the thin non-keratinized epithelium of the floor of the mouth and is also clearly demarcated from it at the mucogingival junction, but the palatal gingiva of the upper arch merges imperceptibly with the pink keratinized epithelium covering the whole of the hard palate.

The gingivae meet the necks of the teeth in a knife-edge margin, which is scalloped around the teeth, coming to a point, the interdental papilla, between the teeth. Between the buccal and lingual surfaces of the interdental papilla is a concavity which is called the interdental col and which skirts around the contact area of adjacent teeth. There is a narrow band of unstippled gingiva, called the free gingiva, which forms a collar around the necks of the teeth. This is free in the sense that it is not tightly bound down to the alveolar bone, as is the attached gingiva, but is more loosely fastened to the necks of the roots or crowns of the teeth. It is separated from the attached gingiva by the shallow free gingival groove, which follows the scalloped outline of the gingival margin. The attached gingiva, therefore, is the area between the free gingival groove and the mucogingival junction. Between the gingival margin and the neck of each tooth is the shallow gingival crevice.

The gingiva is discussed in greater detail in Chapter 6.

The palate

The palate separates the oral cavity from the nasal cavity. It is divided into the hard palate and the soft palate.

The hard palate

The hard palate is formed by parts of the maxillae and palatine bones: the anterior portion by the palatine process of the right and left maxillae and the smaller posterior part by the horizontal plates of the two palatine bones (Fig. 4.3).

The roof of the oral cavity is dome-shaped. It is lined by thick keratinized epithelium which is tightly bound down to the underlying bone and is ideally suited to withstand the friction of mastication. In the midline, immediately behind the anterior teeth, is the small incisive papilla and running backwards from this, along the

midline, is a hard ridge called the median raphe. On either side of the anterior part of the raphe are a series of corrugations, termed rugae, which lie parallel to the anterior teeth. These provide an ideal rubbing surface for the tongue during the mastication of food. Behind the rugae the surface of the hard palate is smooth and on each side of the median raphe a soft pad of glandular tissue lies between the mucous membrane and the bone. The ducts of these glands open on to the surface.

The blood supply to the hard palate is from the greater palatine artery, which emerges on to the surface of the hard palate through the greater palatine foramen. It has a dual nerve supply: most of its area is supplied by the anterior palatine nerve, which also emerges from the greater palatine foramen, but the portion of the palate immediately behind the anterior teeth is supplied by the nasopalatine nerve. Both these nerves are branches of the maxillary division of the trigeminal (Vth cranial) nerve.

The soft palate

The soft palate extends backwards and downwards from the hard palate and, as the name implies, contains no bony tissue. Unlike the hard palate, it is mobile, acting as a flap which can alternately close off the nasopharynx from the oropharynx (as happens during swallowing) or the oral cavity from the oropharynx (as happens during respiration).

The soft palate consists of a sheet of fibrous tissue, termed an aponeurosis, into which are inserted the various muscles responsible for the soft palate's movements. Its lower surface is concave and covered with non-keratinized stratified squamous epithelium, continuous with epithelium of the hard palate. The convex upper surface is lined with respiratory epithelium (ciliated columnar epithelium) which is continuous with that of the nasal cavity. Numerous mucous glands lie between the aponeurosis and both surfaces. Taste buds are present in the epithelium of the oral surface.

The small conical projection which hangs down from the middle of the free posterior margin of the soft palate is the uvula.

The lesser palatine artery, a branch of the greater palatine artery, is the main blood source of the soft palate, and the posterior palatine nerve, a branch of the trigeminal, is the main sensory nerve. This also carries the taste sensation from the taste buds of the soft palate. The artery and nerve reach the soft palate through the lesser palatine foramen.

> The oral cavity consists of these parts.
> The lips
> * orbicularis oris
> * surface features: philtrum, angle, commissures and nasolabial groove.
> The cheeks
> * buccinator.
> The floor of the oral cavity
> * mylohyoid muscle
> * surface features: lingual fraenum, sublingual papillae and folds.
> The tongue
> * surfaces: dorsum, ventral
> * papillae of the tongue
> * muscles: intrinsic, extrinsic.
> Alveolar ridges
> * gingiva: appearance: pink stippled, firm, keratinized
> * free and attached gingiva, gingival crevice and interdental papilla
> * vestibule, mucogingival junction and fraenae.
> The palate
> * hard palate: bones, surface features, blood and nerve supplies
> * soft palate: aponeurosis, movements, uvula, blood and nerve supplies.

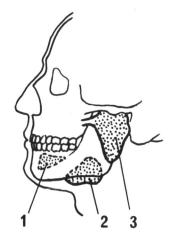

Fig. 4.15 The position of the three main salivary glands: **1** sublingual, **2** submandibular, **3** parotid. The portions of the glands lying deep to the mandible are outlined with a dotted line.

Salivary glands

The oral cavity is bathed in saliva, which is produced by three pairs of large glands, the parotid, the submandibular and the sublingual, and numerous small glands in the lining of the oral cavity itself (Fig. 4.15). Saliva may be serous (watery) or mucous in consistency and is described more fully in Chapter 6.

Parotid gland

The parotid gland is situated below the external auditory meatus, between the mastoid process and the posterior border of the ramus of the mandible. It is the largest of the salivary glands, producing roughly 25% of the total volume of saliva. The saliva which it produces is mainly serous in nature and is carried to the oral cavity by the parotid duct. The duct passes forwards from the gland, on the outer surface of the masseter muscle. At the anterior border of the masseter it turns inwards, piercing the buccinator and buccal pad of fatty tissue, to open on to the buccal mucosa opposite the upper second molar tooth.

Submandibular gland

The submandibular gland lies in the submandibular fossa, below the mylohyoid line on the inner aspect of the body of the mandible. It is the middle of the three glands, both in position and size, and it produces a mixture of serous and mucous saliva. Despite not being the largest gland, it produces approximately 70% of the total volume of saliva. The submandibular duct arises from the posterior part of the gland and initially passes upwards to hook round the posterior border of the mylohyoid muscle. It then travels along the upper surface of that muscle and opens by a small orifice on the sublingual papilla on the floor of the mouth.

Sublingual gland

The sublingual gland is the smallest of the three main glands. It lies beneath the mucosa of the floor of the mouth in the sublingual fossa on the inner aspect of the mandible. It produces approximately 5% of the total volume of saliva of a mainly mucous type, which drains through numerous small ducts opening on the ridge of the sublingual fold.

The smaller saliva glands are situated in the lips cheeks and palate and produce relatively small quantities of saliva. The composition and function of saliva is discussed in Chapter 6.

The salivary glands
Parotid gland
- largest gland
- lies between the ramus and mastoid process
- produces 25% of saliva (mainly serous)
- duct opens on to buccal mucosa.

Submandibular gland
- middle gland by size
- lies in submandibular fossa
- produces 70% of saliva (mixed)
- duct opens on to sublingual papilla.

Sublingual gland
- smallest gland
- lies in sublingual fossa
- produces 5% of saliva (mainly mucous)
- numerous ducts opening on sublingual fold.

Muscles of mastication

The muscles which control the movements of the mandible are collectively referred to as the muscles of mastication. There are four of them on each side (Table 4.9).

Temporalis

This is a fan-shaped muscle situated on the side of the head. It arises from the whole of the temporal fossa and its fibres converge downwards to be inserted into the tip of the coronoid process and the whole of the anterior edge of the ramus. When it contracts, it pulls the coronoid process upwards and backwards, closing the teeth together. Its contraction can be felt by placing the fingertips on the side of the head, above and in front of the ear.

Masseter

The masseter is a strong quadrilateral muscle which originates on the zygomatic arch and is inserted into the roughened outer surface of the

---

Table 4.9 The muscles of mastication

The muscles of mastication are

Those which close the mouth and clench the teeth
- Temporalis.
- Masseter.
- Medial pterygoid.

The one which separates the teeth and opens the mouth
- Lateral pterygoid.

---

ramus. It pulls the mandible upwards and is easily palpated when the teeth are clenched. It is a strong muscle which is used in chewing and grinding.

Medial pterygoid

This is a thick quadrilateral muscle arising from the medial surface of the lateral pterygoid plate. Its fibres pass downwards, backwards and outwards and are inserted into the medial surface of the ramus, between the angle and the mandibular foramen. The medial pterygoid pulls the mandible upwards and forwards and, like the masseter, is important in chewing, clenching and grinding. When the medial and lateral pterygoids contract simultaneously, the mandible is protruded.

Lateral pterygoid

The lateral pterygoid is a short thick muscle which arises from the lateral surface of the lateral pterygoid plate and from the base of the skull lateral to this plate. It passes backwards and outwards to be inserted into the neck of the condyle and the fibrous capsule surrounding the temporomandibular joint. When it contracts, the lateral pterygoid pulls the head of the condyle forwards onto the articular eminence. The reader should refer to the earlier section on the temporomandibular joint movements. When the lateral pterygoid muscles of both sides of the mandible contract together, the effect is to lower the body of the mandible, separate the teeth and open the mouth. However, if the medial pterygoid muscles contract simultaneously with the lateral pterygoids, they prevent the mandible from being depressed and

Table 4.10 The movements of the mandible

This information should be read in conjunction with the section on the temporomandibular joint. The role of the muscles involved in mandibular movements can be summarized as follows

- Depression. The mandible is lowered by gravity and by the action of the lateral pterygoids. However, if the mouth is opened against a resisting force (as, for example, when the teeth are stuck in a toffee) the contraction of three muscles lying below the mandible, the geniohyoid, mylohyoid and digastric, also plays a part.
- Elevation. The mandible is raised by the action of the masseter, temporal and medial pterygoid.
- Protrusion. The medial and lateral pterygoids of both sides, acting together, stick the chin out.
- Retraction. The mandible is pulled back by the temporal muscles.
- Lateral swing. This is the result of the lateral and medial pterygoid muscles of one side only contracting together. When those on opposing sides contract alternately the mandible swings from side to side, as it does during chewing.

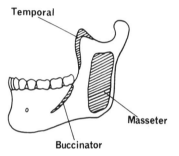

Fig. 4.16 The areas of muscle attachments on the outer aspect of the mandible.

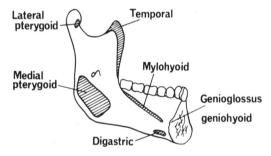

Fig. 4.17 The areas of muscle attachments on the inner aspect of the mandible.

the point of the chin will be protruded. If the lateral and medial pterygoids of one side only contract, the mandible will deviate towards the opposite side. This is a movement which is common in chewing.

The insertions of the muscles of mastication into the mandible are shown in Figures 4.16 and 4.17. The movements of the mandible are shown in Table 4.10. The motor nerve supply to all these muscles is the mandibular division of

the trigeminal nerve, as is described later in this chapter.

Muscles of mastication

Temporalis
- fan shaped
- origin: the temporal fossa
- insertion: tip of the coronoid and anterior edge of the ramus
- raises and retracts the mandible.

Masseter
- strong quadrilateral muscle
- origin: zygomatic arch
- insertion: outer surface of the ramus
- raises the mandible.

Medial pterygoid
- thick quadrilateral muscle
- origin: medial surface of the lateral pterygoid plate
- insertion: inner surface of the ramus
- pulls the mandible upwards and forwards.

Lateral pterygoid
- short thick muscle
- origin: lateral surface of lateral pterygoid plate
- insertion: the neck of condyle and capsular ligament
- pulls the condyle forward on to the articular eminence.

Muscles of facial expression

As the name suggests, these muscles all lie in the superficial tissues of the face: the lips, cheeks, nose, eyelids and forehead. They are collectively responsible for the large variety of facial expressions of which human beings are capable.

The muscles of principal interest to the dental hygienist are those surrounding the lips, most of which are inserted into the orbicularis oris. As previously noted in the section on the lips, the orbicularis oris is a circular muscle which surrounds the mouth and forms the bulk of the lips. It has no origin or insertion; the fibres form a continuous band around the mouth. When it contracts it purses the lips but, by the contraction of the many muscles inserted into it, a wide variety of shapes can be achieved.

The largest muscle inserted into the orbicularis oris is the buccinator, described in the section on the cheeks. Since the buccinator is inserted into the lateral aspect of orbicularis oris, contraction of that muscle will pull the angles of the mouth outwards, producing a sardonic smile. Also inserted into the lateral aspect is a small muscle, superficial to buccinator, termed risorius. This is attached laterally to the under surface of the skin of the cheek and may produce a dimple in that area.

The muscles which are inserted into the upper half of orbicularis oris originate from the facial surface of the facial bones, primarily the maxilla. They include the following.

- Levator anguli oris: inserted into the orbicularis oris close to the angle of the mouth, these muscles raise the corners of the mouth, as in smiling.
- Levator labii superioris and levator labii superioris alaeque nasi. As the name suggests, these raise the upper lip. The latter muscle also inserts into the side of the nose and dilates the nostrils.
- Zygomaticus major and minor. These narrow strips of muscle run from orbicularis oris to the zygomatic process. When they contract, they pull the upper lip upwards and laterally.

The muscles inserted into the lower part of the orbicularis oris originate from the outer surface of the body of the mandible. They include the following.

- Depressor anguli oris. These muscles are inserted close to the angles of the mouth, so contraction will depress the angles, giving an appearance of sadness.

- Depressor labii inferioris. This muscle depresses and everts the lower lip.

A further small muscle of the chin is closely associated with these muscles but, unlike the others, is not inserted into orbicularis oris. It is mentalis, a small muscle which runs from the facial surface of the mandible below the incisor teeth to be inserted into the undersurface of the skin over the point of the chin. Contraction of this muscle will pull the skin of the chin, and therefore the lower lip, upwards. It is this muscle which causes the commonly seen dimple in the chin.

The motor nerve supply to all of the muscles of facial expression, with the exception of the buccinator, is the facial nerve, the VIIth cranial nerve. Buccinator is supplied by the mandibular nerve which is described in detail later in this chapter.

> Muscles of facial expression around the mouth consists of the orbicularis oris with other muscles inserted into it
> - Laterally: buccinator, risorius.
> - Superiorly: levator anguli oris, levator labii superioris, levator labii superioris alaeque nasi, zygomaticus major and minor.
> - Inferiorly: depressor anguli oris, depressor labii inferioris, Mentalis inserted into the skin of the chin.

The nerve supply to the oral cavity

The entire dentition and the associated gingiva are supplied by the trigeminal nerve. This nerve gets its name because it splits into three divisions while still within the cranial cavity: the ophthalmic, maxillary and mandibular nerves (Fig. 4.18). It is principally a sensory nerve and the ophthalmic and maxillary divisions consist of only sensory fibres. However, the mandibular nerve contains both sensory and motor fibres.

The ophthalmic nerve supplies the structures in and around the orbit and is of only peripheral interest to the dental hygienist. The maxillary and mandibular nerves supply, amongst other things, the oral cavity including

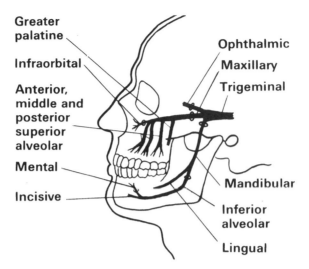

Fig. 4.18 The nerves supplying the oral cavity and surrounding structures. With the exception of the mental and infraorbital nerves, they all lie within or deep to the bones of the skull.

the teeth and gingivae and will, therefore, be described in more detail.

Maxillary nerve

The maxillary nerve leaves the cranial cavity through the foramen rotundum and enters the pterygopalatine fossa, which can be seen on the dried skull as a narrow space behind the body of the maxilla. In the fossa, the nerve divides into its terminal branches.

The infraorbital nerve

The main fibres of the maxillary nerve continue forwards, as the infraorbital nerve, into the orbit, where the nerve lies in a groove in the orbital floor. As it passes forwards, it enters the infraorbital canal and eventually emerges on to the facial aspect of the maxilla, through the infraorbital foramen. It supplies sensation to the area of skin enclosed by the side of the nose, the lower eyelid, the upper lip, the mucous membrane of the upper lip and part of the cheeks.

Alveolar branches

The upper teeth are supplied by the maxillary nerve, via three branches: the posterior, middle and anterior superior alveolar nerves.

- **The posterior superior alveolar nerve** is given off within the pterygopalatine fossa and supplies the upper molar teeth and the buccal gingivae of these teeth.
- **The middle superior alveolar nerve** arises from the infraorbital nerve within the infraorbital canal and supplies the upper premolar teeth and their buccal gingiva.
- **The anterior superior alveolar nerve** is also given off within the infraorbital canal and supplies the upper anterior teeth and labial gingivae.

Palatal nerves

The anterior and posterior palatine nerves arise from the maxillary nerve within the pterygopalatine fossa and pass through the greater palatine canal to the palate. The anterior palatine nerve emerges through the greater palatine foramen to supply sensation to the hard palate and palatal gingiva, with the exception of a small area behind the incisors. The posterior palatine nerve emerges through the lesser palatine foramen and supplies sensation (including taste) to the soft palate.

The nasopalatine nerve supplies the area of the hard palate immediately behind the incisors, including the palatal gingivae of these teeth. It is also a branch of the maxillary nerve, arising in the pterygopalatine fossa. It passes downwards and forwards on the nasal septum

Table 4.11 The nerve supply to the teeth and gingiva

The teeth
- Anterior superior alveolar nerve: upper incisors and canines.
- Middle superior alveolar nerve: upper premolars.
- Posterior superior alveolar nerve: upper molars.
- Incisive nerve: lower incisors, canines and first premolars.
- Inferior dental nerve: lower second premolar and molars.

The gingiva
- Anterior superior alveolar nerve: labial surface of upper incisors and canines.
- Middle superior alveolar nerve: buccal to upper premolars.
- Posterior superior alveolar nerve: buccal to upper molars.
- Nasopalatine nerve: palatal to upper incisors.
- Anterior palatine nerve: palatal to upper canines, premolars and molars.
- Mental nerve: labial to lower incisors, canines and first premolars.
- Buccal nerve: buccal to lower second premolar and molars.
- Lingual nerve: lingual to all lower teeth.

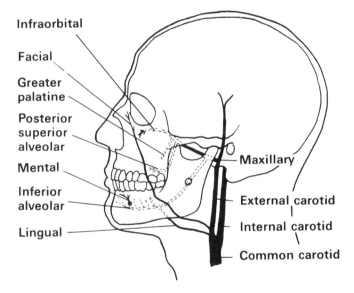

Fig. 4.19 The main arteries supplying the oral cavity and surrounding structures. Those arteries within or deep to the bones are drawn with dotted lines.

to reach the palate through the incisive foramen.

Mandibular nerve

The mandibular nerve leaves the cranial cavity through the foramen ovale and passes downwards in front of the condyle and deep to the ramus. It then enters the mandibular foramen and travels forward through the body of the mandible in the mandibular canal, supplying the posterior teeth. The portion of the mandibular nerve within the mandibular canal is commonly referred to as the inferior dental nerve. At the level of the premolars, it divides into its two terminal branches. The mental nerve emerges through the mental foramen and supplies the labial gingivae of the anterior teeth, the mucous membrane of the lower lip and the skin of the lip and chin. The incisive branch continues on through the bone to supply the lower anterior teeth.

Muscular branches

Between the foramen ovale and mandibular foramen, the mandibular nerve gives off motor nerves to the masseter, medial pterygoid, lateral pterygoid, temporal and mylohyoid muscles and the anterior part of the digastric.

Lingual nerve

This arises from the mandibular nerve soon after it leaves the foramen ovale. It passes downwards and forwards, deep to the ramus, where it is joined by the fibres of the chorda tympani. This is a branch of the facial nerve carrying taste fibres which travel with the lingual nerve to supply the tongue. As the lingual nerve curves forwards it initially lies close to the inner aspect of the body of the mandible at the level of the roots of the third molar and then enters the body of the tongue. It is the sensory nerve of the anterior two-thirds of the tongue and its branches also supply the lingual gingiva of the lower teeth and the floor of the mouth.

Buccal nerve

Before entering the mandibular foramen, the mandibular nerve also gives off the buccal nerve which supplies the cheek and the buccal gingiva of the lower posterior teeth.

The nerve supply to the teeth and gingiva is summarized in Table 4.11. This table should be referred to again when the section on local analgesia is being studied.

Nerve supply to the oral cavity.
- Trigeminal nerve: ophthalmic, maxillary, mandibular branches.
- Maxillary nerve
  - infraorbital branch
  - alveolar branches: anterior, middle and posterior superior alveolar nerves
  - palatine branches: anterior palatine, posterior palatine and nasopalatine nerves.
- Mandibular nerve
  - muscular branches to masseter, medial and lateral pterygoid, temporalis and buccinator.
  - Inferior dental nerve.
  - Mental and incisive nerves.
  - Lingual nerve.
  - Buccal nerve.

Blood supply to the oral cavity

The main artery passing up through the neck on each side to the head is the large common carotid artery, which divides in the neck into the internal and external carotid arteries (Fig. 4.19). The internal carotid principally supplies the contents of the cranial cavity and the external carotid supplies the face and the exterior of the head. The oral cavity receives its blood supply from three branches of the external carotid: the lingual artery, the facial artery, and the maxillary artery.

Lingual artery

This arises from the external carotid in the neck, below the angle of the mandible. It supplies, amongst other structures, the tongue and floor of the mouth.

Facial artery

The facial artery branches off from the external carotid a little above the lingual artery. It runs forward under cover of the body of the mandible and at the anterior edge of the masseter it hooks round the lower border of the mandible on to the face. At this point, its pulse can be felt by placing the fingertip on the notch in the lower border. The artery then passes forwards and upwards through the cheek towards the medial corner of the eye where it terminates. Its branches supply most of the face, including the cheeks and lips.

Maxillary artery

This is one of the two terminal branches of the external carotid, arising behind the neck of the condyle. It runs forwards, deep to the condyle, to enter the pterygopalatine fossa where it divides into its terminal branches. It has several branches which are of interest to dental hygienists.

Inferior alveolar artery

This arises deep to the condyle and travels downwards with the mandibular nerve, entering the mandibular foramen and passing forwards through the body of the mandible in the mandibular canal. It supplies the lower posterior teeth and buccal gingivae and divides into two branches at the level of the premolars: the mental branch leaves the mandible through the mental foramen and supplies the lower lip and chin, and the incisive branch continues on through the bone to supply the anterior teeth and anastomose with the artery of the other side. Before entering the mandibular foramen, the inferior alveolar artery gives off a lingual branch, which runs downwards and forwards with the lingual nerve to supply part of the floor of the mouth.

Superior alveolar arteries

The posterior superior alveolar artery
This arises on the pterygopalatine fossa and supplies the posterior teeth and their buccal gingiva.

Anterior superior alveolar artery
Like the maxillary nerve, the maxillary artery terminates in the infra-orbital branch which travels forwards in the floor of the orbit to enter the infra-orbital canal and emerge on to the facial surface of the maxilla through the infra-orbital foramen. While in the infra-orbital canal it gives off the anterior superior alveolar artery, the blood supply to the upper anterior teeth and labial gingiva.

Palatine arteries

The greater palatine artery arises in the pterygopalatine fossa and passes down through the greater palatine foramen and supplies the hard palate and palatal gingiva. In the greater palatine canal it gives off the lesser palatine artery which emerges through the lesser palatine foramen to supply the soft palate.

Venous drainage

The venous drainage of the maxillary and mandibular areas of the face is similar to the arterial supply. The lingual, facial and maxillary veins correspond roughly to their respec-

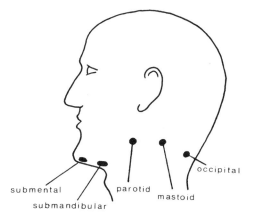

Fig. 4.20 The main lymph glands of the head

tive arteries and drain eventually into the large external and internal jugular veins of the neck.

Lymphatic drainage of the head and neck

Lymph is found in all the tissue spaces of the body and is a clear colourless fluid consisting mainly of tissue fluid and blood plasma. The collection and distribution of lymph (which is the third part of the vascular system) is somewhat similar to that of the blood. At intervals along the lymph vessels, nodes are found. The basic structure of the lymphatics has already been described in Chapter 3.

The lymphatics may drain infected and other pathological material from the tissues, and the nodes act as a filter system. The inflammation observed in nodes filtering infected material is termed lymphadenitis and the enlargement of nodes due to the presence of cancerous cells is termed lymphadenopathy.

Lymph nodes of the head and neck

As illustrated in Figure 4.20, the principal lymph nodes of the head form a ring around the base of the skull. On each side there are the submental, submandibular, parotid, mastoid and occipital lymph glands. Lymph from the various structures of the head drains down into one or other of these glands and from them into either the superficial or deep cervical lymph chains. The cervical lymph chains drain into the thoracic duct on the left side and the right lymphatic duct on the right.

Submental lymph nodes

These are located immediately below the chin. They drain:

- the tip of the tongue,
- the anterior part of the floor of the mouth,
- the anterior gingival tissue and the lower anterior teeth,
- the centre of the lower lip,
- the chin.

The lymph is then carried from the submental nodes to the submandibular group of nodes.

The submandibular nodes

The submandibular nodes lie just below the border of the mandible on each side close to the submandibular salivary glands. They drain the following structures:

- the submental group (as above),
- the nose and upper lip,
- the lateral borders of lower lips,
- the lateral borders of floor of mouth,
- the lateral borders of tongue,
- the teeth and gingiva, with the exception of the lower incisors.

Blood supply to the face and oral cavity consists of the common, external and internal carotid arteries.

External carotid branches to the oral cavity
- lingual artery
- facial artery
- maxillary artery.

Maxillary artery branches
- anterior and posterior alveolar arteries
- infra-orbital artery
- anterior and posterior palatine arteries.

Venous drainage of the face
- lingual, facial and maxillary veins
- external and internal jugular veins.

Lymphatic drainage of the head and neck
- submental, submandibular, parotid, mastoid and occipital lymph nodes
- area drained by the submental node
- area drained by the submandibular node
- superficial and deep cervical lymph chains

Further reading

Atkinson, M. E., White, F. E. (1992) *Principles of Anatomy and Oral Anatomy for Dental Students.* Edinburgh: Churchill Livingstone.

Johnson D. R., Moore W.J. (1997) *Anatomy for Dental Students.* (3rd edition), Oxford University Press.

5

Tooth morphology

The dentition

Humans develop two complete sets of teeth in their lifetime: the primary or deciduous dentition, commonly called the 'baby teeth' or 'milk teeth' and the permanent dentition which replaces the primary one during childhood. There are 20 primary and 32 permanent teeth.

Terminology

For identification purposes, the two dental arches are each divided into right and left halves, making four quadrants: upper right and left and lower right and left. This is represented diagrammatically by a grid in which a horizontal line separates the upper and lower arches and a central vertical line divides right from left. The eight permanent teeth of each quadrant are numbered 1 to 8 working backwards from the midline. The five primary teeth in each quadrant are given the letters A to E in a similar way (Table 5.1).

Table 5.1 Tooth identification
Diagrammatically, the teeth are shown as follows
Permanent dentition
8 7 6 5 4 3 2 1 | 1 2 3 4 5 6 7 8
8 7 6 5 4 3 2 1 | 1 2 3 4 5 6 7 8
Primary dentition
E D C B A | A B C D E
E D C B A | A B C D E

The individual teeth are named as follows.

Permanent teeth

1 Central incisor
2 Lateral incisor
3 Canine
4 First premolar
5 Second premolar
6 First molar
7 Second molar
8 Third molar

Primary teeth

A Central incisor
B Lateral incisor
C Canine
D First molar
E Second molar

The upper canines are often referred to in lay terms as the 'eye teeth' and the third molars are commonly called the 'wisdom teeth'. Alternative terms, used particularly in USA, for premolars and canines are bicuspids and cuspids, respectively.

The biggest disadvantage of the identification system described above is the need to use symbols to indicate the four quadrants of the mouth when identifying individual teeth. For example, the upper right permanent lateral incisor would be identified as 2| and the lower left primary first molar as |D. This creates difficulty when collecting computerized data for research or other purposes and when transmitting data electronically; for example for identification purposes after mass casualties.

International Dental Federation Classification

The International Dental Federation (Fédération Dentaire Internationale, FDI) recommended system of tooth-numbering has been adopted by most countries throughout the world. It uses a different number to identify each specific tooth, avoiding the need for using the grid symbol. Each quadrant is numbered from 1 to 4 for the permanent teeth and 5 to 8 for the primary teeth. The teeth in these quadrants are then given another number: 1 to 8 from the midline backwards in the case of the permanent teeth and 1 to 5 for the deciduous teeth (Table 5.2).

With the increasing use of computers, it is likely that the FDI system will continue to be more widely used and the dental hygienist should be comfortable with its use.

Terminology

- Primary (deciduous) dentition: 20 teeth, replaced by the permanent dentition.
- Permanent dentition: 32 teeth.

Tooth identification.

- The grid method of identifying teeth. The permanent teeth identified by number 1 to 8 from front to back and the primary teeth similarly identified A to E. The appropriate quadrant identified using the symbols ⌞, ⌟, ⌜ and ⌝.
- The names of individual teeth. Central and lateral incisors, canines, premolars and molars.
- The FDI classification of teeth. The teeth identified using a double number; the first identifying the quadrant and the second identifying the position of the tooth. The permanent quadrants are 1 (upper right), 2 (upper left), 3 (lower left) and 4 (lower right). The primary quadrants are 5 (upper right), 6 (upper left), 7 (lower left) and 8 (lower right). All teeth numbered from front to back: 1 to 8 (permanent) and 1 to 5 (primary).

Table 5.2 The FDI tooth identification system

The FDI tooth identification system numbers individual teeth as follows

Permanent teeth	
18 17 16 15 14 13 12 11	21 22 23 24 25 26 27 28
48 47 46 45 44 43 42 41	31 32 33 34 35 36 37 38
Primary teeth	
55 54 53 52 51	61 62 63 64 65
85 84 83 82 81	71 72 73 74 75

General tooth structure

Each tooth is composed of a crown and one or more roots. The bulk of the tooth is made up of dentine, but the crown is covered by a layer of enamel and the roots are covered by a thin layer of cementum (Fig. 5.1). The tooth has a hollow centre which contains the pulp. Each of these tissues is described in greater detail in Chapter 6.

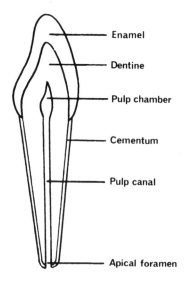

- Enamel
- Dentine
- Pulp chamber
- Cementum
- Pulp canal
- Apical foramen

Fig. 5.1 Diagram of a labiolingual section through a lower incisor tooth.

Crown

This is the portion of the tooth which projects into the oral cavity. Its shape varies from tooth to tooth and is closely related to its function (Table 5.3).

The incisors have chisel-shaped crowns which are ideal for biting into (or incising) food. The canines have pointed crowns which make them ideal for tearing foodstuffs such as meat. These teeth are very pronounced in carnivorous animals such as the dog, from which they derive their name. Premolars and molars are more box-shaped, with rectangular biting surfaces ideally designed for grinding food. These surfaces (the occlusal surfaces) are not smooth, but are made up of a series of elevations (cusps) and grooves (fissures) which improve the efficiency of their grinding action.

Table 5.3 Tooth surface identification

In describing the various tooth surfaces, the following terms are used

- **Mesial**: nearest the midline of the dental arch.
- **Distal**: furthest from the midline.
- **Lingual**: nearest the tongue.
- **Palatal**: nearest the palate.
- **Labial**: nearest the lips.
- **Buccal**: nearest the cheeks.
- **Occlusal**: the surface which comes into contact (occlusion) with the opposing teeth.

Roots

The roots of the teeth are the portions which are contained within the alveolar bone. They are roughly conical in shape, being thickest near the crown and narrowing towards the apex. The fibres of the periodontal ligament which attaches the tooth to bone are inserted into the alveolar bone on the one side and the cementum covering the root on the other.

The incisors and canines have a single root, the premolars have either one or two roots and the molars have either two or three roots.

The dividing line between the crown and root is where the enamel meets the cementum: the enamel–cementum junction. This is not a straight line, but curves towards the apex on the labial and lingual aspects and curves away from the apex on the mesial and distal aspects. These curvatures correspond to the scalloped outline of the gingival margin (see Chapter 4) and are more marked on anterior than posterior teeth.

Pulp

The pulp is the only soft tissue part of the tooth and contains a rich blood and nerve supply. It is divided into the pulp chamber and root canals. The pulp chamber lies within the crown and conforms roughly to its shape. It projects upwards into each cusp of the molar, premolar and canine teeth and towards the mesial and distal angles of the incisors crowns; the pointed projections being termed the pulp horns or cornua. Each root has a root canal leading from the pulp chamber to the apical foramen, through which the pulp connects with the periodontal ligament.

Teeth are made up of a crown and one or more roots.

The tissues of the teeth are
- dentine, which forms the bulk of the tooth
- enamel, which covers the crown
- cementum, forming a thin covering over the root
- pulp, which is the soft central portion of the tooth.

The crown has
- a shape related to function
- surfaces identified by the terms: occlusal, mesial, distal, buccal/labial and lingual/palatal.

The roots are
- conical in shape
- one, two or three in number, depending on the type of tooth
- held in by the fibres of periodontal ligament which are embedded into the cementum.

The pulp is
- the soft central portion of the tooth
- contains a rich nerve and blood vessel supply
- divided into a pulp chamber and one or more root canals.

Individual tooth morphology

When attempting to study the morphology of individual teeth it is extremely helpful, if not essential, to have some extracted teeth available for examination. Although there may seem little point in dental hygienists being able to identify extracted teeth as being upper or lower and right or left, a sound understanding of tooth morphology is essential from a clinical point of view. For example, there is the significance of the palatal pit of upper laterals in relation to caries, the canine fossa of upper first premolars in relation to plaque control and the importance of root morphology in relation to deep scaling.

Permanent incisors

There are eight permanent incisors: two upper centrals, two upper laterals, two lower centrals and two lower laterals. They differ from each other in ways which will be described later, but all have chisel-shaped crowns and a single root (Fig. 5.2).

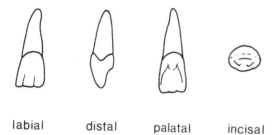

labial   distal   palatal   incisal

Fig. 5.2 Upper left permanent central incisor.

When newly erupted, the incisal edge has three small tubercles, called mamelons, placed mesially, centrally and distally, but these are rapidly worn flat with use. In each case, the distal angle of the crown (between the incisal edge and the distal surface) is more rounded than the mesial angle.

The mesial and distal surfaces are wedge-shaped, being widest at the cervical margin and tapering towards the incisal edge. The labial aspect is roughly rectangular and slightly convex, especially near the cervical margin. Two shallow vertical grooves run from the notches between the incisal tubercles towards the cervical margin. The lingual or palatal aspect is triangular in shape, with mesial and distal marginal ridges running from the mesial and distal angles to converge on the cingulum, a prominence situated close to the gingival margin. Bordered by these prominences is a concavity termed the lingual fossa.

The root of an incisor is approximately one

and a half times the length of the crown and frequently curves distally towards the apex.

Upper central incisor

The crown of the upper central incisor is larger than those of the other incisors. The root is roughly triangular in section, being wider labially than palatally. Otherwise it conforms closely to the general description already given (Fig. 5.2).

Upper lateral incisor

The crown of this tooth is both shorter and narrower than the upper central and its distal angle is more rounded than that of the upper central. It has a well marked cingulum and marginal ridges and there is often a developmental pit or groove between the cingulum and the lingual fossa, making this area particularly prone to tooth decay. There may be developmental grooves on the mesial and distal aspects of the root (Fig. 5.3).

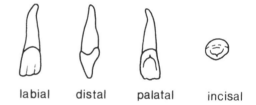

labial   distal   palatal   incisal

Fig. 5.3 Upper left permanent lateral incisor.

The crown of the upper lateral incisor is subject to considerable variation in form. It may be conical in shape (a 'peg-shaped lateral') and the tooth may even be missing from the dentition.

Lower central Incisor

The lower central incisor is considerably narrower mesiodistally than the upper central. The vertical grooves on the labial aspect are faint or absent and the lingual surface is only slightly concave with poorly developed marginal ridges. The root is flattened mesiodistally. This is the smallest of the permanent incisors.

Lower lateral incisor

This is slightly larger than the lower central

incisor, but is otherwise very similar to it. The distal angle tends to be more curved than that of the lower central and the long axis of the root is angled slightly distally in relation to the long axis of the crown (Fig. 5.4).

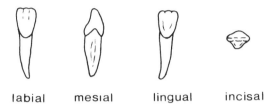

labial   mesial   lingual   incisal

Fig. 5.4 Lower left second permanent incisor.

Permanent canines (or cuspids)

Like the incisors, the canines are wedge-shaped when viewed from the mesial and distal aspects, and have a convex labial surface and concave lingual surface. They also have a single root which often curves distally towards the apex.

Each canine has a single, well marked cusp (hence the term cuspid) from which the incisal edge slopes away mesially and distally towards the points of contact of the canine with the lateral incisor and first premolar respectively. The distal slope is longer than the mesial slope. On the labial surfaces there are two vertical grooves running from either side of the cusp towards the cervical margin. The cingulum and marginal ridges are well marked and there is also, on the palatal aspect, a central vertical ridge running from the cusp to the cingulum.

Upper canine

This is a prominent, strong tooth which, as already noted is often referred to as the 'eye tooth'. Its root is longer than those of all other teeth and is triangular in section, being wider labially than lingually (Fig. 5.5).

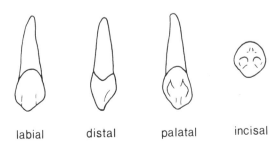

labial   distal   palatal   incisal

Fig. 5.5 Upper left permanent canine.

Lower canine

The lower canine is shorter and thinner than the upper. It has less obvious marginal ridges and cingulum and its root is flattened mesiodistally (Fig. 5.6).

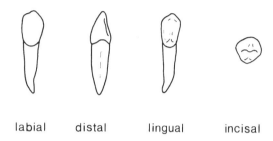

labial   distal   lingual   incisal

Fig. 5.6 Lower left permanent canine.

Premolars (or bicuspids)

These are eight in number, with two in each quadrant. They are also termed bicuspids since they have two cusps: one buccal and one lingual. The buccal cusp is the larger and the two cusps are linked by mesial and distal marginal ridges which circumscribe the occlusal surfaces of the tooth and form a mesial and distal fossa. The occlusal surface is roughly rhomboidal in shape and is longer buccolingually than mesiodistally. A fissure, running mesiodistally, separates the two cusps.

The buccal, lingual, mesial and distal surfaces are all generally convex and each premolar usually has one root, with the exception of the upper first premolar which usually has two.

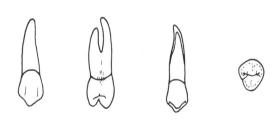

Fig. 5.7 Upper left first premolar.

Upper first premolar

The upper first premolar normally has two roots, one buccal and one palatal, although the two roots may on occasions be fused into one.

Unlike the other premolars, the mesial slope of the buccal cusp of the tooth is longer than the distal slope. Another distinguishing feature of this tooth is that it has a marked depression in its mesial aspect, called the canine fossa, immediately below its point of contact with the canine. It is important to note this, because it may be difficult to remove plaque and calculus from this region (Fig. 5.7).

Upper second premolar

This tooth is similar to the upper first premolar but may be distinguished from it by the fact that it usually has only one root, has no concavity in its mesial aspect and the mesial slope of its buccal cusp is shorter than the distal slope (Fig. 5.8).

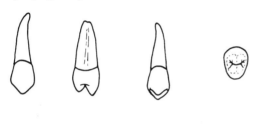

buccal   mesial   palatal   occlusal

Fig. 5.8 Upper left second premolar.

Lower first premolar

This tooth is easily identifiable by its large buccal cusp and very small lingual cusp, which makes it similar to the canine in appearance. The whole of the occlusal surface slopes lingually. The mesial slope of the buccal cusp is shorter than the distal and the tooth normally has a single root, flatted mesiodistally (Fig. 5.9).

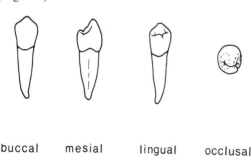

buccal   mesial   lingual   occlusal

Fig. 5.9 Lower left first premolar.

Lower second premolar

The lower second premolar has a well marked lingual cusp which may be divided into two by a fissure passing over on to its lingual aspect. Its occlusal surface is more square in outline than the other premolars. Its cusps are flatter than those of the other premolars and the mesial slope of the buccal cusp is shorter than the distal slope. It has a single root (Fig. 5.10).

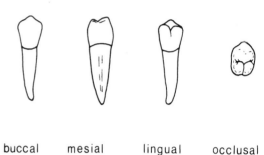

buccal   mesial   lingual   occlusal

Fig. 5.10 Lower left second premolar.

Permanent molars

There are 12 molars in the permanent dentition: three in each quadrant. They have crowns which are shorter than the premolars but which are wider buccolingually and considerably longer mesiodistally. Their occlusal surfaces are roughly rhomboidal in shape. The molars have four principal cusps: a mesiobuccal cusp, a mesiolingual cusp, a distobuccal cusp and a distolingual cusp. The buccal and lingual cusps are separated by a mesiodistal fissure and two fissures, running on to the lingual and buccal aspects of the tooth respectively, separate the mesial and distal cusps. The exact pattern of fissures on the occlusal surface varies with each of the molars and will be described in more detail later. In each case, marginal ridges bound the mesial and distal portions of the occlusal surface.

The buccal and lingual aspects of the molars are convex and have a fissure extending vertically, from between the two buccal or lingual cusps to a point roughly halfway to the cervical margin. The buccal aspect is normally longer and more convex than the lingual.

The upper molars normally have three roots situated mesiobuccally, distobuccally and palatally, while the lower molars usually have two roots placed mesially and distally.

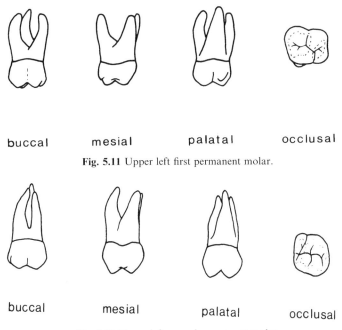

buccal   mesial   palatal   occlusal

Fig. 5.11 Upper left first permanent molar.

buccal   mesial   palatal   occlusal

Fig. 5.12 Upper left second permanent molar.

Upper first molar

This tooth conforms fairly closely to the above description. Its crown is wider buccolingually than mesiodistally. The mesiopalatal cusp is the largest and is joined to the distobuccal cusp by an oblique ridge. A central and a distal fossa are formed between this ridge and the mesial and distal marginal ridges, respectively. A small fifth cusp, called the cusp of Carabelli, may be present on the palatal aspect and occurs in approximately 60% of these teeth.

Of the three roots, the palatal is the largest and is well separated from the other two. The mesiobuccal and distobuccal roots tend to curve towards each other in the apical region (Fig. 5.11).

Upper second molar

This tooth is similar to the upper first molar, but it does not usually have a fifth cusp and it is slightly shorter mesiodistally. Its distal cusps are less well formed and its three roots are less divergent than those of the upper first molar (Fig. 5.12).

Upper third molar

The upper third molar, or wisdom tooth, is the most distal tooth in the upper arch. Its size and form vary considerably and it is rarely as well formed as the upper first and second molars. In common with the lower third molar this tooth is frequently missing; either because it has failed to develop or because it has failed to erupt. The three roots are often fused together and curve distally in the apical region.

Lower first molar

The lower first molar normally has a smaller fifth cusp present between the distobuccal and distolingual cusps: the distal cusp. The mesiodistal fissure separates the fifth cusp from the distobuccal cusp. Its two roots are well developed. The mesial root initially slopes mesially, but the apical portion curves distally and the distal root is much straighter (Fig. 5.13).

Lower second molar

This tooth is very similar to the lower first molar but its crown is somewhat smaller and it does not have the fifth, distal, cusp. It has a typical cruciform fissure pattern. The roots are not as widely separated as those of the lower first molar and both are inclined distally (Fig. 5.14).

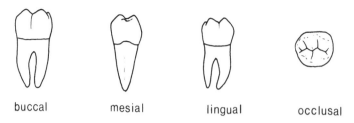

buccal   mesial   lingual   occlusal

Fig. 5.13 Lower left first permanent molar.

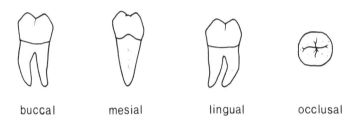

buccal   mesial   lingual   occlusal

Fig. 5.14 Lower left second permanent molar.

Lower third molar

Like its upper counterpart, the lower third molar, or wisdom tooth, varies considerably in size and form and is frequently missing. It is seldom as well formed as the other lower molars. Its two roots are often fused and frequently have a marked distal curvature.

Primary teeth

The primary teeth differ from the permanent teeth in the following ways:

- They are smaller.
- They are usually lighter in colour.
- Their crowns are more bulbous.
- Their roots are proportionally more slender.
- The roots of the primary molars are more divergent than those of the permanent molars. This is to permit them to accommodate the crowns of the premolars, since the permanent teeth develop between them.
- The enamel of the primary teeth is not as hard as that of the permanent teeth.

Primary anterior teeth

Apart from the above points, the primary centrals, laterals and canines are similar to the permanent teeth which succeed them.

Primary molars

Although the primary molars precede the premolars of the permanent dentition, their shape is more like that of the permanent molars. In fact, apart from the general differences listed above, the second primary molars closely resemble the corresponding permanent first molars. The primary first molars are slightly different.

The upper primary first molar has three cusps: mesiobuccal, distobuccal and a crescent-shaped palatal cusp. The lower primary first molar has four cusps: mesiobuccal, mesiolingual, distobuccal and distolingual. These are separated from each other by fissures running mesiodistally and buccolingually.

The primary molars are particularly bulbous on their buccal aspects, near the cervical margin, and in the upper and lower first primary molars this convexity is termed the Tubercle of Zuckerkandl.

Tooth morphology
- Permanent incisors: general morphology – variations of upper centrals, upper laterals, lower centrals and lower laterals.
- Permanent canines: general morphology – variations between upper and lower canines.
- Permanent molars: general morphology – variations of upper first, second and third molars and lower first, second and third molars.
- Primary teeth: morphology of upper and lower first primary molars – similarities between second primary molars and first permanent molars.

Further reading

Atkinson M. E., White F. H. (1992) *Principles of Anatomy and Oral Anatomy for Dental Students*. Edinburgh: Churchill Livingstone.

6

Oral histology and physiology

Oral histology

Histology is the study of the microscopic appearance and development of living tissues and dental histology is the specialized microscopic examination of the dental tissues: enamel, dentine, cementum, pulp, periodontal ligament, alveolar bone and gingiva.

Development of the dental tissues

The development of the teeth and their supporting structures is a very complex process. The various stages are outlined below, simplified as far as possible. It will be seen that enamel develops from epithelial tissue whereas the other dental tissues are all of connective tissue origin. This seems logical since epithelium is the covering tissue of body and enamel covers the crown – the exposed part of the tooth.

Early stages

Dental lamina

Although the primary teeth do not normally erupt until after birth, they begin to develop long before birth (Fig. 6.1). By the sixth week of intrauterine life, the fetus has already developed a primitive oral cavity. Two horseshoe shaped thickenings, corresponding to the two dental arches, start to form in the epithelium of the

oral cavity: one in the roof and the other in the floor. These are called the dental laminae and it is from these that the dentition develops.

Enamel organs

Ten epithelial 'buds' begin to grow into the connective tissue from each dental lamina. They are called the enamel organs and each one is responsible for the development of one of the 20 primary teeth. This is referred to as the bud stage of enamel organ formation.

Cap stage

As the enamel organs grow deeper into the connective tissue and increase in size, they become concave on their deeper aspects, resembling skull caps. The connective tissue lying within the concavity becomes more densely cellular and is known as the dental papilla. It will be seen that this eventually forms the pulp of the tooth. At the same time, a layer of fibrous tissue, called the dental follicle, develops as a capsule around the enamel organ.

Bell stage

Each enamel organ continues to increase in size, becoming more concave, until the outline of the concavity starts to resemble the crown of the tooth being formed. This is referred to as the bell stage because of the similarity of the enamel organs to cow bells. About this time,

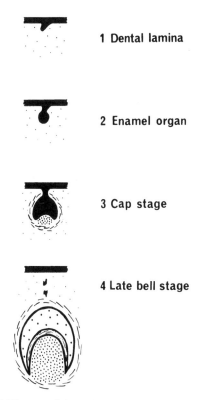

1 Dental lamina

2 Enamel organ

3 Cap stage

4 Late bell stage

Fig. 6.1 Diagram of the early stages of tooth development.

the dental lamina joining them to the oral epithelium begins to disintegrate.

Enamel formation (amelogenesis)

The cells which form enamel are called ameloblasts. They develop from the inner enamel epithelium cells, which become greatly elongated, with their nuclei placed at the end of the cell nearest the stratum intermedium (Fig. 6.2). Shortly before the formation of enamel starts,

the cells of the dental papilla begin to lay down dentine (see below). The ameloblasts then start to deposit enamel between themselves and the newly formed dentine. Initially the enamel is not fully calcified but, within a short time, more calcium salts are added until it reaches its full density. This is called enamel maturation.

This process begins at the deepest part of the concavity of the 'bell', the area which corresponds to the cusps or incisal edge of the developing tooth, and gradually spreads towards the rim of the 'bell' until all the cells of the inner enamel epithelium have been converted into ameloblasts and the outline of the crown has taken shape. As the ameloblasts retreat from their original position, they lay down an increasing thickness of enamel between themselves and the dentine, until the full width of enamel is formed. The enamel in the region of the incisal edge or cusps is the first to reach its full thickness and that in the cervical region is last.

Dentine formation (dentinogenesis)

It has already been noted that dentine formation begins shortly before the formation of enamel. Soon after the inner enamel epithelium cells change into ameloblasts, the layer of cells in the dental papilla adjacent to them also begin to elongate (Fig. 6.2). They become odontoblasts, the cells responsible for dentine deposition, which are not quite as elongated as ameloblasts. In laying down the dentine, the odontoblasts initially form the organic matrix of collagen fibres and ground substance, called pre-dentine. Calcium salts are then deposited in the matrix, producing the completed dentine.

Like enamel, dentine first forms in the deepest part of the concavity of the enamel

---

Table 6.1 Layers of the bell stage of the enamel organ

By the late bell stage the enamel organ has differentiated into four distinct layers

- The inner enamel epithelium: a layer of cuboidal cells.
- The stratum intermedium: a layer of rather non-descript cells.
- The stellate reticulum: a zone of scattered, star-shaped cells.
- The outer enamel epithelium: a layer of cuboidal cells, which is continuous with the inner enamel epithelium around the rim of the bell.

The functions of these various layers are not known but, once this stage has been reached, tooth development proper is about to begin.

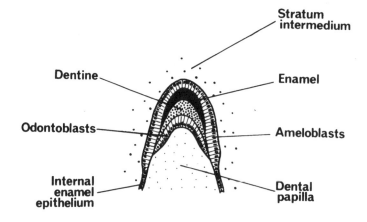

Fig. 6.2 Diagrammatic illustration of a developing tooth shortly after the start of dentine and enamel formation. The area depicted is the deepest part of the enamel organ. Note the elongation of the inner enamel epithelium cells to form ameloblasts and the fact that dentine formation slightly precedes enamel formation.

organ and the process gradually spreads towards the rim. As the odontoblasts move inwards from their original position, forming an increasing thickness of dentine, each one leaves behind a thin strand of cell protoplasm called the odontoblastic process. This becomes enclosed within a microscopic tube of dentine, called the dentinal tubule.

Pulp formation

As the formation of the crown of the tooth progresses, numerous blood vessels and nerves develop within the dental papilla and, by the time the full thickness of dentine is formed, it encloses the pulp chamber, containing the highly vascular and richly innervated pulp.

Root formation

Crown formation is completed before eruption begins, but the roots develop during eruption and are not entirely formed until some time after the tooth is fully erupted. Once enamel formation is finished, the rim of the enamel organ begins to grow deeper into the tissues, mapping out the shape of the root or roots. The four distinct layers seen in the enamel organ do not develop in this downgrowth which is called Hertwig's sheath (Fig. 6.3). Nor do the innermost cells become ameloblasts, remaining

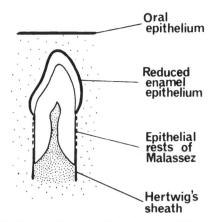

Fig. 6.3 Diagram illustrating the formation of the root.

cuboidal in shape. However, the connective tissue cells next to the inner surface of Hertwig's sheath change into odontoblasts and these in turn start to lay down the dentine of the root in the same way as the dentine of the crown was formed. The odontoblasts move inwards, away from Hertwig's sheath, forming a progressively thickening layer of dentine until the full thickness is reached, by which stage a thin root canal is left in the centre of the root. This whole process begins at the rim of the enamel organ, so that the cervical portion of the root is completed long before the apical part and, when the root is fully formed, the thin root canal connects the pulp chamber with the connective tissue around the apex.

Cementum formation

As the dentine of the root forms, Hertwig's sheath begins to disintegrate, allowing the connective tissue cells surrounding it to come into contact with the dentine. These cells develop into cuboidal-shaped cementoblasts, the cells responsible for laying down cementum. Initially they deposit the organic matrix, called pre-cementum, which consists of collagen fibres and ground substance. Into this, calcium salts are deposited, forming the completed cementum, in a manner similar to the formation of dentine from pre-dentine. Gradually the cementoblasts lay down a progressively thickening layer of cementum and, when its full thickness has been reached, a layer of precementum persists on its outer surface throughout the life of the tooth.

Development of the periodontal ligament

While the root is forming, so, too, is the alveolar bone. Between the two lies the dental follicle, which surrounds the entire enamel organ and the developing tooth, and it is from this that the periodontal ligament is derived. The fibroblasts within the follicle form bundles of collagen, which are arranged roughly perpendicular to the surface of the root and, as the cementum forms on the root surface, the inner ends of the bundles become embedded in it. Meanwhile the opposite ends become embedded in the developing alveolar bone. Initially, three distinct layers are visible in the periodontal ligament: an outer and inner layer of regularly arranged fibre bundles and an intermediate, more irregular layer. These three distinct layers persist until eruption is complete, when the intermediate layer disappears.

Hertwig's sheath, which started to disintegrate as the root formed, does not disappear completely, but the remnants persist as a meshwork of epithelial cells in the periodontal ligament, called the epithelial cell rests of Malassez.

Reduced enamel epithelium

When dentine and enamel formation begins, the ameloblasts become cut off from the blood supply of the dental papilla and have to rely on the capillary plexus in the dental follicle for their nutrition. The stellate reticulum begins to reduce in width and its cells become more closely packed together, until they become indistinguishable from the cells of the outer enamel epithelium. Having laid down the full thickness of enamel, the ameloblasts become shorter and they, too, can no longer be distinguished as a separate layer, so that the completed enamel is covered by a layer of polyhedral epithelial cells a few cells thick, called the reduced enamel epithelium. The reduced enamel epithelium protects the crown while it remains unerupted within the tissues and is important in the process of tooth eruption.

Development of the permanent teeth

What has been described so far is the formation of the primary teeth. The same basic process applies to the permanent teeth, but their initial development differs slightly. The enamel organs of the permanent incisors, canines and premolars (i.e. the teeth with primary predecessors) develop from a cord-like epithelial downgrowth from the dental lamina, which grows deeper into the tissues on the lingual aspect of the deciduous enamel organ. The enamel organs of the permanent molar teeth, which have no deciduous predecessors, develop from a backward proliferation of the dental lamina. As this grows through the connective tissue, behind the developing deciduous second molar, the enamel organs of each of the three permanent molars bud off from it in turn.

Once the permanent enamel organs have formed, the process of development continues in the way already described.

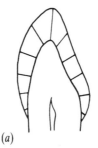 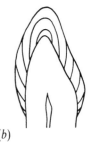

(a)   (b)

Fig. 6.4 Diagrams of labiolingual sections through the crown of a lower incisor tooth: (a) direction of the enamel prisms, (b) direction of incremental lines of the enamel.

Stages in the development of the teeth

Dental lamina: two horseshoe shaped thickenings which form in the epithelium of the oral cavity.

Enamel organs
- Bud stage: ten epithelial 'buds' which grow into the connective tissue from each dental lamina.
- Cap stage: the buds become concave on their deeper aspects, resembling caps.
- Bell stage: the concave buds start to resemble the crown of the tooth.

Amelogenesis: The cells which form enamel are called ameloblasts and develop from the inner enamel epithelium cells.

Dentinogenesis: a layer of cells in the dental papilla elongate to become odontoblasts, which are responsible for dentine deposition.

Pulp formation: numerous blood vessels and nerves within the dental papilla develop into the pulp.

Root formation: the rim of the enamel organ grows into the tissues, mapping out the shape of the root. The adjacent connective tissue change into odontoblasts which lay down the root dentine.

Cementum formation: the connective tissue cells surrounding the root develop into cuboidal-shaped cementoblasts, which form cementum.

Enamel

Enamel covers the whole of the crown of the tooth and is thickest in the region of the cusps or incisal edges, where it is up to 2.5 mm thick, tapering down to the fine edge at the cervical margin.

Chemical composition

Enamel is the hardest and most densely calcified tissue of the body. Its composition is as follows: 96% inorganic salts - a complicated calcium salt, called calcium hydroxyapatite, often referred to simply as apatite - and 3% water and 1% organic matrix, which is similar to the keratin of keratinized epithelium.

Structure

Various features can be seen when enamel is examined with a microscope: some are listed below.

Enamel prisms

Enamel is built up of vast numbers of microscopic rods or prisms, which lie roughly perpendicular to the enamel surface (Fig. 6.4). There are millions of prisms in each tooth and when the surface of the enamel is examined microscopically the prisms show an arrangement which resembles that of fish scales. As the prisms pass from the enamel-dentine junction to the surface they are not completely straight, but have a wavy arrangement which is said to strengthen the enamel. In certain areas, especially in the region of the cusps, the prisms are particularly irregularly arranged and such areas are known as 'gnarled enamel'.

Incremental lines

Amelogenesis does not progress at a steady rate, but tends to go through a series of alternating active and resting phases. The incremental lines correspond to the various resting phases and are visible through the light microscope as a series of dark lines, lying roughly parallel to the enamel surface (Fig. 6.4). The more marked of these are referred to as the brown striae of Retzius and one particularly noticeable line, corresponding to the disturbance of enamel formation which occurs at the time of birth, is called the neonatal line. It is present only in the deciduous teeth and the first permanent molars, since these are the only teeth which have begun to calcify before birth.

Enamel lamellae

These are thin longitudinal 'cracks' in the enamel, which are filled with organic material. Some occur during development of the enamel and others form after eruption (Fig. 6.5).

Enamel tufts

Enamel tufts run from the enamel-dentine junction a short distance into the enamel, not usually further than one-third of its thickness.

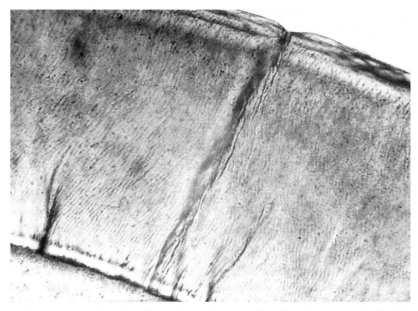

Fig. 6.5 A ground section of enamel showing enamel lamella and two enamel tufts. The lines of the prisms can also be seen throughout the enamel.

They are more numerous than lamellae and their function is unknown.

The amelodentinal junction

The junction between enamel and dentine does not appear as a straight line when viewed in section. It has a scalloped appearance, an arrangement which is thought to increase the strength of the bond between the two tissues.

Function of enamel

The extreme hardness of enamel is important in preventing the teeth from wearing away from the friction of mastication. Few other substances could withstand such hard work for upwards of half a century. However, enamel is also quite brittle and breaks easily if not adequately supported by dentine, as happens when caries attacks the tooth.

Enamel is an insensitive tissue and prevents hot, cold or other painful stimuli from affecting the tooth. The importance of this is quickly recognized if the enamel protection is lost, either through caries or through trauma, or when gingival recession exposes the dentine of the root.

The structure of enamel
- **Enamel prisms**: microscopic enamel rods passing in a wavy line from the enamel-dentine junction to the surface.
- **Incremental lines**: lines caused by resting phases during development.
- **Enamel lamellae**: thin 'cracks' in the enamel filled with organic material.
- **Enamel tufts**: short projections from the enamel-dentine junction into the enamel.
- **The amelodentinal junction**: the scalloped join between the enamel and dentine.

Dentine

Dentine makes up the main bulk of the tooth. In the crown it is covered by enamel and in the root it is covered by a thin layer of cementum.

Chemical composition

Dentine is softer than enamel, but is harder than both cementum and bone. It is light yellow in colour and has the following composition:

70% inorganic salts, mainly calcium hydroxy-apatite, and 30% water and organic matrix. The organic portion is made up of collagen fibres and a mucopolysaccharide ground substance.

Structure

The main features of dentine, which may be seen with the help of a microscope, are described below.

Dentinal tubules

Dentine contains millions of microscopic tubules which run from the pulp cavity outwards to the enamel-dentine or dentine-cementum junction (Fig. 6.6). They do not lie in a straight line, but resemble an S in shape: the curvatures are well marked on the sides of the tooth, but less so in the area of the incisal edge or cusps, where they are almost straight. The tubules contain the long slender protoplasmic process of the odontoblasts, which line the whole of the pulpal surface of the dentine.

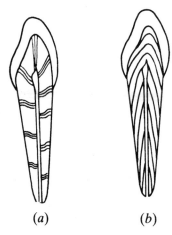

(a)   *(b)*

Fig. 6.6 Diagrams of labiolingual sections through a lower incisor: (a) direction of the dentine tubules, (b) direction of the incremental lines of the dentine.

Incremental lines

Like enamel formation, dentine production proceeds rhythmically, in alternating active and resting phases, which give rise to a series of incremental lines, lying at right angles to the dentinal tubules and almost parallel to the outer surface of the dentine (Fig.6.6). In dentine the more prominent lines are known as contour lines of Owen. The primary teeth and first

permanent molar teeth have a particularly noticeable incremental line marking the interference with dentine formation at the time of birth; this is the neonatal line and is similar to that of enamel.

Interglobular dentine

When dentine is forming, inorganic salts are deposited in the predentine matrix. Initially small distinct globules of calcium hydroxyapatite are formed called calcospherites, and gradually these increase in number and size until they fuse into a large homogeneous mass. Sometimes, however, the calcification process is not completed and the distinct globules remain. These areas are called interglobular dentine.

Dentinal nerve endings

The pulp is a richly innervated tissue and some nerve endings extend into the dentinal tubules for a very short distance. Dentine sensitivity is discussed later in this chapter.

Structure of dentine
- **Dentinal tubules**: microscopic tubes running from the pulp towards the surface containing a process for part of the way.
- **Incremental lines**: changes in the density of the dentine caused by resting phases during dentinogenesis.
- **Interglobular dentine**: globules in the dentine caused by incomplete calcification.
- **Dentinal nerve endings**: these extend from the pulp into the dentine for a short way.

Age changes in dentine

Unlike enamel, dentine is a vital tissue which changes throughout life. The different changes that may take place are termed regular secondary dentine, irregular secondary dentine, translucent dentine and dead tracts.

Regular secondary dentine

When the tooth has completely formed, dentine deposition does not stop, but continues at a much slower but variable rate, gradually redu-

tubules, gradually occluding them. When viewed through the light microscope, normal dentinal tubules show up as dark lines in the dentine, but when they are occluded with dentine the dark lines are no longer visible. Because these areas have a more uniform appearance, they are called translucent dentine or sclerotic dentine.

Dead tracts

When the irritation is much stronger, the odontoblastic processes may be completely destroyed, leaving the dentinal tubules empty. Because the tubules are empty, they appear blacker than normal when viewed through a microscope. Overheating of the neck of the tooth with a hygienist's polishing cup or brush may well have this effect and care should be taken to avoid doing so (Fig. 6.7).

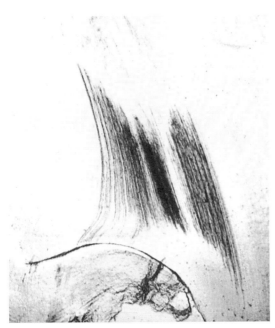

Fig. 6.7 A ground section of dentine showing dentinal tubules with a number of dead tracts.

cing the size of the pulp cavity. The dentine laid down after tooth formation is finished is called regular secondary dentine. It is separated from the original dentine by a dark line and has fewer and more irregular dentinal tubules. It should be stressed that regular secondary dentine develops under normal conditions, i.e. it is a physiological, not a pathological, change.

Reparative or irregular secondary dentine

Reparative or irregular secondary dentine is similar to regular secondary dentine in that it forms after the tooth development is completed but, unlike regular secondary dentine, it is a response to rapid loss of tooth substance by, for example, extensive wear, caries or cavity preparation, i.e. it is a pathological change. Here it is often referred to as reparative dentine since it is more rapidly laid down than regular secondary dentine, is even more irregular and has fewer dentinal tubules.

Translucent dentine

As well as being able to deposit secondary dentine on the pulpal surface of the dentine, the odontoblasts can react to irritating stimuli by laying down more dentine within the dentinal

---

Age changes in dentine
- Regular secondary dentine: formed throughout life slowly reducing the size of the pulp.
- Reparative or irregular secondary dentine: rapidly formed after severe irritation of the pulp.
- Translucent dentine: calcification of the dentine tubules causing it to appear clear when viewed through a light microscope.
- Dead tracts: empty dentinal tubules caused by necrosis of the odontoblastic process.

Cementum

A thin layer of cementum covers the whole surface of the root. It is the attachment tissue of the tooth with the fibres of the periodontal ligament inserted into it on the one side and into the bone on the other. Two types of cementum are recognized: cellular cementum which contains cells called cementocytes, and acellular which does not (Fig. 6.8). Other than the presence or absence of cells, the two types are identical. The first formed cementum is usually of the acellular type and that formed later is usually cellular. Therefore, acellular cementum usually extends from the amelocemental junction to the apical foramen. Cellular cementum tends to cover the apical third and normally lies on top of the acellular type. The reason for the two kinds of cementum is not known.

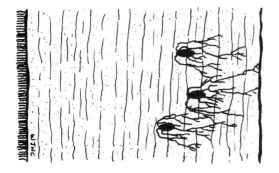

Fig. 6.8 Diagram of a longitudinal section through cementum, showing a layer of acellular cementum covered by cellular cementum. There are three lacunae with their canaliculi directed towards the periodontal ligament.

Chemical composition

Cementum is softer than dentine and is similar in many ways to bone. It has the following composition: 50% inorganic salts, mainly calcium hydroxyapatite, and 50% organic matrix; thin collagen fibres lying parallel to the root surface and mucopolysaccharide ground substance. As well as the thin fibres of the matrix, there are the larger Sharpey's fibres, which are the embedded portions of periodontal fibres.

Structure

Cementocytes

It has already been seen that cementum is laid down by cementoblasts. Cementocytes are simply cementoblasts which have become enveloped by cementum as formation proceeds. Each cementocyte lies within a cavity called a lacuna and has numerous thin processes which spread out from the lacuna in narrow channels called canaliculi. The processes are directed mainly towards the outer surface of the cementum, enabling the cementocytes to derive their nutrition from the periodontal ligament. They frequently appear to anastomose with those of other cementocytes. Often the cementocytes die off and the empty lacunae and canaliculi appear black when viewed through a microscope.

Incremental lines

Like each of the other calcified tissues, cementum is not deposited at a uniform rate and the series of resting phases is marked by incremental lines which are roughly parallel to the surface of the root.

Sharpey's fibres

These are the larger collagen fibre bundles of the periodontal ligament, which are inserted into the cementum, perpendicular to its surface.

Functional changes

Cementum is not a static tissue, but alters in response to the functional requirements of the tooth.

Continued deposition

Throughout life the thickness of cementum increases as more is deposited on the root surface by the cementoblasts and it is estimated that the thickness trebles between the ages of 11 and 76 years. This allows for various important changes.

- Newly formed periodontal fibres can be embedded in the cementum, replacing those which have aged.
- Alteration of the inserted fibres allows the tooth to move bodily through the alveolar bone as happens during eruption, growth and during orthodontic treatment.
- The deposition of more cementum at the apex of the root helps to compensate for attrition of the occlusal surface or incisal edge.

Resorption

Most teeth also have small areas in which the cementum has been resorbed and then later repaired by further deposition. The resorption is carried out by large multinucleated cells similar to osteoclasts and is generally caused by inflammation or excessive forces, such as may result from traumatic occlusion or too rapid orthodontic movement.

Structure of cementum
- **Composition**: 50% inorganic and 50% organic.
- **Cementocytes**: embedded cemento-blasts lying within cellular cementum.
- Incremental lines: lines marking resting phases in cementum formation.
- **Sharpey's fibres**: periodontal ligament fibres which are inserted into cementum or alveolar bone.

Pulp

The pulp consists of a loose areolar tissue enclosed within the dentine. It is divided into the pulp chamber, lying within the crown, and a root canal in each root of the tooth.

Structure

There is little difference between pulp and any other loose connective tissue (see Fig. 2.6). It consists of fibres, cells and structures such as blood vessels and nerves.

Fibres

Pulp contains a loose meshwork of collagen and reticular fibres which are randomly distributed and give support to the blood vessels and nerves. There are no elastic fibres, other than those within the walls of the blood vessels.

Cells

The fibroblasts, histiocytes, plasma cells and lymphocytes, described in Chapter 2, are all present in pulp, but there are also odontoblasts, which are unique to pulp. These cells line the pulpal wall of the dentine, with their thin odontoblastic processes occupying the dentinal tubules, but not usually crossing the full thickness of the dentine (Table 6.2).

Table 6.2 The shape of the odontoblasts

The shape of the odontoblasts varies with their location as follows
• Pulp chamber: elongated columnar cells.   • Root canals: cuboidal cells.   • Apical foramen: flattened cells.

Anatomical structures

The pulp has a particularly rich blood and nerve supply. Its rich capillary network is fed by several small arteries and is drained by small veins, all of which pass through the apical foramen.

The nerves of the pulp are of two types: sympathetic and sensory (Table 6.3).

Table 6.3 The nerves in the pulp chamber

The nerves in the pulp chamber are
• **Sympathetic nerves:** controlling the dilatation of the blood vessels.   • **Sensory nerves:** the only nerve endings found in the pulp are pain receptors, which means that all stimuli, such as heat, pressure and touch, are transmitted as pain.

Like the blood vessels, the nerves reach the pulp through the apical foramen. Little is known of the lymphatics of the pulp other than that they exist, and they, too, drain through the apical foramen (Table 6.4).

Structure of the pulp
- Cells: including fibroblasts, histiocytes, plasma cells, lymphocytes and odonto-blasts.
- Anatomical structures: blood vessels, lymphocytes, nerves supply both sympathetic and sensory nerves.

Periodontal ligament

The periodontal ligament is the connective tissue surrounding the root of the tooth and attaching it to the alveolar bone. It is continuous with the gingival connective tissue around the neck of the tooth, with the alveolar bone marrow spaces, through the openings in the bone of the tooth socket, and with the pulp, through the apical foramen. It is very narrow, being between 0.1 and 0.3 mm wide.

Structure

The periodontal ligament contains each of the

Table 6.4 Age changes in the pulp

The dental hygienist soon comes to realize that the teeth of older patients are much less sensitive than those of adolescents or young adults. This is explained by two changes that take place in the pulp with age

- The pulp becomes less vascular and more fibrous.
- The pulp is reduced in size by the formation of secondary and reparative dentine.

These changes also make the pulp less susceptible to damage, which is important to the dentist, who must take these factors into consideration when planning restorative procedures.

Table 6.5 The principal periodontal ligament fibres

Functional groups of the principal periodontal ligament fibres are

- **Oblique**: attached into the cementum at a point more apical than their attachment into bone. This is the major group of periodontal ligament fibres.
- **Crestal**: running from the alveolar crest towards the cervical cementum.
- **Horizontal**: lying horizontally between the bone and cementum.
- **Apical**: radiating from the cementum around the apex to the bone at the base of the socket.
- **Inter-radicular**: running from the bifurcation or trifurcation of the roots to the crest of bone between the roots.

---

elements of any connective tissue including fibres, cells and anatomical structures but, unlike the pulp, it is densely fibrous.

Fibres

The fibres are almost entirely collagenous and are of two main types.

- **Interstitial fibres**. These are randomly arranged throughout the periodontal ligament, supporting the blood vessels and nerves.
- **Principal fibres**. These are much more dense and are the fibre bundles which run from cementum to bone, holding the tooth firmly in its socket. They have a wavy arrangement which, since collagen is inelastic, is said to allow for microscopic movement of the tooth. The principal fibres are arranged into several functional groups (Table 6.5, Figs 6.9 and 6.10).

Other groups of fibres which support the tooth in its socket are described in the section on gingiva, namely the circular, free gingival and trans-septal fibres.

Cells

Although each of the cells of connective tissue

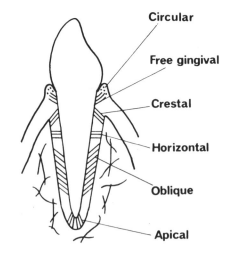

Fig. 6.9 Diagrammatic illustration of the free gingival and circular fibres of the gingiva together with the crestal, horizontal, oblique and apical fibres of the periodontal ligament. Note that the width of the periodontal ligament has not been drawn to scale.

is found in the periodontal ligament, by far the most numerous are the fibroblasts. There are also cementoblasts, lining the outer surface of the cementum, and osteoblasts and osteoclasts bordering the alveolar bone. Forming islands of

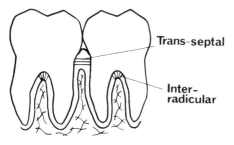

Fig. 6.10 Diagrammatic illustration of the trans-septal and the inter-radicular fibres of the periodontal ligament.

epithelial cells are the epithelial cell rests of Malassez, which, as described in the section on development and are the remnants of Hertwig's sheath (Fig. 6.11).

Anatomical structures

Blood vessels
The periodontal ligament has a much richer blood supply than other equally fibrous tissues. Its sources are threefold: branches from the gingival connective tissue, branches of the apical vessels before they enter the pulp and branches from the bone marrow spaces. The last group reaches the periodontal ligament through openings in the bone of the tooth socket, called Volkmann's canals, and are the major source of supply. The venous drainage follows the same three pathways.

Nerves
The nerves to the periodontal ligament accompany the blood vessels and various types of nerve endings are found, including pain and touch receptors. Even the lightest of pressure on a tooth is transmitted and the messages sent from the periodontum to the brain are extremely important in controlling mastication. This will be readily appreciated by anyone who has tried to eat soon after being given a dental local anaesthetic.

Lymphatics
Little is known of these, but it is assumed that they follow the same three pathways as the blood vessels and nerves (Table 6.6).

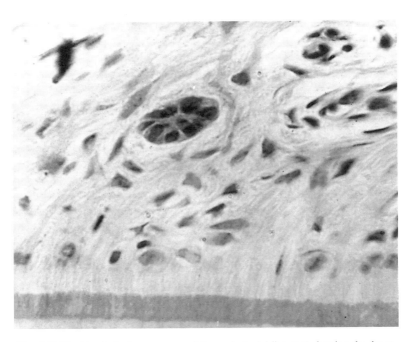

Fig. 6.11 The histological appearance of the periodontal ligament showing the dense bundles of collagen fibres inserted into the cementum. Between the fibres are numerous fibroblasts and an epithelial cell rest of Malassez.

Table 6.6 The periodontal ligament
Functions of the periodontal ligament

- **Supportive**: it holds the tooth firmly in its socket.
- **Sensory**: its rich nerve supply is important in controlling mastication.
- **Protective**: it prevents the apical vessels being compressed and damaged by downward pressure on the tooth.
- **Formative**: the cementoblasts and osteoblasts of the periodontal ligament continue to form cementum and bone, respectively, throughout the life of the tooth.
- **Nutrient**: cementum gains its nutrition from the periodontal ligament.

Structure of the periodontal ligament
- **Collagenous fibres**: interstitial fibres and principal .
- **Anatomical structures**: blood vessels and nerves including sympathetic and sensory.
- **Cells**: fibroblasts, cementoblasts, osteoblasts, osteoclasts, epithelial rests of Malassez.

Alveolar bone

The two alveoli are horseshoe-shaped processes of maxilla and mandible, designed to support the teeth. When the teeth are lost, the alveoli undergo resorption.

Structure

Like any other bony tissue, the alveoli consist of outer and inner cortical plates composed of compact bone, with cancellous bone between the two. Also between the two cortical plates are the tooth sockets; the bone between adjacent sockets is called the interdental septum.

Lamina dura

Each tooth socket is lined by a thin plate of bone, termed the lamina dura, which is visible on a dental radiograph and is often of diagnostic importance. Into the lamina dura are inserted the ends of the periodontal fibres which, like those inserted into the cementum, are called Sharpey's fibres. The lamina dura is pierced by large numbers of bony canals called Volkmann's canals (mentioned previously) and, for this reason, is often referred to as the cribriform plate. The roots of the upper poster-

ior teeth project up into the maxillary sinus and are separated from it by only the lamina dura and mucosa of the sinus and, in some cases, the plate of the bone is missing, with only the lining of the respiratory epithelium covering the roots.

Alveolar crest

The rim of the tooth socket is termed the alveolar crest and it can be seen, from a dried bone specimen of the maxilla or mandible, that the alveolar crest is scalloped in outline, matching the gingival contour.

Cortical plates

The thickness of the facial and lingual alveolar cortical plates varies considerably from one area to another and from person to person. It tends to be thin on the labial aspect of the anterior teeth and may even be completely missing in places. On the dried skull such a wedge-shaped defect, where a root has no covering of bone, is often visible and is called a dehiscence. These dehiscences are of some importance with regard to the progress of periodontal disease and they may be the reason for areas of localized severe gingival recession.

Bone cells

As throughout the skeleton, the bone of the alveoli is not static but is continually being remodelled by osteoblasts and osteoclasts. Osteoblasts are irregular-shaped cells which deposit bone and osteoclasts are large multinucleated cells which resorb it. Both these cells are present in the tooth socket and by their action teeth move bodily through the bone, either during growth or during orthodontic treatment. The bone of the socket on the side towards which the tooth is moving is resorbed by osteoclasts, while more bone is deposited on the opposite side by osteoblasts.

> Structure of alveolar bone
> - **Lamina dura**: a thin plate of bone lining the tooth socket.
> - **Alveolar crest**: the rim of the socket.
> - **Cortical plates**: the compact bone on the facial and lingual sides of the socket.
> - **Osteoblasts**: bone forming cells.
> - **Osteoclasts**: bone resorbing cells.

Gingiva

Gingiva is the mucous membrane covering the alveolar ridge and forming a cuff around the neck of each tooth. Microscopically it consists of stratified squamous epithelium, supported by a thin layer of densely fibrous connective tissue (Fig. 6.12). The anatomy of gingiva has already been described in Chapter 4.

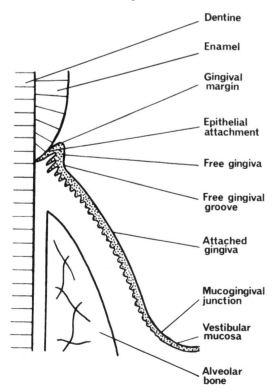

Dentine
Enamel
Gingival margin
Epithelial attachment
Free gingiva
Free gingival groove
Attached gingiva
Mucogingival junction
Vestibular mucosa
Alveolar bone

Fig. 6.12 Diagram of a vertical section through the labial gingiva of a lower tooth.

Structure

Attached gingiva

The attached gingiva is tightly bound down to the underlying alveolar bone by collagen bundles, which give it its stippled appearance. Because the fibrous connective tissue merges with the periosteum, this type of covering is called mucoperiosteum. Its epithelium is keratinized and is thicker than that of the vestibule and the floor of the mouth. Unlike those areas, it has large dermal papillae, increasing the area of the germinal layer of cells.

Free gingiva

The epithelium of the free gingiva is even thicker than that of the attached gingiva, being thickest at the gingival margin, which is not surprising in view of the friction which the gingival margin withstands during mastication. It also has even larger dermal papillae and, in the healthy individual, is well keratinized (Table 6.7).

Interdental papilla

The epithelium of the labial and lingual peaks of the interdental papilla is thick and keratinized, with long dermal papillae, in complete contrast to the interdental col. There the epithelium is very thin and poorly keratinized with a flat germinal layer. This is of considerable clinical significance in relation to the aetiology of chronic periodontal disease.

Gingival crevice

Between the free gingival crest and the cervical margin of the crown is a shallow sulcus, 0.5–1 mm deep, called the gingival crevice. The main histological features of the gingival crevice are shown in Figure 6.13. The gingival epithelium facing the tooth is termed the crevicular epithelium coronally (area 2) and junctional epithelium (area 1), adjacent to the tooth.

The junctional epithelium is that part of the gingiva which attaches the gingival connective tissue to the tooth surface. It forms a band 2–3 mm deep around the tooth, is approximately 15–30 cells thick coronally and tapers to a single cell apically. The cells are non-keratinized and very loose-knit, with wide intercellular spaces.

Table 6.7 The collagen fibres of the free gingiva

The collagen fibres of the free gingiva are arranged in three main groups

- **Circular fibres:** these form a collar around the neck of the tooth, holding the free gingiva tightly against it.
- **Free gingival fibres:** these originate from the cementum of the cervical portion of the root and fan outwards into the free gingiva.
- **Trans-septal fibres:** these run from the cervical cementum on the distal side of one root to the cementum on the mesial aspect of the next tooth.

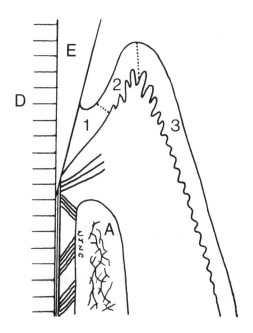

Fig. 6.13 Diagram of the dentogingival area: **A** alveolar bone, **D** dentine, **E** enamel, **1** junctional epithelium, **2** crevicular epithelium, **3** oral gingiva.

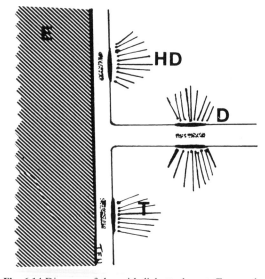

Fig. 6.14 Diagram of the epithelial attachment: **E** enamel, **HD** hemidesmosome, **D** desmosome, **T** tonofibrils.

Structure of gingiva
- **Attached gingiva**: tightly bound down to the alveolar bone.
- **Free gingiva**: the gum tissue forming the wall of the crevice or sulcus.
- **Interdental papilla**: that part of the gingiva between the teeth.
- **Gingival crevice**: a shallow sulcus between the free gingiva and tooth.

The junctional epithelium adjacent to the enamel (in a patient without recession) forms the epithelial attachment which is mediated by a basal lamina and intercellular organelles, the hemidesmosomes. The hemidesmosome is shown in Figure 6.14 and these and the basal lamina are also found between the basal epithelial layer and underlying connective tissue.

This form of attachment is very dynamic and allows gliding movement of the junctional epithelial cells along the tooth surface, such as would occur during eruption, or in response to chronic irritation from bacterial plaque.

Gingival changes with inflammation

Gingivitis is so common that it is rare to find a dentition without some degree of gingival inflammation. The interdental col and junctional epithelium with their thin non-keratinized epithelium are the most susceptible areas to bacterial irritation and are difficult to keep clean.

It has been shown that with inflammation the junctional epithelium migrates on to the cementum. The cells become separated by masses of polymorphs which migrate through the junctional epithelium. Crevicular fluid exudate through the junctional epithelium into the crevice (or pocket) increases and the crevicular epithelium becomes ulcerated and hyperplastic. With severe inflammation, the oral gingival epithelium becomes thin and may lose its layer of keratin.

Gingival physiology

Cellular turnover

All areas of the gingival epithelium are replaced by continuous cell turnover which varies greatly. It has been estimated that the junctional epithelium has a cellular turnover up to 25 times greater than the oral gingival epithelium. Furthermore, as the area for desquamation into the gingival crevice is relatively small, the rate of desquamation of the junctional epithelium has been estimated to be 50 to 100 times faster than the oral gingival epithelium.

Permeability of crevicular tissue

The permeability of the crevice appears to be limited to the junctional epithelium. Wide intercellular spaces have been demonstrated in this tissue, and these spaces enlarge when inflammation is present.

Gingival crevicular fluid

Crevicular fluid is an exudate which escapes through the junctional epithelium into the crevice. Its flow is very small or absent in health, but increases with increasing gingival inflammation. It can be measured using small filter paper strips and the amount of flow gives a good guide to the degree of inflammation (Fig. 6.15).

The fluid contains the majority of serum constituents as well as polymorphs. Immunoglobulins can be detected in the fluid. It is thought to have a variety of beneficial effects in combating infection in a similar manner to serum exudating from an open wound. Polymorphs in the crevice have been shown to be

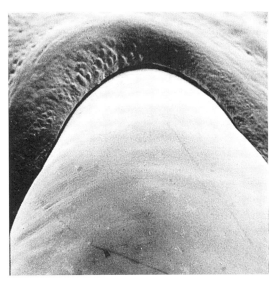

Fig. 6.15 A scanning electron micrograph of the gingival area.

actively phagocytosing bacteria. The immunoglobulins include antibodies, antitoxins and opsonins. The fluid also has a physical flushing action, washing the crevice.

Depth of gingival crevice

The crevice can be divided into two parts, namely the clinical crevice and the histological crevice. The histological crevice is a shallow furrow of 0.5 mm or less in depth, lined by the crevicular epithelium. The clinical crevice is defined as the depth to which a periodontal probe can be inserted with light pressure. This tears the junctional epithelium, so forming a traumatic crevice. The depth depends on many factors, but rarely exceeds 2 mm in healthy gingiva. A number of studies have shown that the tip of a blunt periodontal probe penetrates a small way into the junctional epithelium in health. When inflammation is present, it may pass completely through into the connective tissues.

Oral physiology

Physiology is the study of how the various tissues and organs of the body function. Oral physiology confines itself to the study of the structures related to the mouth.

Saliva

Origin

The major salivary glands are the parotid gland, submandibular gland, and sublingual gland. There are also numerous small minor glands in the lining of the oral cavity. These have been described already in Chapter 4. Saliva is produced by a number of sources as shown in Table 6.8

Table 6.8 Origins of saliva

The proportion of the total volume of saliva produced by

- Parotid gland: 25%.
- Submandibular gland: 70%.
- Sublingual gland: 5%.
- Minor salivary glands: small amounts.

The rate of flow of saliva varies considerably throughout the day, being greatest when eating and least during sleep when flow almost stops. An average of 0.5 – 1 litre is produced daily (Table 6.9).

The exact proportions of these dissolved substances vary with several factors.

- **The individual**. The saliva produced by each individual differs in its exact composition from that of others.
- **The gland of origin**. Each gland produces saliva of a different composition from the others. For example, the parotid produces a mainly serous or watery saliva, the sublingual produces a thick mucous saliva and the submandibular produces a mixture of the two.
- **The stimulus**. The flow of saliva is increased by various stimuli, such as the sight, smell and thought of food and it has been shown

Table 6.9 Dissolved constituents in saliva

Many dissolved constituents may be found in saliva. Saliva consists of 99.5% water and 0.5% of other dissolved substances, described below

Proteins. A wide range of proteins occur in saliva.
- *Mucoids*. These are a group of proteins which are often collectively called mucin and give saliva its mucous consistency. They are also referred to as glycoproteins, since they consist of long protein chains with shorter carbohydrate side chains. It will be seen in Chapter 9 that these glycoproteins form part of the intercellular portion of plaque.
- *Enzymes*. Many different enzymes are present in saliva, some of which are produced by the glands and some of which are the products of the bacteria and leukocytes present in the oral cavity. The best known of these enzymes is salivary amylase, which is produced by the glands and is discussed in the section on the alimentary canal (Chapter 3). Another is lysozyme, which is thought to be involved in controlling bacterial growth in the oral cavity, since it can destroy bacteria.
- *Serum proteins*. Since saliva is formed from serum, it is not surprising that small quantities of serum proteins are found in it. These include albumin and globulins.

Waste products. Similarly, small quantities of the waste products in serum, urea and uric acid occur in saliva.
- **Inorganic ions.** The principal ions found in saliva are calcium and phosphate, which are particularly important in the formation of calculus (see Chapter 9). Smaller quantities of sodium, potassium, chloride, sulphate and other ions are also present. Bicarbonate ions form an important buffer in saliva.
- **Gases.** When first formed, saliva contains the dissolved gases oxygen, nitrogen and carbon dioxide in similar proportions to serum. This means that the concentration of carbon dioxide is relatively high and it is only kept in solution by the pressure within the glands and ducts. Once saliva reaches the mouth, much of the carbon dioxide is given off.

Additives within the mouth. Various substances are not present in saliva as it passes through the ducts, but become mixed with the saliva in the oral cavity.
- **Micro-organisms.** When initially formed, saliva is sterile, but vast numbers of micro-organisms are present in it within the mouth. Many strains of bacteria are present and some of these have had a good deal of attention in the past because of their possible association with dental disease. Yeasts are usually present (e.g. *Candida albicans*) and viruses are often present (e.g. *Herpes simplex* virus).
- **Leukocytes.** It is assumed that the neutrophil leukocytes found in saliva reach it through the gingival crevice, since they are not present in saliva collected from the ducts and few are present in the saliva of babies before the teeth erupt.
- **Dietary substances.** Obviously, saliva within the mouth often contains the remains of food or drink recently swallowed.

Table 6.10 The functions of saliva

The functions of saliva are as follows

- **Mastication and deglutition.** The mucoids of saliva are needed to form the slippery bolus of food which will slide easily down the pharynx and oesophagus.
- **Oral clearance.** The importance of saliva's washing action in cleaning the mouth is emphasized on waking from sleep when the saliva flow is reduced, especially if the mouth has been lying open. Also, it has already been mentioned that saliva contains the enzyme lysozyme, which may be important in controlling bacterial growth within the mouth. Patients suffering from disorders which reduce their salivary flow often have rapid deposition of plaque, with rampant caries and severe periodontal disease.
- **Speech.** The tongue needs saliva as a lubricant during speech, a fact soon recognized by nervous public speakers. Nervousness inhibits saliva flow and, unless a glass of water is handy, it may be difficult to talk.
- **Taste.** Only dissolved substances can stimulate the nerve endings in the taste buds.
- **Water balance.** A reduction in the flow of saliva produces the sensation of thirst with the consequent increased intake of fluids.
- **Digestion.** Although salivary amylase is able to break down carbohydrates such as cooked starch, it is relatively unimportant in the overall digestive process. However, the significance of salivary amylase in the aetiology of caries should not be overlooked.
- **Excretion.** Since saliva contains small amounts of urea and uric acid, it has been suggested that it has a minor excretory function. However, it is likely that most of the urea and uric acid are resorbed into the blood in the intestines.
- **Buffering action.** A buffer is a substance which helps to maintain a neutral pH. It neutralizes both acids and alkalis. Saliva has this ability due mainly to the presence of the bicarbonate ions but, in view of the short time most substances are held in the oral cavity and the acidity in the stomach, it is not clear how important this feature is in relation to digestion. It is, however, of great significance to the dental hygienist in relation to the Stephan curve, which is described in Chapter 10. The loss of buffering capacity in people who suffer from dry mouths leaves them vulnerable to rapidly developing dental caries.

that different stimuli can alter its composition. For example, dry foods, such as dry biscuits and toast, produce a serous saliva, whereas meat produces a very mucous saliva.

- **Changes occurring within the mouth.** It has already been seen that a large number of cells and other substances are added to saliva once it enters the oral cavity.

In view of these variables, it is meaningless to discuss the exact proportions of the various substances (Table 6.10).

Functions of saliva
- Mastication and deglutition.
- Oral clearance.
- Speech.
- Taste.
- Water balance.
- Digestion.
- Excretion.
- Buffering action.

Taste

Taste buds
Taste buds are the specialized receptors of the sensation of taste. They are microscopic in size and there are said to be roughly 9000 of them in the mouth. They are found over the whole dorsum of the tongue and in the oral lining of the soft palate, but in children they also occur on the hard palate and surface of the cheeks, which explains the marked reduction in the sensitivity to taste with advancing age.

Basic tastes
It has already been mentioned that only solutions can be tasted. In other words, unless a substance dissolves to some extent in saliva, it has no taste. Experiments have shown that all flavours are made up of four basic tastes: sweet, sour, salt and bitter, to which some add the more doubtful tastes of alkaline and metallic. It has also been shown that certain regions of the tongue are more sensitive to one of these tastes

---

Table 6.11 Perception of flavour

Various factors influence our perception of flavour which act in association with taste

- **Texture of foodstuffs**. The importance of the sensation of touch to flavour is well illustrated by the fact that new bread is enjoyed mainly for the softness of its centre and the crispness of its crust. This may be the reason why wearers of upper dentures with a plate covering the palate complain of loss of taste.
- **Irritation**. Irritation of the oral mucosa accounts for much of the pungency of pepper, mustard, ginger and curry.
- **Smell**. The sensation of smell is closely linked to that of taste, which is why foodstuffs lose so much of their flavour when we suffer from a cold.

---

than the others (Fig. 6.16 and Table 6.11).

The tip is most sensitive to sweet.

The sides are most sensitive to salt and sour.

Around the sulcus terminalis is most sensitive to bitter.

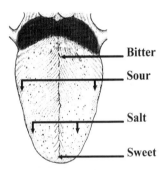

Fig. 6.16 Taste buds most sensitive to the four basic tastes of salt, sweet, bitter and sour are grouped in particular areas on the dorsal surface of the tongue.

Nerve pathways

The routes taken by the stimuli as they travel from taste buds to brain have already been described in the relevant sections of Chapter 4. However, they are recapitulated here for the sake of completeness.

Anterior two-thirds of the dorsum

The taste fibres from this area run initially in the lingual nerve, but leave it before it joins the mandibular nerve. They pass via the chorda tympani to the facial nerve, the VIIth cranial nerve, which carries them to the brain.

Posterior one-third of the dorsum

The taste fibres from this area travel to the

brain in the glossopharyngeal nerve, the IXth cranial nerve.

Soft palate

Initially the taste fibres from the soft palate are carried by the posterior palatine nerve but, before it joins the maxillary nerve, they leave it and run in a small nerve, called the nerve of the pterygoid canal, to the facial nerve, which carries them to the brain.

Mastication

Mastication is the process of chewing foodstuffs. It involves the concerted action of the teeth, tongue, cheeks and lips. We have already seen that the temporomandibular joint allows the mandible two basic movements: vertical opening and forward protrusion. Using these two basic movements various actions can be performed: incising, tearing and grinding (see Table 6.12).

Lips and cheeks

Apart from closing off the oral cavity, once food has been placed in it for mastication, the lips, which are very sensitive to temperature and touch, help prevent unsuitable materials from being eaten. During mastication the muscles of the lips and cheeks push the food from the vestibule back into the oral cavity proper and, to a certain extent, the cheeks are used to store food which is waiting to be masticated. This is a much more important feature in some animals, such as hamsters.

Table 6.12 Mastication

Tooth movements during mastication allow the following actions

- **Incising**. The vertical opening and closing, with the mandible in a slightly protruded position, is the action used for incising, as in biting into an apple. It is principally the anterior (incisor) teeth which are used and they are suitably chisel-shaped.
- **Tearing**. The pointed canine teeth are well designed for tearing fibrous foods such as meat. With the mandible slightly protruded and swung slightly to one side, the two canines of that side are used to pierce the meat and, by pulling the head away from it, the meat is torn and shredded. Knives and forks have made these teeth largely redundant in humans, but they are prominent and important in carnivorous animals.
- **Grinding**. If both temporomandibular joints act together the mandible is protruded, whereas if they act alternately it swings from side to side. Both these movements are used during the grinding of food and the molars and premolars are aptly designed for this purpose.

Tongue and hard palate

The rough surface of the dorsum of the tongue and the rugae of the hard palate, both of which are covered with thick keratinized epithelium, provide a suitable surface for rubbing and pulping foods. They are well supplied with temperature, touch and taste nerve endings which can once again check the suitability of the materials being chewed, before they are swallowed.

Eruption and shedding of teeth

Eruption is the movement of the tooth from within the tissues of the jaw, where it is formed, into the oral cavity. For descriptive purposes, it is often divided into two stages, sometimes called active and passive eruption.

- **Active eruption**: during this phase, the tooth moves bodily through the tissues, emerges into the oral cavity and comes to rest in its correct occlusal relationship with its opposite number.
- **Passive eruption**: when it reaches the occlusal plane, only two-thirds of the crown is visible in the mouth. The remainder is still covered with gingival tissue. Passive eruption is the gradual rootwards shift of the gingival margin, until it comes to rest at the enamel-cementum junction. This stage has also been referred to as coronal exposure and gingival maturation.

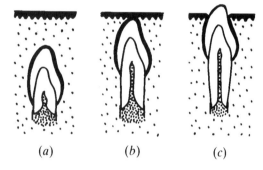

(a)	(b)	(c)

Fig. 6.17 Diagrammatic illustration of the eruption of a tooth: (a) soon after eruption begins, (b) fusion of the reduced enamel epithelium with the oral epithelium, (c) emergence of the tip of the tooth into the oral cavity.

Eruption of the primary teeth

It has been noted that when the crown is fully formed it is covered by the reduced enamel epithelium (Fig. 6.17). As the root starts to form, the crown begins to move through the tissues towards the oral mucous membrane. Eventually the reduced enamel epithelium comes into contact with the oral epithelium and becomes continuous with it. The tip of the tooth emerges into the mouth through the area of epithelium, with no bleeding, since the epithelial continuity has not been broken.

Gradually, more of the root forms and more of the crown pushes through into the oral cavity until it reaches the occlusal plane. At this stage, the oral epithelium is continuous with the reduced enamel epithelium which forms a cuff around the hidden one-third of the crown but, by the time the gingival margin has receded to

---

Table 6.13 Theories of eruption

Why teeth erupt is unclear, but several theories have been put forward

---

- **Root growth**: it is suggested that the crown may be thrust into the oral cavity by the developing root.
- **Bone growth**: bone being deposited below the developing tooth might push the crown towards the mouth.
- **Pulpal proliferation**: it may be that the proliferation of cells in the developing pulp builds up pressure which drives the crown away from the underlying follicle and bone.
- **Blood pressure**: the increased vascularity in the developing pulp might raise the blood pressure, producing a similar effect to pulpal proliferation.
- **Periodontal fibres**: it has also been suggested that the obliquely arranged collagen fibres of the developing periodontal ligament pull the tooth towards the oral mucosa.

All of these theories have little evidence to support them. In fact, the evidence that is available is mostly negative and it may be that eruption results from a combination of several factors.

---

the enamel–cementum junction, the remainder of the reduced enamel epithelium has been replaced by the stratified squamous oral epithelium, forming the gingival crevice and epithelial attachment.

Eruption of the permanent teeth

The same basic process is involved in the eruption of primary and permanent teeth, especially those permanent teeth without predecessors, but the eruption of the permanent incisors, canines and premolars is closely linked to the shedding of the primary teeth. Initially the permanent incisors and canines develop lingually and apically to the primary teeth but, as they erupt and resorb the primary roots, they come to lie immediately below them. The premolars first develop between the roots of their predecessors but, with the vertical growth of the alveolus, they come to be immediately below the primary apices and then erupt vertically upwards (Table 6.13).

Shedding of the primary teeth

The shedding of the primary teeth is brought about by two factors. The principal one is that the roots are resorbed by cells surrounding the erupting permanent teeth and, on the odd occasion that a permanent tooth fails to develop, the primary tooth is retained in the mouth long after it should have been shed. To a lesser extent the primary teeth are lost because,

with the growth of the jaws, the forces of mastication become too great for them to withstand. Consequently, the primary tooth which is retained because its successor is absent, is normally lost in due course.

Histology of root resorption

The developing permanent tooth is surrounded by its fibrous follicle and is separated from the primary root by a thin plate of bone. As the tooth begins to erupt, the bone is resorbed by the action of large, multinucleated cells called osteoclasts, the crown being protected by its reduced enamel epithelium. Once through the bone, the multinucleated cells carry on eating their way into the cementum and dentine of the primary root and, as the permanent tooth continues to erupt, the primary root is gradually resorbed. Eventually the primary crown is left with no root and falls away from the tissues.

Eruption dates

The stages at which the individual teeth erupt are very variable and even the order in which they erupt varies. For example, the first tooth to erupt is normally the primary lower central incisor at 6 months, but occasionally babies are born with teeth fully erupted and others may be well over 6 months without teeth. There is little to be gained from memorizing a long list of eruption dates and the dates given in Table 6.14 are mainly for reference purposes. It is more

Table 6.14 Chronology of the formation of the dentition

Tooth	Calcification started	Eruption date	Root completed
Primary teeth			
Incisors	Before birth	6–9 months	Roughly
First molars	Before birth	12 months	12–18 months
Canines	Before birth	18 months	after eruption
Second molars	Before birth	24 months	of the tooth
Permanent teeth			
First molars	Before birth	6 years	
Lower centrals	Soon after birth	7 years	
Upper centrals and lower laterals	Soon after birth	8 years	
Upper laterals	6–12 months	9 years	Roughly
Lower canines	6–12 months	10 years	2–3 years after
First premolars	18 months	11 years	eruption of the
Second premolars	2 years	12 years	tooth
Upper canines	6 months	13 years	
Second molars	3 years	13 years	
Third molars	8 years	18–21 years	

In this considerably simplified table, the teeth are arranged in order of eruption.

important to grasp the general picture of the manner in which the primary dentition is established and how the permanent dentition replaces it.

The primary dentition

The primary teeth all start to form before birth. On average they begin to erupt at 6 months and the dentition is fully established by 2½ years. The order in which they erupt is usually: A, B, D, C and E; and the roots are fully formed 1–1½ years after eruption. When newly erupted, the teeth are arranged in close contact with each other but, by the age of 6 years, when the permanent teeth start to replace them, they are well spaced, because of the growth of the jaws.

The permanent dentition

At 6½ years, the first permanent molars erupt behind and in series with the primary teeth. Shortly afterwards the primary lower central incisors are shed and replaced by their permanent successors and between then and 13 years all the other primary teeth are replaced. At 13 years of age the second molars erupt and, finally, between the ages of 17 and 21 years the third molars erupt. When they first appear in the mouth, the permanent teeth are crowded

together but, with continuing growth of the jaws, they straighten themselves out, although in many cases some degree of crowding remains.

The order of eruption of the permanent teeth is different for the upper and lower arches. The upper teeth erupt in the following order: 6, 1, 2, 4, 5, 3, 7, 8. The order of the lower teeth is: 6, 1, 2, 3, 4, 5, 7, 8. The overall sequence is as listed in Table 6.6.

Further reading

Atkinson M. E., White F. H. (1992) *Principles of Anatomy and Oral Anatomy for Dental Students*. Edinburgh: Churchill Livingstone.

Berkovitz B. K. B., Holland G. R., Moxham B. J. (1992) *Color Atlas and Textbook of Oral Anatomy*. 2nd edition. London: Mosby.

Jenkins G. N. (1986) *The Physiology and Biochemistry of the Mouth*. 4th edition. Oxford: Blackwell Scientific Publications.

Hassell T. M. (1993) Periodontal tissues – structure and function. *Periodontology 2000. Volume 3*. Copenhagen: Munksgaard.

Schroeder H. F., Listgarten M. A. (1971) *Fine Structure of the Developing Epithelial Attachment of Human Teeth*. 2nd edition. Basel: Karger.

Scott 1. H., Symons N. B. B. (1992) *Introduction to Dental Anatomy*. 9th edition. Edinburgh: Churchill Livingstone.

Ten Cate A. R. (1994) *Oral Histology: Development, Structure and Function*. 4th edition. London: Mosby.

7

Microbiology, cross-infection and immunity

Microbiology

Microbiology is the study of micro-organisms, i.e. living organisms which are so small that they can be seen only with a microscope. They may be broadly divided into two groups.
- Pathogenic micro-organisms, which are harmful to human beings and may produce disease.
- Commensal micro-organisms, which are not usually harmful to human beings but may cause disease when the tissue resistance is lowered.

Classification of micro-organisms

Those that are of interest to the dental hygienist fall into three principal categories: fungi, bacteria and viruses.

Fungi

Fungi are primitive forms of plant life which vary considerably in size, from the macroscopic mushrooms and toadstools to the microscopic yeasts. In general they consist of branched filaments which form a tangled mass termed a mycelium. They multiply by forming oval buds which subsequently become detached and produce a separate mycelium.

Candida (Monilia) albicans is a common commensal of the mouth. It is often found in the saliva, but normally causes no damage to the oral tissues. However, under certain conditions, it may become pathogenic, causing candidiasis.

Bacteria

These are minute unicellular organisms which vary greatly in both size and shape (Fig. 7.1) but, in general, are large enough to be visible with the light microscope. They multiply by simple division and may be either motile or non-motile (Table 7.1).

Table 7.1 Classification of bacteria

Bacteria are classified according to their shape

- **Cocci** are spherical bacteria which may grow in clusters (staphylococci) or chains (streptococci).
- **Bacilli** are elongated, rod-shaped organisms.
- **Filamentous bacteria** are long thread-like organisms.
- **Fusiform bacilli** are similar to filamentous organisms, apart from the fact that they have tapered ends which give them a cigar shape.
- **Vibrios** are curved or comma-shaped.
- **Spirochaetes** are spiral or corkscrew-shaped.

All of these types of bacteria are present in dental plaque and most of them feature in the chapters on oral pathology.

Under adverse conditions some bacteria are able to form spores, which have a tough protective coating making them very resistant

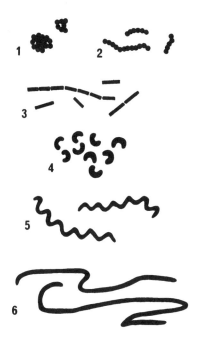

Fig. 7.1 Diagrammatic representation of the various types of bacteria: **1** staphylococci, **2** streptococci, **3** bacilli, **4** vibrios, **5** spirochaetes, **6** filamentous bacteria.

to harmful agents. Once the conditions become more favourable, the spores revert to their normal form, which makes this feature particularly important with regard to sterilization.

Various staining techniques are used to make bacteria more readily visible when viewed through a microscope: one of the most important is Gram's method. Using Gram's stain, bacteria may be divided into two groups: *Gram-positive bacteria*, which stain blue; *Gram-negative bacteria*, which stain red. This feature is mentioned again in describing the bacterial changes which take place as plaque accumulates on the surfaces of the teeth.

Viruses

Viruses are much smaller than bacteria, the majority being visible only with the electron microscope. Unlike fungi and bacteria, viruses depend entirely on living cells for their survival and can only multiply within living cells. They cannot, therefore, be grown on artificial culture media, such as broths.

Herpes simplex is a common commensal virus of the mouth. However, like *Candida albicans*, it can become pathogenic under

certain circumstances, giving rise to either acute herpetic gingivostomatitis or, more commonly, a cold sore. These are described in more detail in Chapter 13.

> **Micro-organisms of importance to the hygienist**
> - **Fungi**: primitive forms of plant life consisting of branched filaments forming a tangled mass termed a mycelium.
> - **Bacteria**: minute unicellular organisms usually large enough to be seen with the light microscope. Types include cocci, bacilli, filaments, fusiforms, vibrios and spirochaetes.
> - **Viruses**: very small organisms which can only be seen with the electron microscope.

Sterilization

Sterilization is the process by which objects are rendered free of micro-organisms and in dental practice there are two main reasons for sterilizing the instruments used:

- The prevention of wound infection, especially by commensal micro-organisms, which would be harmless on the surface of intact epithelium but can infect an open wound.
- The prevention of cross-infection, preventing the transmission of pathogenic organisms from one individual to another.

In this respect, it is essential for dental hygienists to set themselves the highest standards. There are numerous methods by which sterility may be achieved and the choice of a suitable method depends on both the efficiency of the technique and its effect on the material being sterilized.

Heat

The effectiveness of heat as a method of sterilization increases with the temperature and is enhanced by the presence of moisture. The higher the temperature, the shorter is the time required for sterilization.

Dry heat

There are two methods of applying dry heat to achieve sterilization.

Naked flame

Although all micro-organisms are killed immediately by exposure to a naked flame, this method has limited application in dental practice in view of the potential for thermal damage.

Hot-air oven

This is an insulated box with a thermostatically controlled heat source. As already noted, dry heat is less effective than moist heat as a sterilizing method and a temperature of 160°C for 1 hour is required to kill spores. Although this is a satisfactory way of sterilizing suitably lubricated handpieces, at 160°C gauzes and cotton wool rolls singe. The long time required for sterilization prevents the technique from being widely used.

Moist heat (autoclave)

This technique is very reliable and has become the method most widely used in dental practice and the hospital service. An autoclave works on the same principle as a pressure cooker. It is a strong cylinder with an airtight door which can be securely closed. The water it contains is brought to the boil and the pressure within the cylinder is controlled by means of a safety valve and pressure gauge. By raising the pressure, the water boils at a higher than normal temperature. The items for sterilization are contained in a tray above the water level and are sterilized by the steam which is given off, not the boiling water itself. The autoclave is normally operated at an increased pressure of 3 bar (30 lb per sq in) which raises the boiling temperature to 134°C: 3 minutes at this temperature kills all organisms including spores. The autoclave is suitable for sterilizing a wide range of instruments including handpieces, cotton wool and instruments made with rubber or plastic (Fig. 7.2).

Gamma radiation

This is a very effective method of sterilization used commercially, which is suitable for a wide range of materials since it does not damage them. It has the added advantage that items

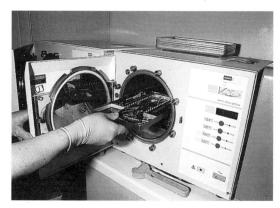

Fig. 7.2 A small autoclave suitable for use in a dental surgery.

may be sterilized within airtight polythene or cardboard containers. The size and cost of the apparatus required makes it unsuitable for dental practices, but it is the method by which prepacked disposable syringes, needles, sutures and other items are sterilized by the manufacturers. Since these items are sealed within their containers, they remain sterile until opened for use.

Boiling water

There is no place in modern dental practice for using boiling water as a means of attempting sterilization and it is of historical interest only. Boiling at 100°C for 5–10 minutes will kill most micro-organisms, but certain important spores and viruses can survive long periods of boiling. Whereas it was once the most commonly used method of sterilization in the dental surgery, its use is now contrary to General Dental Council instructions.

> Methods of sterilization
> - Hot air oven: operates at a temperature of 160°C for 1 hour.
> - Autoclave: uses the pressure cooker principle at a pressure of 3 bar (30 lb per sq in) at 134°C.
> - Gamma radiation: used commercially for sterilization.

Disinfectants

A disinfectant is a chemical compound that is

able to destroy most micro-organisms with which it is in contact, given sufficient time. Often it is impractical to sterilize a surface completely and disinfection is sufficient to prevent cross-infection with pathogenic organisms. The importance of these compounds has expanded as the risks and information about cross-infection have increased in recent years.

There are three main areas where disinfectants are used in the dental surgery. The most important is the cleaning of gloved hands. Even if gloves are changed between each patient, there will always be occasions when it is necessary to touch non-sterile items, such as notes or X-rays, and gloves should be disinfected before and after such a procedure.

The second important area is the cleaning of the dental unit and associated equipment, such as light handles and dental chair. These require disinfection before a patient enters the surgery and after he or she leaves. The third important area is the removal of organisms from equipment that cannot be sterilized by more effective means, such as autoclaving. Ultrasonic handpieces are a good example of this group. The main chemicals used as disinfectants in the dental surgery are described below.

Chlorhexidine

This is a bis-biguanide salt, usually the gluconate, although the acetate and hydrochloride salts also have some uses in disinfection. Proprietary names include Hibitane® and Savlon®. It has a wide range of uses, as will be described below, including hand and glove, surface spray and surface wipe disinfection.

Advantages

It has a broad range of anti-microbial activity and is effective against both Gram-positive and negative organisms. It has a low toxicity, is pleasant to use and has the advantage of residual effect on the skin which continues to increase each time it is applied. It has little damaging effects on rubber or plastics and is non-corrosive. It is often combined with 70% alcohol for use as a surface disinfectant.

Disadvantages

Some organisms, including some bacteria, fungi and viruses, are resistant to it. Prolonged

contact may cause dermatitis in sensitive individuals and irritation of mucous membranes or eyes can occur. Its activity is greatly reduced in the presence of organic material such as tissue fluid or serum.

Quaternary ammonium compounds

These are a group of cationic surfactants which include such well known proprietary compounds as Cetavlon®, Cetrimide® and Roccal®. Cetrimide® is also found in Savlon® together with chlorhexidine. Their main uses are surface disinfection.

Advantages

They have low toxicity and are pleasant to use. They are non-corrosive and have no effect on rubber or plastics. As with most disinfectants, eye contact should be avoided.

Disadvantages

They have a relatively narrow range of activity, being more effective against Gram-positive organisms and will not destroy spores or viruses. They are very rapidly inactivated by organic matter and therefore have little place in the dental surgery as disinfectants.

Chlorinated solutions

This group includes the common household bleaches. Proprietary brands are Alcide®, Clorasol® and Milton®.

Advantages

They are effective against a wide range of organisms and are not inactivated by organic matter. They are effective, therefore, where blood has been spilled. They can be used in a number of different dilutions, depending upon the level of disinfection required, and are cheap to use.

Disadvantages

They are very irritant and toxic and unpleasant to use, causing eye and chest irritation if inhaled. They will corrode metals and bleach most fabrics. Because of these properties they are not suitable for hand disinfection and must be thoroughly removed from any equipment before use. With storage they lose their effectiveness, so need to be made up daily.

Phenolics

This group includes a wide range of antiseptics with such proprietary names as Dettol®, and Jeyes® fluid. They are frequently combined with other chemicals.

Advantages

Some have a wide range of antibacterial activity and many are non-corrosive.

Disadvantages

Some of this group are toxic and may be absorbed by rubber and some plastics. They may cause skin irritation and are unpleasant to use because of their strong smell. They have limited use in the dental surgery.

Iodophor compounds

These iodine-containing compounds include povidone-iodine, used by many oral surgeons for hand disinfection. Proprietary names include, Betadine® and Videne®.

Advantages

They have a wide range of activity and are especially useful against viruses. They are non-corrosive and are safe to use with rubber or plastics and therefore highly recommended as surface disinfectants. They are retained on surfaces after drying and have a residual antimicrobial action.

Disadvantages

They have a bright orange colour and will stain materials badly. They are irritant to the eyes and some individuals may have a rare sensitivity to iodine. They are often unstable, especially at high temperatures.

Aldehyde compounds

This group includes those used for the chemical disinfection of instruments when more conventional methods are not possible. Commercial names include Cidex® and Gigasept®.

Advantages

They have a wide range of activity which may be increased by prolonged soaking in the chemicals. They are the most potent of all the currently available disinfectants. They are non-corrosive.

Disadvantages

They are highly irritant and sensitization may occur. Glutaraldehyde especially should be handled with great care as it evaporates quickly and the vapour is toxic; therefore they are not suitable as surface disinfectants. Because of their poor shelf-life they need to be freshly mixed before use.

> **Types of surface disinfectants**
> - Chlorhexidine, e.g. Hibitane®.
> - Quaternary ammonium compounds, e.g. Cetavlon®.
> - Chlorinated solutions, e.g. household bleach.
> - Phenolics, e.g. Dettol®.
> - Iodophor compounds, e.g. povidone-iodine.
> - Aldehyde compounds, e.g. glutaraldehyde.

Hand disinfectants

The first and most important fact that must be recognized when cleaning any surface is that liquid soap and water, used carefully to wash the area, will remove the great majority of organisms. Hand or glove washing should be the activity that is given priority in any regimen designed to prevent cross-infection. The addition of a chemical disinfectant to the procedure will achieve an even higher level of asepsis. The main hand disinfectants are listed here.

Chlorhexidine

The leading proprietary brand is Hibiscrub®, a 20% chlorhexidine gluconate solution in a surfactant. It is pleasant to use and the antibacterial effect increases with continued use during the working day.

Iodine

Betadine®, a povidone-iodine handwash, is used by many oral surgeons. It has the advantage of leaving a biocidal residue after it has dried. Care must be taken as it has a dramatic bright orange colour which will stain any clothing on which it falls.

Surface disinfection

The chemical used to disinfect a surface will depend upon the nature of the contamination. The recommended procedure is to spray the working surface with detergent solution and wipe down. This is adequate where blood spills have not occurred.

Hypochlorite

This is used when blood spills have occurred. A solution containing 10 000 parts per million available chlorine should be used. In general this corresponds to a 1:10 dilution of household bleach. Because of the irritant nature of hypochlorite it is best used as a wipe; spray use should be avoided.

Chlorhexidine

Dispray® contains 2.5% chlorhexidine gluconate in 70% alcohol, therefore it should not be used near a naked flame. It is a convenient and quick method of disinfecting work surfaces.

Instrument and material disinfection

Delicate instruments that cannot withstand autoclaving may be soaked in a surface disinfectant, whilst the same procedure may be adopted with items such as impressions.

Instruments

These should be soaked in freshly activated 2% alkaline glutaraldehyde such as Cidex® for at least 1 hour, then rinsed thoroughly before use. It is often convenient to leave the items overnight.

Impressions

Alginates may be sprayed with 10% hypochlorite solution and left for 2 minutes before being poured. Elastomeric materials may be immersed in glutaraldehyde for 1 hour.

The control of cross-infection

The avoidance of cross-infection in hygienist practice is a subject of paramount importance. The well-being of patients should not be put at risk as a result of receiving dental treatment. Equally, it is the responsibility of all staff in a dental practice to ensure the absolute safety of others working there and the purpose of this chapter is to outline working methods aimed at reducing the risks of cross-infection. It is important that dental hygienists have a clear understanding of, and practical familiarity with, safe procedures in the avoidance of cross-infection. An essential element in the prevention of cross-infection is the taking of a competent case history. Although in many countries this is legally the responsibility of the supervising dental surgeon, the dental hygienist should be able to identify patients who are a high risk or at risk and therefore be in a position to take appropriate precautions. Some of the commoner infectious diseases from which the hygienist and patient are at risk are shown in Table 7.2.

The following advice covers the treatment of patients suffering from viral hepatitis and human immunodeficiency viruses (HIV), but it should be remembered that all patients are potentially an infection risk and procedures should routinely be used to allow for this possibility.

Hepatitis viruses

The term 'viral hepatitis' covers infection by various viruses, of which hepatitis B virus is the most important. Viral hepatitis is currently divided into five well recognized types A, B, C, D, E, and a catch-all grouping of non-A non-B, which has been used for many years to describe a type of hepatitis for which no specific causative agent could be identified. Recently a G virus has been identified. Hepatitis A virus (HAV) and hepatitis B (HBV) have been recognized since the 1940s although the disease of hepatitis B was only first described in 1965. Hepatitis C virus (HCV) was described in 1989. Hepatitis D virus (HDV) or delta hepatitis is recognized as an infection which is dependent

Table 7.2 Common infectious diseases from which the hygienist and patient are at risk

Infectious agent	Infection route	Incubation period
Viral		
Chicken pox	BSA	10–20 days
Common cold	BSA	2–3 days
Glandular fever	BSA	4–7 weeks
Herpes	BXS	Up to 2 weeks
Hepatitis A	BAO	2–7 weeks
Hepatitis B	BSA	1–5 months
Hepatitis C	BSA	1–5 months
Hepatitis D	BSA	1–5 months
Hepatitis E	BSA	1–5 months
Hepatitis G	BSA	Unknown
Human immunodeficiency viruses (HIV)	XBA	Up to 15 years
Influenza	SA	1–3 days
Measles	SA	9–11 days
Bacterial		
Legionella	A	2–10 days
Staphylococcus	SA	4–10 days
Streptococcus	BSA	1–3 days
Syphilis	BX	2–12 weeks
Tetanus	O	7–10 days
Tuberculosis	SA	Up to 6 months
Fungal		
Candida	S	2–3 days

Key: A = airborne droplets, B = blood, O = open wound, S = saliva, X = sexual contact.

on the presence of HBV and was first described in 1983. Hepatitis D may occur as a co-infection with HBV or as a superinfection in an HBV carrier. Hepatitis E virus (HEV) is similar to HAV with a faecal–oral mode of transmission. Recent research on hepatitis E reveals that it is more common in men than women but there appears to be a quite high fatality rate (10% to 20%) in women who develop hepatitis E in the third trimester of pregnancy.

There are reports of hepatitis G in the literature but as yet little is known about the pathogenesis of this problem. Further information on the classification is shown in Table 7.3.

The hepatitis B virus

This is a major cause of acute and chronic liver pathology arising from infection and leading to cirrhosis and primary hepatocellular carcino-ma. It is estimated that globally there are more than 300 million carriers of the virus and 90% of these live in less well developed countries. It is endemic in China, South East Asia, many of the Pacific islands, Africa, parts of the Middle East and the Amazon region of Latin America. However, in the USA, Western Europe and Australia it is estimated that less than 1% of the population are virus carriers.

Recent figures from the USA indicate that the majority of patients infected with HBV have been infected subclinically and have no aware-ness of their infectivity. About 6–10% of young adults infected with HBV become carriers. Of these, 25% will progress to develop liver cirrhosis.

Hepatitis risk groups

The importance of the carrier in the spread of HBV cannot be overstated. A carrier is defined as a person who is HBsAg-positive on at least two occasions 6 months apart. Infectivity, however, is best correlated to HBeAg positivity which will indicate a more infectious and contagious state and hence at more risk of transmitting the disease. Patients may be divided into low- and high-risk groups by serology. The low-risk patient will have HBsAg present in their blood and also have HBe antibody. Patients who have been diagnosed as HBsAg-positive should be re-tested annually. Patients in the high-risk groups will have HBsAg present but no core antibody, or have HBeAg present but no core antibody.

Risk of infection

Research undertaken in the USA has shown that dentists who have not been immunized are three times more likely to acquire HBV infec-tion than the general population and interest-ingly non-immune surgeons are 6 times more likely to acquire the infection than is the case in the general population. In addition, 76% of saliva samples from known carriers are HBsAg-positive and gingival crevicular fluid and nasal secretions have all tested positive for HBsAg in this group. As many patients mouths have inflamed gingival margin and as some dental procedures allow blood to mix with saliva this will become loaded with HBV. This is why the saliva is considered a potentially infectious fluid and subject to universal precautions.

Table 7.3 Hepatitis viruses

The main hepatitis viruses are

- **Viral hepatitis A**. This virus is spread by the faecal–oral route and outbreaks usually result from food or water contamination. It is not a significant problem in the dental surgery but vaccination is available for those at risk such as travellers to countries where the virus is prevalent.
- **Viral hepatitis B**. Approximately 1 person in 500 is a carrier of the hepatitis B virus. Half of these carriers have never had clinical symptoms of the disease and are therefore unaware of the possibility of carrier status. It has been estimated that 250 hepatitis B carriers are unknowingly treated within the general dental service every working day.
- **Viral hepatitis C**. Hepatitis C has become a major risk for health care personnel involved in procedures involving blood or serum. It is also a major cause of post-transfusion hepatitis where blood is not screened or treated. HCV is a small RNA virus and there are 8 recognized genotypes and within each genotype there are several subtypes, so it is possible for patients to be infected with more than one strain of the virus. This may explain how the virus is so resistant to treatment and also the difficulty in producing a vaccine. The only agent currently available for the treatment of hepatitis C is alpha interferon administered by subcutaneous injection.
- **Viral hepatitis D**. This is caused by a defective transmissible virus or agent which requires the presence of hepatitis B for its own replication. Superinfection with hepatitis D in a hepatitis carrier is often associated with very severe liver damage.
- **Viral hepatitis E**. Similar to HAV with a faeco–oral mode of transmission.
- **Viral hepatitis G**. Known to be transmitted parenterally.

Hepatitis B vaccines

The latest vaccines against HBV are produced by recombinant DNA technique using yeast cells. The genetically engineered vaccines currently available in the UK are H-B-Vax 11 (Pasteur Merieux) or Engerix B (SmithKline Beecham). The deltoid muscle is the preferred site of injection and involves three injections: the first two 1 month apart and the third 6 months later. Side-effects included mild fever (2%) and a sore arm (15%). A blood test 2 months after vaccination is complete is necessary to identify the small number of subjects who are still not protected. It should be noted that immunization takes up to 6 months to confer protection and the duration of immunity is thought to last for 3–5 years. Antibody levels should, therefore, be checked every 3 years with a booster every 5 years.

For those who are accidentally infected commonly via a needlestick type injury, specific hepatitis B immunoglobulin (HBIG) is available for use with the vaccine. This can be obtained via a local Accident and Emergency Department (and administered within 48 hours) and where further advice can be obtained when necessary. It must be emphasized that a clinician or an assistant who is a carrier can still undertake dental care.

Transmission of hepatitis B is most likely to occur by accidental inoculation with a blood-contaminated instrument. There is no evidence that aerosol inhalation will transmit hepatitis, but transmission after blood splashes in the eye has been reported. The prevention of cross-infection is by the use of effective control measures and is described later.

Human immunodeficiency viruses

Acquired immune deficiency syndrome (AIDS) is a blood-borne disease of low infectivity that is caused by the human immunodeficiency viruses (HIV1 and HIV2). The epidemiology of the disease is similar to the hepatitis B virus. It must be remembered that the risk of transmission of this virus from patients to medical, dental or other staff, even after needlestick injury, is low.

The disease is transmitted by inoculation with contaminated blood or blood products. Individuals who are likely to become infected are shown in Table 7.4. In the medical and dental professions transmission could occur by accidental inoculation with a blood-contaminated instrument from an infected patient but experience has shown that this is exceptionally rare, even after needlestick injuries relating to AIDS patients. In addition, the virus has been

---

Table 7.4 Patients at high risk of cross-infection

While all patients are a potential cross-infection risk, those in the following groups constitute high-risk patients

- Those with hepatitis surface or core antigen but without core antibody.
- Patients with AIDS, shown by a severe opportunistic infection not associated with primary immunodeficiency or immunosuppressive drugs, or patients with Kaposi's sarcoma.
- Patients with suspected AIDS who have persistent generalized lymphadenopathy, unexplained weight loss or prolonged unexplained fever.
- The sexual contacts of patients with known HIV infection.
- Patients who are HIV antibody-positive, their partners and children (this includes some haemophiliacs and others who may have received donated body tissues and/or fluids).
- Intravenous drug abusers.
- Homosexual men and their partners.
- Prostitutes, both male and female.
- Patients who have had acute hepatitis in the last 6 weeks.
- Patients with chronic active hepatitis or cirrhosis.
- Patients who are or have recently been in prison.

---

detected in the saliva of some HIV-positive patients. Therefore, it is prudent to take special care during procedures, especially when handling contaminated syringes and sharp instruments, to avoid self-inoculation. It must be remembered that whilst patients with AIDS are usually extremely ill, HIV-positive patients without clinical AIDS may appear healthy.

Patients who are shown not to have hepatitis antigen in their blood can be removed from the risk groups. Those suspected of being HIV carriers or to have AIDS, for whom the HIV antibody test is negative, provided that a year has elapsed since the last exposure to risk, may also no longer be considered a cross-infection risk. This also applies to those who are or have been in prison. They should also be shown to be negative to hepatitis B tests.

Treatment of patients to minimize cross-infection risk

All members of clinical and support staff are expected to participate in patient care. The essential point to remember is that treatment of infection risk patients should not differ from that given to other patients: all patients should be managed as potential infection risk. Only the staff who are directly involved in dental procedures on these patients need be informed in advance that a patient is a cross-infection risk. Special precautions are not required for these patients in the waiting room and emergency treatment should not be withheld from

patients who are a suspected cross-infection risk. It should be remembered that patients suffering from HIV infection due to their immune system suppression are at risk from contacting infections from other patients in the practice, and the following precautions are for their benefit as well as your own.

For examination, gloves should be routinely worn and cuts and abrasions covered. The mouth should be examined carefully for oral manifestations of HIV infection by the clinician responsible for the treatment, as this will indicate progression of the disease. The dental hygienist should wear gloves, gowns, masks and eye protection. An instrument pack should include all relevant hand instruments, aspirator tip, rotary instruments and three-in-one syringe tip. To avoid blood splashes, ultrasonic or air scalers must not be used: high-volume aspiration and disposable equipment should be used.

The handpiece, three-in-one syringe and aspirator tubes should be sterilizable or if this is not possible, should be protected with disposable surgical sleeves and a disposable container should be used for the mouthwash. After use, dental equipment, including the dental chair and spittoon, should be cleaned with detergent solution and dried. Treatment timings should take these procedures into account.

Blood spills should be wiped with paper and covered with 1% sodium hypochlorite solution or sodium dichloroisocyanurate tablets or granules for 5 minutes and the area again wiped

Table 7.5 Treatment of a penetrating or needlestick injury

- Wash the injury thoroughly with soap under running water without scrubbing, and allow to bleed profusely. Apply Betadine® and cover, if necessary, with a suitable dressing. Check the medical status of the patient concerned and complete an accident form if appropriate.
- Where the injury has been caused by a sharp from an identified infection-risk patient, advice should be sought from the principal of the practice who should undertake the necessary administrative arrangements and refer the injured person to the haematology department of a local hospital. If the injured person is not immune and the patient is hepatitis B-positive, 5 ml of immunoglobulin must be given intramuscularly within 48 hours. The injured person should be followed up and given a hepatitis B vaccination course starting within 1 month.

and all waste placed in a yellow bag for contaminated material. After treatment, disposable material should be incinerated and contaminated instruments should be autoclaved.

Personal protection

All dental hygienists are strongly advised to be vaccinated against hepatitis B and tested on a regular basis for an appropriate level of protective antibody. At the start of each session hands should be thoroughly washed and dried with a disinfectant detergent (e.g. Betadine® or Hibiscrub®) and any cuts covered with waterproof sticking plasters. A pair of rubber gloves should be worn for the remainder of the session and these should be washed immediately after putting them on and when otherwise contaminated. They should be replaced if punctured or torn. A specially toughened glove – Biogel D® – has been developed for use on several patients with washing in between. Latex gloves should be used for all procedures except where operators are sensitive to the material, when low-allergen gloves may be worn. To permit effective hand-washing, taps in the surgery should be able to be operated by elbow, foot or electronically and not touched by hands, whether gloved or ungloved. Towels should be hung with the leading edge away from the wall and after using a towel the final act should be to pull it down so as to expose a clean surface for the next person.

The most dangerous injury in the surgery is a needlestick and great care should be taken to avoid them. A similar injury may be caused by the tip of a mechanical scaler when left on the handpiece after use. In the unfortunate event of a penetrating or needlestick injury the procedures shown in Table 7.5 should be adopted.

Spectacles must be worn by the patient and by the hygienist when scaling, polishing, root planing or creating an aerosol when using an ultrasonic or air scaler. Masks should be worn when the operator has a cold or a recurrent cold sore and their use is also highly recommended when polishing or creating an aerosol. Reusable or disposable gowns, laboratory coats or uniforms should be worn during clinical work and they should be changed when soiled with blood. Clinical clothes should not be worn outside clinical areas, especially where food or drink is being consumed.

Sterilization is achieved by autoclaving or dry heat and these must be the methods of choice for all suitable instruments after the removal of debris using an open tray system. Every effort should be made to use disposable items. Instruments or items of equipment which cannot be autoclaved can be disinfected by glutaraldehyde 2% solution for 30 min or 1% sodium hypochlorite for 10 min. All sharp instruments, whether used or not, must be disposed of in a sharps bin. As well as obvious items such as needles, scalpel blades, suture needles and local anaesthetic cartridges, this also applies to steel burs and polishing cups and brushes. Sharps bins must be sealed and replaced when not more than two-thirds full to avoid accidental injury to persons handling them.

Disinfection of dental equipment

The bracket table handle, the light switch, control buttons and the light handle should not be touched when hands are contaminated. These surfaces should be wiped with a cloth and detergent solution or be sprayed with a disinfectant spray between patients and then dried, as should the working surface of the bracket table. The dry bracket table should be covered with paper before receiving instruments for the next patient. Tray systems should be used wherever possible. When any of the above are visibly contaminated with blood they should be wiped with a 1% sodium hypochlorite solution and then dried. If, after flushing, a spittoon is visibly contaminated with blood, it should be wiped with 1% sodium hypochlorite solution.

Handpieces and air scalers must be lubricated and autoclaved after each patient and the heads of conventional handpieces should be removed before autoclaving. This lubrication is essential to prevent damage to the handpiece internal mechanism during autoclaving. Before a sterile handpiece or air scaler is attached to its tubing, the foot switch should be activated and the water supply flushed through into the spittoon for 20 s to remove any organisms present in the tubing. Triple syringe tips should be removed and autoclaved after the treatment of each patient. Before the treatment of the next patient, the syringe should be flushed with water for 20 s before an autoclaved tip is reattached. Aspirator tubing should be flushed through with 1% sodium hypochlorite solution at the end of each day.

Working practices

Heavy-duty rubber gloves must be worn by personnel cleaning operative areas or when cleaning contaminated instruments before autoclaving. Aerosol dispersal must be kept to a minimum by using a wide-bore aspirator whenever possible. When an air scaler or ultrasonic scaler is to be used, the patient should rinse with a 0.2% chlorhexidine solution (Corsodyl®) for 1 minute before treatment is started to reduce the number of oral organisms and thereby reduce the aerosol microbial burden.

All rotary instruments should be cleaned, ideally in an ultrasonic bath, or failing that, using a bur cleaner, and then sterilized by autoclave or hot air oven. Steel burs and polishing cups and brushes generally should be considered as disposable.

Hands should be washed before and after using X-ray apparatus, light units or similar equipment, as well as patient notes. Where practicable, auxiliary equipment should be wiped with a cloth moistened with disinfectant solution.

Daily working regime

Before laying out any sterile instruments or equipment, clean the following using chlorhexidine/alcohol spray: all working surfaces, light switch and handles, chair control, triple syringe, handpieces housing, aspirator housing, spittoons and patient's bib.

Set out instruments, rubber cups, prophylaxis points, handpieces, aspirator tips, three-in-one tips and saliva ejectors. Place cotton wool rolls and pellets into small disposable pots, using sufficient only for the patient to be treated. Read any notes and mount any radiographs required before treatment. Always wash gloved hands before handling notes or before placing them back into the patient's mouth. Once you are operating, avoid non-clean contacts. Do not answer the phone, for example, without first washing hands, in order to avoid contamination of the telephone handpiece. If further items are required, e.g. prophylaxis paste, light curing units, ensure your hands are clean before handling the items.

After treatment clean all visible debris from instruments, burs and equipment and sterilize before further patient use and ensure that sufficient sterile instruments are available for all the patients to be seen in a session. Never leave burs or scaler tips in handpieces: thus accidental injury to passers-by can be prevented. Dispose of sharps in the sharps bin only, not in the waste bin, and dispose of all dirty napkins, towels etc. in the waste bin. Disinfect the whole area as previously detailed before treating the next patient. When writing up notes ensure that neither they nor your pen becomes contaminated with material from the patient's mouth.

Cross-infection control is based upon
- Good working practices.
- Use of effective sterilization and disinfection methods.
- Treating all patients as potentially infectious.
- Use of barrier techniques.
- Limit aerosols by efficient aspiration.
- Vaccination against hepatitis B.
- Disposal of sharps in a dedicated container.
- Early treatment of needlestick injuries.

Table 7.6 Types of acquired immunity

Acquired immunity may be either naturally or artificially acquired

- Natural immunity follows an infection. In some cases, such as chickenpox and measles, it lasts for life and in others, like influenza and the common cold, the period of immunity is much shorter.
- Artificial immunity is acquired by vaccination, which is a simulated infection. Although the vaccine injected is either killed or harmless, the immunity produced is effective against the natural infection. The body's response with both types of active immunity is usually termed the immune response.
- Passive artificial immunity involves the injection of antibodies into the blood stream of an individual who has come into contact with an infection to which they have no immunity. In the past the injected antibodies were usually obtained from animals, often horses, but modern techniques of genetic engineering may soon permit the production of antibodies in the laboratory.

The immune system

Immunity is the response of the body to micro-organisms and foreign materials. The immune system is composed of specialized cells and tissues whose role is defence of the host. The system acts to identify the cells and tissues of the host and distinguish then from non-self material. Immunity may either be innate, i.e. inborn, or acquired, i.e. developed after birth.

Innate immunity

Innate immunity is present at birth and is the first line of defence against invading organisms. It is not specific against any particular organism and is often called non-specific immunity. Innate immunity has three components: physical, chemical and cellular.

Physical barriers in the mouth consist of the oral epithelium such as the gingiva and mucosa, and secretions such as saliva which continually wash and cleanse the mucosa surfaces. Humoral factors are present in blood and in saliva and in gingiva crevicular fluid. These are immunologically active factors including immunoglobulins and complement. Cellular components include the neutrophils and mast cells.

One particular form of innate immunity is found in new-born babies. Antibodies from the mother's serum cross the placenta and enter the fetal circulation, conferring a degree of immunity for the first 3–6 months of life.

An important part of innate immunity and one that is involved in activating the acquired immune response are the human leukocyte antigens (HLA). These are part of our genetic makeup called the major histocompatibility complex (MHC). Many of the genes in the MHC are involved in the immune system. The HLA system is involved in recognition of antigen by T lymphocytes. In addition certain HLA genes have been shown to confer greater susceptibility to particular diseases. A dental example is localized juvenile periodontitis.

Acquired immunity

Some parts of the immune response are not present at birth but develop later. As this acquired response develops in reaction to the entry of foreign material into the body, it is specific and has memory. It is sometimes called adaptive. Details of acquired immunity are shown in Table 7.6.

The immune response

The acquired immune system is able to recognize and react specifically to foreign material (usually called an antigen), but does not normally react to the body's own component. Antigens are substances which have a large molecular size, usually proteins, which are foreign to the body. The body's immune system is able to mount a number of defensive actions. Bacteria entering the tissues, for example, may be killed, but if toxins are produced, these will require to be neutralized. Thus, different responses will occur depending upon the type of antigen.

Two main types of immunological defence reactions can be triggered by antigens entering the body: the humoral and the cell-mediated. Both responses are usually involved simultaneously but it is simpler to consider them separately. The overall outline of the system is shown in Figure 7.3.

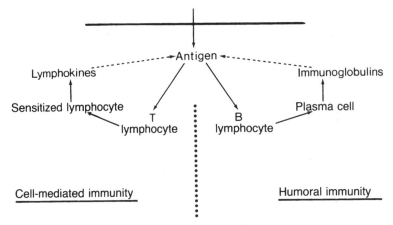

Fig. 7.3 Diagrammatic representation of the immune response.

Humoral immune response

In this type of reaction the antigen is attacked by specific proteins released from immune cells. These proteins are called antibodies or immunoglobulins. The immunoglobulins are types of serum globulins (see Chapter 3), called gammaglobulins, and each one is specific to the antigen which triggered its formation.

The antigen is phagocytosed by macrophages which process the antigen and instruct a lymphocyte (the B lymphocyte in this case). The B lymphocyte, once stimulated by the antigen, changes into a plasma cell and produces immunoglobulins which react with the antigen. This type of response is referred to as humoral because the immunoglobulins can be released some distance from the site of infection and are carried in the blood to the area.

Cellular immune response

In this response the T lymphocyte is activated to produce local factors including cytokines, which may be produced by a whole range of body tissues if they are damaged (see Table 7.7). The T cell is attracted to the site of the antigen and interacts directly to destroy it. The cytokines have a whole range of effects, one of which is damage to cell membranes. Although this may destroy foreign microbes, the potential also exists for damaging the body's own cells. The cytokines also initiate and increase the body's inflammatory responses as well as attracting and activating B cell lymphocytes.

Table 7.7 Properties of cytokines

General properties of cytokines

- Released by a variety of cells, e.g.: lymphocytes, monocytes, leukocytes.
- Have a variety of effects depending upon the source cell.
- Have a direct effect on the cell that releases them.
- May have remote effects acting like a hormone.
- Induce the release of other cytokines.
- May act in synergy with other cytokines to produce enhanced effects.

Components of the immune response

It can be seen that the immune response consists of certain cells, proteins and tissues which function together to provide protection from foreign material entering the body. The commonest sources of danger are the millions of organisms, both commensal and pathogenic, which exist in our environment, but a splinter of wood embedded in the skin will provoke the same defences.

The cells

The lymphocyte is the most important cell in the immune response. There are two types of lymphocyte: the B cell, which arises initially in the collections of lymphoid glands (bursa) surrounding the gut, and the T cell, which arises from the thymus. The origins of these cells are not really of significance to the dental hygienist, but they explain the choice of the letters B and T. Once produced, the B and T lymphocytes colonize the lymphoid tissue scattered throughout the body and produce clones of cells with similar defensive abilities.

Other cells are also important. Neutrophil polymorphs act to phagocytose the antigens and damaged tissue. Large macrophages found throughout the body also phagocytose antigens, process them and instruct the B and T cells, so initiating the immune response. The mast cell is also important. These are found attached to the walls of small blood vessels, and in certain immunological reactions they release histamines and other similar substances, which cause many of the vascular changes seen in hay fever and other allergic conditions.

The proteins

The proteins involved in immune reactions are very complex and only an outline of their functions will be discussed.

Complement
Complement is a series of proteins and enzymes present in the blood, which is activated by the combination of immunoglobulins and antigens. Its main function is to assist in the destruction (lysis) of organisms or to promote their phagocytosis, a function called opsonization. In addition, complement factors trigger the inflammatory response.

Antibodies
Immunoglobulins (antibodies) are produced by plasma cells and released into the blood stream. Their functions range from helping polymorphs to phagocytose bacteria, to neutralizing toxins. Once the body has been stimulated to produce immunoglobulins, long-lived memory cells remain in the circulation, which can be triggered to initiate the production of large amounts of plasma cells and hence immunoglobulins, should the antigen be encountered again. This is why, once some diseases have been suffered, we obtain lifelong immunity (but not, regrettably, to caries or periodontal disease).

Immunoglobulins
The immunoglobulins are given alphabetical letters - G, M, A and E to distinguish them. Immunoglobulin G is the commonest antibody in serum and can cross the placenta and protect the fetus and baby in the early months of life. Immunoglobulin M is a very large protein which is extremely efficient at killing bacteria. Immunoglobulin A is present mainly in body secretions such as saliva, milk and tears. It defends mucosal surfaces, such as in the oral cavity, from bacterial invasion. Immunoglobulin E is found in serum and on the surface of mast cells. It is responsible for many of the features of allergic reactions.

Cytokines
Cytokines are produced by activated T cells when stimulated by contact. They perform various functions, including attracting other lymphocytes including the B cells, attracting and activating macrophages and damaging bacterial cell walls. However, they also cause local damage and this is believed to be one of the sources of tissue damage in periodontal disease.

Tissues

The tissues of the immune system produce the various cells. The main ones are the bone marrow and the lymph nodes scattered throughout the body.

> Components of the immune response
> - **Cells**: T and B lymphocytes, polymorphonuclear leukocytes, macrophages, mast cells.
> - **Proteins**: complement, immunoglobulins (IgG, M, A, E), cytokines.
> - **The tissues**: bone marrow, lymph nodes.

Pathogenicity of organisms

As stated at the beginning of this chapter, micro-organisms may be divided into pathogenic and commensal types. Pathogenic micro-organisms are capable of producing agents called toxins, which are harmful to the tissues. These are of two types: exotoxins and endotoxins.

Exotoxins are given off by the organism and circulate freely throughout the body. They are extremely potent, causing a great deal of damage in small quantities. A typical feature of diseases caused by exotoxins is that the micro-organisms remain localized in one area while the exotoxins cause widespread damage, as happens in diphtheria and tetanus.

Endotoxins are produced within the organism and are only released when it dies and breaks up. They are less potent than exotoxins and, if they produce generalized symptoms, it is because of the invasiveness of the organism. In other words, the micro-organisms themselves disperse throughout the body. Tuberculosis and syphilis are examples of such diseases. Endotoxins may also be produced as a result of the breakdown of the cell of necrotic commensal organisms.

Commensal organisms do not produce potent toxins but are capable of producing low-grade damage as in, for example, periodontal disease. The commensal organisms colonizing the tooth surface irritate the gingiva and provoke the inflammatory and immune responses in a number of ways. The main methods are by the presence of enzymes, endotoxins and other antigens in the plaque bacteria.

Enzymes help to damage the crevicular epithelium and make it more permeable to the infiltration of other microbial by-products such as endotoxins. They are also proteins and as such are antigenic and therefore provoke the immune response. The endotoxins are produced when cell wall components are released from plaque organisms after they are lysed. These infiltrate through the junctional epithelium and are very potent initiators of both the inflammatory and immune responses. The organisms, their enzymes and endotoxins can, therefore, all be seen to be powerful inducers of the immune response, of both cell-mediated and humoral type.

Role of the immune response in periodontal disease

Initially the immune response appears to play a protective role, preventing plaque micro-organisms from penetrating the gingival tissues. However, whilst being a defensive mechanism for the whole body, the immune response is capable of being locally harmful. This is illustrated by the intense local reaction which may result from injecting certain antigens subcutaneously. This reaction may prevent spread of the antigen, but is locally damaging.

With continued, low-grade, long-term stimulation of the humoral and cell-mediated responses, plaque products will initiate and cause the progression of periodontal disease, with the body's own mechanisms being responsible for most of the breakdown of the periodontal tissues.

Abnormalities of the immune response

Hypersensitivity

Hypersensitivity is the technical term for allergy and can be defined as an immune reaction which produces tissue damage in the host. The immunological reactions which result in tissue damage are identical with those which destroy micro-organisms. As already noted, the immune response, whilst being a defensive mechanism, can under certain circumstances cause tissue damage. Hypersensitivity does not imply an exaggerated immune response, but merely a response which happens to cause tissue damage to the host.

Examples of hypersensitivity are asthma, hay fever and allergic reactions to certain drugs, including penicillin. In relation to drugs, the hypersensitivity reaction to the first exposure to the drug may produce relatively mild symptoms, such as nausea, pyrexia or skin rashes. However, the secondary exposure to the same drug is likely to have a much more severe systemic effect, known as anaphylaxis. Such a reaction can even result in death.

Autoimmunity

Autoimmunity means the production of an immune response to the host's own tissues. There is a failure of the immune system to recognize 'self' proteins. This is usually due to these proteins becoming slightly altered by relatively simple compounds or elements being attached to them. An example of this is the contact dermatitis which occasionally results from substances such as iodine coming in contact with the skin. The same effect can result from antigens coming in contact with tissue cells and attaching themselves to the cell membrane. There is as a result, an immune reaction against the intact tissue cell, which has the antigen as an integral part of it. It is this type of reaction which causes rheumatic fever. An exotoxin secreted by bacteria lodged in the throat circulates in the blood and becomes attached to the synovial membrane of joints and valves of the heart. The resulting immune response causes an inflammatory reaction in these tissues. Autoimmunity is also associated with certain relatively uncommon oral conditions, such as pemphigus.

Further reading

British Dental Association (1993) *The Control of Cross Infection*. BDA Advisory Service, Advice Sheet A12.

Chief Dental Officer (1993). Letter to all dentists in England. *Cross Infection Control*. Department of Health, PL/CDO (93) 3.

Croser D., Chipping J. (1989) *Cross Infection Control in General Dental Practice a Practical Guide for the whole Dental Team*. London: Quintessence Publishing.

Expert advisory group on AIDS (1990) *Guidance for Clinical Health Care Workers: Protection against Infection with HIV and Hepatitis Viruses*. HMSO, ISBN 0 11 321249 6.

Field E. A. (Ed.) (1994) Hand hygiene, hand care and hand protection for clinical dental practice. Recommendations of the European panel for infection control in Dentistry. *British Dental Journal* **176**, 129–134.

Marsh P., Mártin M. (1992) *Oral microbiology*. 3rd edition. London: Chapman and Hall.

Peakman M., Vergani D. (1997) *Basic and Clinical Immunology*. New York: Churchill Livingstone.

Stucke V. A. (1993) *Microbiology for nurses*. 7th edition. London: Bailliere Tindall.

8

General pathology

Acute inflammation

Acute inflammation is the fundamental reaction of the body to injury. Many different agents may cause the injury, but they all produce the same basic response. As long ago as the first century AD, Celsus described the cardinal signs of inflammation as *rubor, tumor, calor* and *dolor*, which anyone who has suffered from a boil will recognize as redness, swelling, heat and pain. A century later a fifth cardinal sign was added by Galen which was *loss of function*.

Causes of acute inflammation

The many and varied causes of injury and, therefore, acute inflammation may be classified as shown in Table 8.1.

Stages of acute inflammation

Vascular response

After injury, the arterioles in the affected area at first constrict, causing a blanching of the area for a short time, and then dilate. The vasodilation allows more blood to enter the area (i.e. hyperaemia), making it red and hot. This vascular response can easily be demonstrated by running the fingernail firmly across an area of skin. At first a white line will appear and this will gradually be replaced by a red line.

Emigration of the white blood cells

The rate of flow of blood through the affected tissues becomes much slower and eventually

Table 8.1 Inflammation

Some causes of acute inflammation

- **Physical agents**: including mechanical trauma, heat, extreme cold, ionizing radiation and electricity.
- **Chemical agents**: a wide range of chemicals may cause injury to the tissues including all strong acids and alkalis.
- **Micro-organisms**: acute inflammation is frequently a feature of infection of the tissues by micro-organisms.
- **Antigens**: the immune response was discussed in some detail in the previous chapter.
- **Interruption of blood supply**: if cells are cut off from their supply of oxygen and nutrition, they die. This is referred to as necrosis and it causes acute inflammation in the surrounding tissue.

stops. The neutrophil polymorphonuclear leukocytes, instead of passing rapidly by, come to lie close to the endothelial cells lining the blood vessels. This is called margination of the white cells. Soon they push pseudopodia between adjacent endothelial cells and gradually work their way through into the tissues, the endothelial gap closing behind them. Neutrophil leukocytes are both mobile and phagocytic, allowing them to scavenge around on the tissues, picking up any minute foreign particles such as bacteria or cell debris. The neutrophils are the first line of defence and they are gradually replaced by the larger monocytes, termed macrophages, in the tissues; these clear up the debris from the whole area. The emigration of the white blood cells is often referred to as the cellular exudate.

Fluid exudate

While the cells are passing into the tissues, fluid is also exuding from the blood vessels into the tissues, as a result of three changes.

- The blood pressure within the capillaries is increased by the vasodilation of the arterioles.
- The capillary walls become more permeable.
- The osmotic pressure in the tissue is increased by the breakdown of large protein molecules into numerous smaller osmotically active fragments.

The fluid exudate has the following roles.
- It carries antibacterial substances such as antibodies into the tissues. These may include drugs, such as antibiotics, given to combat the cause of the inflammation.
- It dilutes any irritant substance in the tissues.
- It carries fibrinogen from the blood into the tissues where it is converted into fibrin. This in turn helps to localize the irritant by forming a fibrin clot around it. It also aids the process of phagocytosis and may help to unite torn tissues.

The fluid exudate produces another cardinal sign of inflammation: swelling, caused by the build-up of pressure in the tissues. Loss of function which results from the pain is caused by the release into the surrounding tissues of inflammatory mediators.

Results of acute inflammation

The changes which follow acute inflammation depend on two factors: whether or not removal of the cause occurs, and the amount of tissue damage. If the cause is removed, the sequelae will depend on the amount of tissue damage.

Resolution

Where little tissue damage has occurred, the area is cleared by the phagocytic action of the macrophages. The causative agent, cell debris, necrotic leukocytes and fibrin are all removed in this way. The excess fluid is drained by the lymphatics and the tissue returns to normal. This is termed resolution.

Suppuration

When much tissue damage has been produced by the causative agent, return to normal is not possible. In this case pus is formed and the lesion is called an abscess. Pus consists of dead leukocytes, fibrin, micro-organisms, tissue debris and exuded fluid. It tends to track in the route of least resistance and eventually discharges through the body surface. Dental abscesses very often track through the alveolar bone to discharge through the attached gingiva, but they may also discharge on to the face or through the periodontal ligament. Once the abscess has discharged and drained it will heal up if the cause has been removed.

However, if the cause remains, the inflammatory response will continue alongside the tissue's attempts at repair. This produces a lower grade of inflammation, called chronic inflammation.

Acute inflammation has the following features
- The cardinal signs are rubor, calor, dolor, tumor and loss of function.
- The stages include a vascular response, emigration of white blood cells and production of a fluid exudate.
- The changes which follow acute inflammation depend on whether the cause is removed and the amount of tissue destruction which has occurred.
- Resolution can occur when there is little tissue damage and the cause has been removed.
- Suppuration occurs when there is much tissue damage and pus forms.
- If the cause still remains after this stage then chronic inflammation will develop.

Chronic inflammation

Clinically, the features of chronic inflammation are not as pronounced as those of acute inflammation. For example, it will be seen that in chronic gingivitis the gingivae are not as red as in acute gingivitis, and chronic gingivitis is normally fairly painless, while acute gingivitis can be exceedingly painful.

Causes of chronic inflammation

It has already been mentioned that chronic inflammation occurs when the causative agent persists, that is it is not easily removed from the tissues. In this respect, insoluble particles like silica and asbestos are well suited to causing it. Also, micro-organisms which are inadequately eliminated by the body defences cause a prolonged chronic inflammatory response, which may be classified as follows.

- **Specific**: caused by single identifiable organism (e.g. tuberculosis and syphilis).
- **Non-specific**: caused by a number of different micro-organisms (e.g. chronic gingivitis).

Features of chronic inflammation

In chronic inflammation, the inflammatory process, already described, continues alongside the tissue's attempts at repair. Repair of tissues is achieved by the formation of granulation tissue, which is therefore a prominent feature of many chronic inflammatory lesions.

When a tissue has been damaged the defect is filled by fluid exudate and a fibrin clot is formed. Endothelial cells from the adjacent blood vessels begin to form side-shoots which grow into the fibrin clot, eventually forming new blood vessels. When looking at chronic inflammation under the microscope many chronic inflammatory cells will be seen including lymphocytes, plasma cells and macrophages which are present to combat the antigenic material. Fibroblasts are also present, laying down collagen and thus forming the structure of granulation tissue, which can be likened to a battle ground where the chronic inflammatory cells can wage war against the infection. It is common, in chronic periodontal disease, to find defects in the alveolar bone filled with granulation tissue.

In some chronic inflammatory lesions, the repair process seems to be excessive, resulting in hyperplasia. The reason for this is not known, but chronic gingivitis may often produce gingival hyperplasia.

Features of chronic inflammation

The features of chronic inflammation are less pronounced than acute inflammation.
They may be specific or non-specific.
The key feature of chronic inflammation is the presence of granulation tissue infiltrated by chronic inflammatory cells.
This represents the body's attempts at repair while infection is still present.
Granulation tissue is commonly present in patients with chronic gingivitis.

Neoplasia

Neoplasm is literally new growth of tissue. It implies an abnormal and excessive growth which often presents as a tumour mass. The term 'tumour' was at first applied to any swelling, no matter what the cause, but is now more usually used only for benign or malignant swellings. However the suffix -oma, which denotes a tumour, is still used for other swellings, for example, haematoma, which is a swelling produced by bleeding into the tissues.

Classification

Neoplasms are classified in two main ways: according to their behaviour and according to their tissue of origin.

Behaviour

They may be divided into two groups: benign and malignant neoplasms. As the name suggests, the malignant ones are far more serious and dangerous than the benign and they are called 'cancer' by the layperson. The main differences between the two types are as follows.

- **Growth:** benign neoplasms are slower growing than malignant ones and the growth of the benign type may stop altogether after a time, whereas the growth of malignant ones does not. It is therefore unusual to find very large benign tumours.

- **Shape:** benign neoplasms tend to be more round or regular in outline than their malignant counterparts.
- **Capsule:** benign tumours are often enclosed within a fibrous capsule. The malignant variety is not.
- **Histology:** the microscopical appearance of a benign neoplasm closely resembles the tissue of origin, whereas the microscopical appearance of malignant neoplasm is so erratic that it is often difficult to tell what the tissue of origin is. The term 'well differentiated' is used to describe a neoplasm which closely resembles its parent tissue and one which is dissimilar from its parent tissue is said to be 'poorly differentiated'.
- **Invasion:** malignant neoplasms infiltrate into the host tissue, whereas benign ones do not. Microscopically, this infiltration extends well beyond the visible limits of the neoplasm, which is important when the tumour is being excised.
- **Metastases:** these are groups of cells which become detached from the main neoplasm and are carried by the lymphatics or blood vessels to another part of the body, where they lodge and form secondary growths. This is a feature only of malignant tumours and is of enormous importance regarding the prognosis or probable outcome of the lesion.
- **Ulceration:** this is not a usual feature of benign lesions and any ulcer which fails to heal within a few weeks must be suspected of being malignant.
- **Outcome:** the final and possibly most significant difference between the two types is related to their outcome. Whereas benign neoplasms seldom cause any problem, the malignant ones have a very high mortality rate.

Tissue of origin

Both benign and malignant tumours may be of either epithelial or connective tissue origin and they are classified according to their tissue of origin.

The commonest type of benign epithelial neoplasm is called a papilloma. It can occur on any epithelial surface and is warty in appearance and painless. Papillomas occasionally occur in the mouth, especially on the tongue, lips and buccal mucosa. Benign epithelial neoplasms also occur in glandular tissue, where they are called adenomas.

Benign connective tissue neoplasms are named according to the type of connective tissue from which they originate. Examples are fibrous tissue: fibroma, bone: osteoma, adipose tissue: lipoma, muscle: myoma.

Malignant epithelial neoplasms are called carcinomas and they are more common than the connective tissue cancers. They may be further subdivided according to the type of epithelium from which they originate. A squamous cell carcinoma can occur on any stratified squamous epithelium, including that of the mouth. Its appearance varies from a white patch to a hard nodular mass and either type may ulcerate. In other words, it is impossible to describe the exact appearance of a squamous cell carcinoma and any unusual growth or ulcer should be suspected, until proved otherwise.

Malignant connective tissue neoplasms are called sarcomas. They are less common than carcinomas, but tend to be much more serious when they occur, since they spread more quickly. Sarcomas are subdivided according to their tissue of origin as shown in Table 8.2.

Table 8.2 Malignant tumours

Classification of malignant tumours of connective tissue

- **Fibrous tissue**: fibrosarcoma.
- **Bone**: osteosarcoma.
- **Lymphoid tissue**: lymphosarcoma.
- **Muscle**: myosarcoma.
- **Blood**: leukaemia is caused by malignancy of the white blood cells.

Precancerous state

It has been observed that, before a malignant lesion develops in an area, early cell changes can be seen. Histologically, the cells begin to look irregular without showing frank malignant change. This is referred to as a precancerous or premalignant state.

Precancerous changes can occur in any area and it is to test for this type of change in the epithelium of the uterine cervix that cervical smears are taken. It can also occur in the oral cavity, where it is termed leukoplakia. Microscopically there is epithelial dysplasia, with an atypical appearance of the cells and hyperkeratinization. The clinical picture is white shiny patches on the mucous membrane, produced by the excessive keratinization. This is discussed more fully in Chapter 13.

Causes of malignancy

Despite the vast amount of research into the aetiology of cancer, remarkably little is known of the cause. It is known that several factors will lead to malignancy, but how or why this happens is yet to be explained. Some of these factors are as follows.

Chemical carcinogens

A carcinogen is an agent which produces cancer and it has long been realized that certain chemicals have this property, for example coal tar and mineral oils. Such chemicals can cause carcinoma of the skin if there is frequent long-standing contact. Tobacco smoke contains many chemical carcinogens.

Physical carcinogens

The link between ionizing radiation and cancer is well established and is the reason why so much care is needed when using X-ray machines. Ultraviolet radiation can also be harmful to the skin and people like farmers in sunny climates may develop patches of dyskeratosis on the face after long exposure to strong sunlight.

Chronic disease

A number of chronic diseases can occasionally lead to malignancy. These include any chronic ulcer, cirrhosis of the liver, lichen planus and ulcerative colitis.

Heredity

It is probable that heredity plays a part in quite a few cancers, with breast cancer being a good example. It is definitely known that some obscure malignancies do have an hereditary predisposition.

Neoplasms can be benign or malignant.

- They can be classified according to behaviour and tissue of origin.
- Premalignant change in epithelium in the mouth is termed leukoplakia.
- Cancer is a multifactorial disease but various chemical and physical carcinogens have been identified.

Further reading

Spector W. (1989) *An Introduction to General Pathology*. 3rd edition. Edinburgh: Churchill Livingstone.

Walter J. B., Israel M. S. (1987) *Principles of Pathology for Dental Students*. 6th edition. Edinburgh: Churchill Livingstone.

9

Plaque, calculus and stains

Introduction

Once a tooth erupts, various materials gather on its surfaces; these substances are frequently called tooth-accumulated materials or integuments. Those of most interest to the hygienist are the acquired salivary pellicle, dental plaque, calculus, materia alba, food debris and extrinsic stains, which are discussed in this chapter.

Salivary pellicle

Salivary pellicle is a thin organic layer which forms rapidly on teeth after cleaning. It is composed of precipitated mucoproteins that originate from salivary glycoproteins. These are unstable in solution and are attracted to the apatite of the enamel crystallites. The pellicle is approximately 0.1 μm thick and initially does not contain micro-organisms, although it soon becomes colonized by plaque-forming bacteria.

This acquired pellicle covers the whole of the clinical crown except areas subject to attrition. When non-abrasive toothpastes are used it may achieve a considerable thickness and become stained. It cannot be removed by forceful rinsing and stains lightly with disclosing agents. Its significance or role in inflammatory periodontal diseases is unknown.

Dental plaque

Dental plaque is the film of organisms that develops on teeth, gums and oral appliances and restorations. Plaque is always present on the teeth, even after careful cleaning, as there are many sites that are not readily cleanable. Plaque reforms rapidly after cleaning and is relatively little influenced by dietary factors, although sucrose intake will speed up its formation.

Plaque formation

Plaque formation is usually preceded by salivary pellicle deposition, although plaque organisms can sometimes be detected adhering directly to enamel. The salivary pellicle is initially colonized by bacteria, most commonly Gram-positive streptococci (Fig. 9.1).

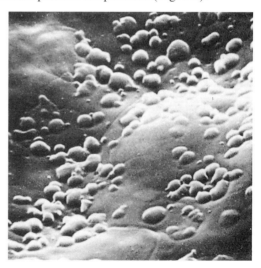

Fig. 9.1 Early plaque colonies as viewed in the scanning electron microscope. Coccal organisms can be seen on enamel. Replica technique ×1750.

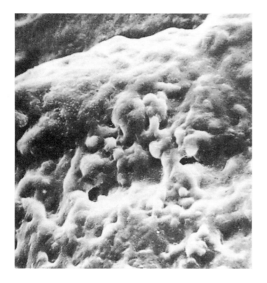

Fig. 9.2 The same area as shown in Fig. 9.1 two weeks after ceasing of all oral hygiene measures. A complex mass of organisms can be seen. Replica technique ×450.

Plaque formation occurs most rapidly in the cervical area adjacent to the gingival crevice, and in other sheltered sites, such as occlusal fissures and surface pits. There is some evidence that plaque which forms in uncleanable sites,

such as periodontal pockets, is of a different composition from smooth-surface supragingival plaque. This is presumably because of the anaerobic environment and persistent presence of mature plaque deposits.

Initially the supragingival film of plaque is only visible with the help of disclosing agents, but as it accumulates, it becomes steadily more obvious without staining. As it becomes thicker, it also covers a larger area of the tooth (Fig. 9.2).

The presence of sucrose in the diet has a marked effect on two aspects of plaque formation. Streptococcal organisms metabolize the sucrose to produce extracellular polysaccharides, mainly glucans which facilitate the attachment of further organisms to the enamel surface. The growth of the plaque mass is also enhanced with increased sucrose intake.

Plaque composition

Plaque is made up of approximately 70% micro-organisms and 30% interbacterial substances, including extracellular polysaccharides and host cells.

The types of micro-organisms present have

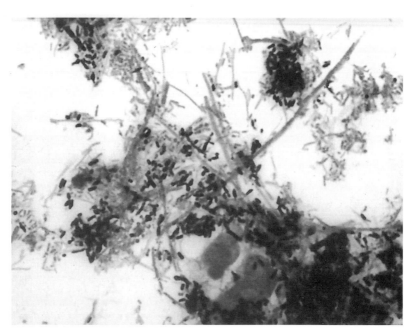

Fig. 9.3 A smear of 3-week-old plaque showing a wide range of organisms, including Gram-negatives and fusiforms (courtesy of Dr CWI Douglas).

Table 9.1 Plaque formation

The stages that supragingival plaque goes through following a thorough cleaning of a tooth surface are as follows

Immediately after cleaning: within a short time salivary pellicle is deposited on the teeth.

3–8 hours: there is a colonization by Gram-positive cocci and small rods. These organisms include the following:

- *Streptococcus sanguis*, a very common plaque organism dominant in early plaque formation. It is commonly found in the lesions of bacterial endocarditis (see Chapter 14).
- *Streptococcus mutans* is found in dental plaque, though not usually in large numbers unless there is a large amount of sucrose in the diet. It produces a sticky extracellular polysaccharide coat of dextrans and mutans, and is able to produce lactic acid from glucose or sucrose. It is believed to be one of the most important organisms in the initiation of enamel caries, and immunization with antigens from *S. mutans* is able to prevent dental caries in monkeys.
- *Streptococcus mitior (mitis)* is usually the commonest streptococcus found in plaque. Like *S. sanguis* it is often found in the cardiac lesions of bacterial endocarditis.
- *Streptococcus salivarius* is found mainly in saliva and on the dorsum of the tongue. It is not found in dental plaque in large numbers.
- *Actinomyces viscosus* and *A. naeslundii* are two Gram-positive rods that are often found in early plaque.

24 hours: a clinically detectable layer of plaque has now formed. Bacteria which are attached to the salivary pellicle grow and form microcolonies. Other organisms are attracted to and adhere to the pioneer' organisms. Recent studies indicated that the early growth of plaque is mainly accounted for by the multiplication of adherent organisms. At the end of 24 hours the flora becomes increasingly complex and Gram-negative anaerobic cocci can be detected.

3 days: the number of organisms present continues to increase, with the Gram-negative cocci and rods assuming greater prominence. The anaerobes also increase in numbers and fusobacteria and filaments can be detected.

- **7 days**: the final phase of plaque maturation sees a continued decrease in the percentage of Gram-positive cocci and rods present. The complex flora contains spirilla, spirochaetes, fusiform bacilli and vibrios as well as large numbers of Gram-negative cocci, bacilli and filamentous organisms (Fig. 9.4).

been shown to vary with the individual, the site examined and the age of the plaque. A quantity of $1\,mm^3$ of mature dental plaque weighing about 1 mg may contain more than 10^8 bacteria (Fig. 9.3). However, a recently cleaned tooth will contain a very sparse flora on individual bacterial colonies. Supragingival plaque has been shown to go through the stages shown in Table 9.1.

Subgingival plaque usually develops from the supragingival plaque deposits. However, the conditions in the pocket influence the type of colonizing organism. The environment is anaerobic and nutrients are supplied from the crevicular fluid. In all, 90% of culturable organisms are anaerobic, including *Bacteroides melaninogenicus*, *Fusobacterium nucleatum*, actinomyces and spirochaetes (Fig. 9.4, Table 9.2).

Calculus

Dental calculus is the mineralized bacterial plaque deposit on the teeth or other solid oral structures such as restorations or appliances. It consists of 70% inorganic salts and 30% microorganisms and organic material. Calculus is invariably covered by a film of plaque, which also occupies its porous structure. Because of this, the presence of calculus makes effective oral hygiene impossible and therefore its removal to prevent or assist in the control of inflammatory periodontal disease is of great importance (Table 9.3).

Calculus is usually classified according to its relationship to the gingival margin. Supragingival calculus is seen on the visible clinical crowns of teeth above the gingival margin. Calculus below the crest of the gingiva in

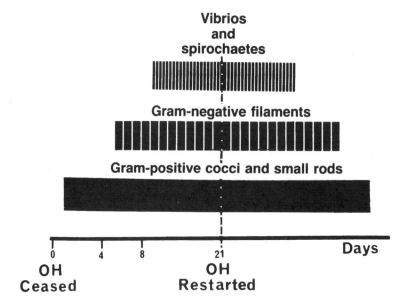

Fig. 9.4 The microbial changes in dental plaque after cessation of oral hygiene measures (after Löe *et al.* 1965).

Table 9.2 Interbacterial substances in dental plaque

Although micro-organisms are the principal constituents of plaque, additional components can be identified by microscopy

- **Proteins**. The proteins in plaque are derived from the glycoproteins of saliva.
- **Carbohydrates**. The carbohydrate portion of plaque is of dietary origin and is absent from the plaque of individuals being fed on a carbohydrate-free diet. Small molecular weight carbohydrates, principally sucrose, diffuse into the plaque. Streptococci in plaque metabolize these and produce sticky extracellular polysaccharides, fructans and glucans.
- **Epithelial cells**. Disintegrating epithelial cells can often be found on the tooth surface surrounded by plaque deposits.
- **Leukocytes**. White blood cells of varying degrees of vitality can be found in plaque. Often entrapped micro-organisms are found within the cytoplasm of the leukocytes.
- **Erythrocytes**. These are seen in plaque samples taken from deposits adjacent to ulcerated gingiva.
- **Food debris**. Very occasionally small shreds of food, such as muscle fibres, can be found in plaque samples taken from interproximal areas.
- **Enzymes**. Many bacterial enzymes have been demonstrated, including collagenase which is capable of depolymerizing collagen fibres and fibrils. Hyaluronidase enzyme breaks down hyaluronic acid, an important tissue cementing polysaccharide found between epithelial cells. Many proteases are found which contribute to the breakdown of non-collagenous proteins in the ground substance and increase capillary permeability.
- **Toxins**. Endotoxins found in plaque are lipopolysaccharide constituents of the cell walls of Gram-negative bacteria. They are powerful mediators of both the inflammatory and immune responses.
- **Acids**. Organic acids such as lactic and pyruvic acid are formed by the action of bacteria on small molecular weight carbohydrates.
- **Antigens**. These trigger the immune responses and consequently cause tissue damage.

Table 9.3 Composition of calculus

Calculus consists of 70% inorganic salts and 30% micro-organisms and organic material

Inorganic salts: two-thirds of the inorganic salts are in a crystalline form. The major minerals are calcium and phosphorus with small amounts of magnesium, sodium, carbonate and fluoride together with traces of other elements. The four principal crystalline forms are:.

- Calcium hydroxyapatite.
- Magnesium whitlockite.
- Octacalcium phosphate.
- Calcium brushite.

The first three of these inorganic salts are varieties of the hydroxyapatite crystal lattice, which is the principal salt in bone, cementum, dentine and enamel. The proportion of these salts varies with the individual and the age of the calculus sample, as well as the location, whether supragingivally or subgingivally. Brushite is more common in supragingival calculus, whilst whitlockite is often found subgingivally. These variations account for some of the different appearances and physical properties of calculus often observed.

Micro-organisms: calculus contains a broad spectrum of organisms with filamentous microbes predominating.

Surface zone: the organisms resemble those of mature plaque with Gram-negative cocci, rods and filamentous bacteria.

Internal zone: the predominant organisms are Gram-positive filaments of the Actinomyces type. Most of the organisms within calculus are non-viable.

Organic substances: the organic interbacterial substances in calculus are similar to those of plaque. The bulk consists of proteins and carbohydrates, with lipids accounting for a small amount. Protein-carbohydrate complexes are found, together with amino acids, small molecular weight carbohydrates, desquamated epithelial cells and leukocytes.

Table 9.4 The main theories of calculus formation

There are two main theories concerned with the way in which plaque becomes mineralized: the precipitation theory and the nucleation theory

Precipitation theory. Various changes can cause the precipitation of salts from a solution and this theory suggests that one or other of these changes might cause precipitation of the mineral ions of saliva. The main mechanisms suggested are as follows:

- Increased pH. Salts will be precipitated out of a solution when it becomes more alkaline. The pH of saliva may be elevated on reaching the mouth as a result of loss of carbon dioxide or by the production of ammonia by plaque bacteria.
- Increasing the concentration of ions in the solution, leading to their precipitation. Colloidal proteins in saliva bind calcium and phosphate ions and maintain a supersaturated solution. With stagnation of saliva the colloids settle out and calcium phosphate salts then precipitate. In addition, the release of the enzyme phosphatase from dental plaque or desquamated epithelial cells increases the production of phosphate in saliva from organic phosphates.

Nucleation theory. This is currently considered to be the more likely theory. It is proposed that some element in the organic matrix acts as a seeding agent. These seeding agents induce foci of calcification which enlarge and fuse to form a larger mass. This process is termed epistaxis. The seeding agents in calculus formation are not known, but certain bacteria such as *Streptococcus salivarius, Leptothrix buccalis* and *Actinomyces* strains are thought to be capable of bringing the mineral ions of saliva into the correct relationship with each other for the formation of salt crystals. This crystal then acts as a nucleus for further crystal formation in a manner similar to the seeding of an oyster with a grain of sand to form a pearl.

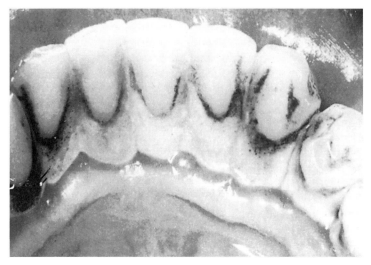

Fig. 9.5 Supragingival calculus lingual to the lower incisors. Staining from cigarette tar deposits may be seen at the periphery of the calculus.

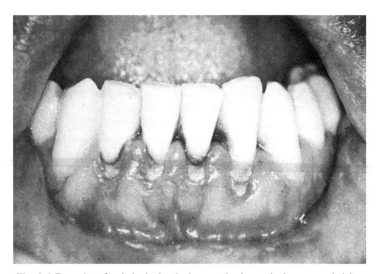

Fig. 9.6 Deposits of subgingival calculus on the lower incisors revealed by recession of the gingiva.

periodontal pockets is termed subgingival (Table 9.5).

Formation of calculus

The formation of calculus is always preceded by plaque accumulation which serves as an organic matrix for the subsequent mineralization of the deposit. The precipitation of mineral salts in plaque can start any time from the 2nd to the 14th day of plaque formation, but some individuals can begin to calcify plaque in about 8 h. Initially, small crystals develop close to bacteria; gradually the intermicrobial matrix becomes entirely calcified and eventually the bacteria also become mineralized. The calcification occurs in layers, which vary in their degree of calcification and have resting lines between them (Table 9.4, and Figs 9.5 and 9.6).

Attachment of calculus

Calculus may be attached to enamel or root in a number of ways which affect the difficulty of

Table 9.5 Types of calculus

Calculus is classified according to its relationship to the gingival margin as follows

- **Supragingival calculus**. This refers to calculus above the crest of the gingiva on the clinical crowns of the teeth. This is white or pale yellow in colour, unless stained by tobacco tar or food pigments (Fig. 9.5). It is relatively soft and is easily removed from the tooth surface with a scaler. Supragingival calculus occurs most commonly on the buccal aspect of the upper molar teeth and the lingual aspect of the lower anterior teeth. This is probably due to the fact that the ducts of the major salivary glands open into the mouth in these areas. The minerals in supragingival calculus are derived from saliva.
- **Subgingival calculus**. This is much darker, harder and more difficult to remove than supragingival calculus. It is brown to black in colour (Fig. 9.6) and more evenly distributed throughout the mouth. It forms apically to the crest of the gingiva in periodontal pockets and may be present as small discrete deposits or form a band running round the tooth. Determination of the location and extent of subgingival calculus requires the careful use of a calculus probe. The minerals in subgingival calculus are derived from the gingival crevicular fluid exudate in periodontal pockets and not from saliva. The dark colour is thought to be caused by the breakdown products of blood lost from the ulcerated pocket epithelium.

removal, as described below:

- By means of the acquired pellicle. The pellicle may also calcify, so the calculus crystals come into close contact with the tooth minerals.
- By penetration into enamel, cementum or dentine. Small surface irregularities may be penetrated by calculus crystals, so that the calculus is locked into the tooth. The root surface may be particularly susceptible to this due to the hollows and depressions left by resorption lacunae, Sharpey's fibre pits and small carious lesions.
- In spaces left by cemental tears.

Significance of calculus

Calculus of itself would probably cause little damage to the periodontal tissues. However, its presence is invariably associated with periodontal disease. This is because it is always covered with a layer of plaque, provides a nidus for further accumulation of plaque and holds plaque against a large area of gingiva. Calculus may also contain toxins derived from plaque that are irritant to the gingival tissues.

Subgingival calculus is probably the product of periodontal pockets rather than the cause. Its presence is much more significant than supragingival deposits as it indicates that the disease has progressed from gingivitis to periodontitis.

Stains

Dental stains are pigmented deposits on or in the tooth surface. Staining of teeth may be either extrinsic (on the surface of the tooth) or intrinsic (within the substance of the tooth) (Tables 9.6 and 9.7).

Tooth-accumulated materials
- Acquired salivary pellicle: a thin, structureless, protein film that forms rapidly on clean tooth surfaces from salivary mucins.
- Dental plaque: aggregations of microbes and their by-products that form on the teeth, gums and other solid oral structures.
- Calculus: calcified microbial plaque which may be supragingival or subgingival.
- Materia alba: a soft, white mixture of organisms, desquamated epithelial cells, leukocytes and salivary proteins. It is very loosely adherent to the tooth surface and may be removed with a water spray. It is often considered to be unconsolidated dental plaque.
- Food debris: food retained on the teeth. Food debris, unless impacted between the teeth, is usually rapidly removed by the action of the oral musculature and saliva.
- Extrinsic stains: a variety of substances may stain the external surfaces of teeth.

Table 9.6 Intrinsic staining of teeth

Treatment of intrinsic staining is not usually within the scope of the dental hygienist but patients will frequently ask questions about the cause of these problems. The more common causes of intrinsic staining are as follows

- Pulp necrosis.
- Hypoplastic enamel.
- Tetracycline ingestion during tooth formation.
- Fluorosis.
- Dental caries or restorations.
- Systemic upset during tooth formation.

These are discussed elsewhere in the text

Table 9.7 Causes of extrinsic staining of teeth

Extrinsic staining of teeth results from the pigmentation of the usually colourless salivary pellicle and may be removed by polishing the teeth. They can be divided into metallic and non-metallic stains

Metallic stains: various metals are capable of staining the teeth should they come in contact with them. Metals or their salts may be inhaled into the oral cavity by industrial workers, or introduced in medicines. Examples are the brown or black stain of mercury. Iron-containing medicines can cause a black iron sulphite stain. With improved industrial working conditions which are now subject to stringent health regulations, metallic staining of the teeth is now rarely seen.
- **Non-metallic stains**: these are very common and various types have been described:
- *Black stain*: this is usually seen as a thick black or dark brown line adjacent to and following the contour of the gingival margin, approximately 1 mm from the soft tissues. It is often firmly attached. It is more common in children and its cause is unknown.
- *Tobacco stain*: this is probably the commonest stain observed in patients. It varies in colour from light brown to black and occurs more frequently on the lingual and palatal aspects of the teeth. It is the result of tobacco smoking, and the combustion products, principally tar, stain the pellicle and penetrate deficiencies such as pits and fissures producing a very tenacious deposit. Generally the severity of tobacco stain depends more upon the standard of oral hygiene than the quantity of tobacco smoked.
- *Green stain*: this is similar in its distribution to black stain and is also more common in children and adolescents. It usually occurs on the labial surface of maxillary anterior teeth. The stain has been attributed to chromogenic bacteria causing discoloration of the pellicle.
- *Yellow stain*: this is a generalized dull yellow staining of the tooth which results from discoloration of dental plaque by dyes in foodstuffs.
- *Chlorhexidine stain*: an important disadvantage of using chlorhexidine to control plaque is the unsightly black staining which often occurs.

Further reading

Grace A. M., Smales F. C. (1989) *Periodontal Control. An effective system for diagnosis, selection, control and treatment planning in general practice.* London: Quintessence.

Lindhe J. (1989) *Textbook of Clinical Periodontology.* 2nd edition. Copenhagen: Munksgaard.

Loe H., Theilade E., Jenkins S. B. (1965) Experimental gingivitis in man. *J. Periodontol.*, **36**, 177.

Loe H., Kleinmann D. U. (1986) *Dental Plaque Control Measures and Oral Hygiene Practices: proceedings from a state-of-the-science workshop.* Oxford: IRL Press.

Marsh P. D., Martin M. V. (1992) *Oral microbiology.* 3rd edition. London: Chapman Hall.

Rateitschak K. H., Rateitschak E. M., Wolf H. F., Hassell T. M. (1989) *Color Atlas of Dental Medicine Volume 1: Periodontology.* 2nd edition. New York: Thieme Medical Publishers Inc.

10

Dental caries

Introduction

Dental caries is a disease of the mineralized portion of the tooth. It is caused by acid produced by the action of plaque micro-organisms on fermentable carbohydrates found in the diet. Other factors can hasten or slow its progress, these including poor oral hygiene, poor salivary flow and the presence of fluoride in tooth substance. It is one of the most common diseases in the world and there are few people who have not suffered from it. The incidence of coronal caries (that affecting the crown) in western countries has been in steady decline over the past 30 years. This fall is usually attributed to the widespread use of fluoride toothpastes.

Classification of dental caries

Caries attacks the enamel, cementum and dentine, gradually eating into and destroying the tooth (Fig. 10.1). The clinical picture varies with the site and the extent of the lesion and four basic types are described: *pit and fissure caries, and smooth-surface caries* which may start on enamel; *root caries* on exposed root cementum or dentine and *recurrent or secondary caries* which occurs at the margins of restorations.

In addition to these four basic types, there is *rampant caries*, which is the rapid destruction of teeth which often occurs in teenagers who 'snack' between meals or in patients who suffer from xerostomia as a result of radiotherapy to

the head and neck. This may even effect the proximal regions of lower incisors. *Nursing caries* is a variant of rampant caries affecting the primary dentition. In marked contrast *arrested caries* is occasionally seen where a carious lesion has stopped progressing due to a change in the environment of the tooth, i.e. the cavity becomes more easily cleanable and less plaque retentive.

The earliest evidence of caries developing in enamel is known as the white spot lesion. The change in the appearance of the enamel in this early lesion is due to an increase in porosity which alters the way in which light is reflected. At this stage the enamel is still hard and no cavity has formed as only a small amount of mineral has been lost. However, this early lesion due to the increased porosity, may take up stain and consequently turn brown in colour. This brown colour may come from elements of the diet such as tea or coffee. Both brown and white lesions may be present in the mouth for several years without progressing. Alternatively, they sometimes progress quickly and multiple white spot lesions seen in a young person should be a matter of concern for the clinician.

Pit-and fissure caries

While caries on smooth surfaces can be easily visualized, pit and fissure caries can be more difficult to see. The fissure which appears clinically caries-free may show signs of early lesion formation. However a 'sticky' fissure

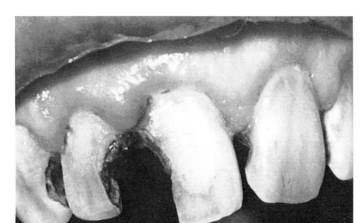

Fig. 10.1 Carious cavities in upper anterior teeth

may be retentive to a probe, not due to caries, but to the shape of the fissure. This is one reason why a sharp probe is not recommended to detect fissure caries, but only to clear the fissure of plaque to enable the fissure to be visualized and discoloration or frank cavitation detected. Indeed a sharp probe may even damage demineralizing enamel, especially when heavy pressure is applied. The various stages leading from the earliest signs of caries to the complete breakdown of the tooth are as shown in Figure 10.2. and described in Table 10.1

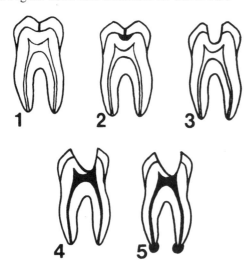

Fig. 10.2 Diagram of stages of carious breakdown of a lower molar tooth. **1** small pit, **2** bluish white area, **3** open carious cavity, **4** pulpitis, **5** apical abscess. These stages are described in the text.

Smooth-surface caries

Smooth-surface caries is found most commonly at the interproximal contact points, but it can occur on any smooth surface of the tooth. It appears initially as a chalky white area that gradually becomes roughened due to the breakdown of the enamel. Eventually an open cavity is formed and the subsequent stages are the same as described for pit-and-fissure caries.

Attention is now being given to early carious lesions, since there is evidence that, in the early stages, caries is reversible. A conservative approach is recommended for caries and often the hygienist will be asked to offer dietary advice and apply topical fluorides to encourage remineralization of smooth-surface enamel. Fluoride applications can return early caries lesions to a normal translucent appearance provided cavitation has not occurred.

Root surface caries

Since root caries attacks areas of exposed cementum and dentine, the first two stages described in pit-and-fissure caries are not relevant. Cementum and dentine begin to break down, softening rapidly so that early cavitation is a common feature of root caries The later stages are as described for pit and fissure caries. This type of caries tends to occur more frequently in older people, because gingival recession is more common in this age group. This type of caries will present a major

Table 10.1 Stages of dental caries

The stages of dental caries are

- **Small pit.** The first indication of tooth destruction is the appearance of a small black pit which is just big enough for a probe to catch in it. This is the initial break in the enamel and it extends as far as the enamel-dentine junction.
- **Bluish-white area.** Because dentine is softer than enamel, the caries destroys it more quickly, undermining the enamel. The caries shows through the translucent enamel as a bluish-white area surrounding the initial pit.
- **Open cavity.** As the caries spreads in the dentine, it leaves a progressively larger area of enamel unsupported and eventually the enamel collapses, leaving an open carious cavity. The caries at the base of the cavity may be either soft and cream-coloured (the rapidly spreading type, more common in children) or hard and dark (the slower-spreading caries typically found in adults).
- **Pulpitis.** With the continuing spread of the lesion, the pulp eventually becomes involved and infected, producing pulpal inflammation, known as pulpitis.
- **Apical abscess.** This is an extension of the pulpitis, through the apical foramen into the periodontal ligament around the apex. At this stage the pulp will have died and the tooth will be non-vital.

treatment challenge in the future for dental team members as the number of elderly people in the population increases.

The different types of caries are
- Pit and fissure caries.
- Smooth surface caries (including root caries).
- Recurrent or secondary caries.
- Rampant caries.
- Nursing caries.
- Arrested caries.

Pain with carious lesions

The degree of pain accompanying a carious lesion varies across the full range, from extreme pain to none at all. Classically, the pain felt at each stage is as follows.

- The small pit and the bluish-white area are completely painless.
- The open cavity, because of the exposed dentine, is often painful to heat and cold and, occasionally, with sweet foodstuffs. However, pain is not invariably present and some large cavities are entirely painless. This may be because the dentine is insulated by a layer of caries and food debris, or it may be because the pulp has already died.
- Pulpitis presents as a severe throbbing

pain that is made worse by heat and tends to be eased by cold. It was described in Chapter 8 that one of the features of inflammation is swelling. The pulp cannot swell, because it is enclosed in hard calcified tissue, and so as pressure builds up it causes a throbbing pain. This explains why heat worsens the pain and cold reduces it.

- An acute apical abscess causes a throbbing pain due to pressure increasing in the periapical tissues. It is increased by pressing the tooth. Eventually pus discharges, either through the open pulp or through the alveolar bone, and the abscess becomes chronic and painless. In many cases the acute phase does not occur and, therefore, neither does any pain.

To summarize, although pain is frequently what drives the patient to seek treatment, many large cavities, with pulp necrosis and chronic apical abscesses, are found which have been entirely painless throughout their progression.

Radiographic appearance of dental caries

Small, interproximal cavities are difficult to diagnose, because the close contact between adjacent teeth makes it impossible to see or probe them. For this reason, radiographs may be taken periodically to check for the presence

---

Table 10.2 The zones of enamel early caries

Four layers are usually seen.

- **Surface layer.** Microscopic examination shows that there is an intact superficial layer of enamel covering the altered enamel below. This layer is between 20 and 100 μm thick. The reason for such a layer persisting relatively unaffected in the early stages is not really understood, but it could be due to the surface layer being fluoride rich and is probably the reason why such lesions can be successfully reversed by remineralization. The pore volume here is 1%. Obviously, as the caries progresses, this intact layer is breached.
- **The body of the lesion.** This is the largest zone, within which the mineral content of the enamel is reduced by up to 25%. The pore volume is 5% at the periphery and up to 25% at the centre of the body of the lesion. The Striae of Retzius are enhanced in this part of the lesion.
- **The dark zone.** The dark appearance it is believed is the result of the demineralized spaces or pores being of varying sizes and quinoline which the section is mounted in is a large molecule which cannot enter the small spaces which are consequently filled with air and so appear dark and give the whole zone a dark appearance when viewed under the microscope. The pore volume is between 2 to 4%. The mineral content in this zone is reduced by 6%.
- **The translucent zone.** This is the earliest change in enamel at the front of the advancing lesion. It appears structureless and its mineral content is reduced by roughly 1.0%.and the pore volume is 1%. Sound enamel has a pore volume of only 0.1%.

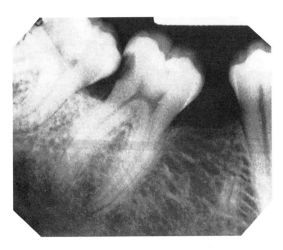

Fig. 10.3 A radiograph of lower right posterior teeth showing a carious cavity on the distal of the second molar tooth. The first molar is missing but the tip of the anterior (mesial) root has been retained.

of caries, which will show up on the radiograph as a dark area in the tooth (Fig. 10.3). Bitewing radiographs are of great importance but it should be remembered that when an interproximal cavity is noted, the lesion has already spread to involve the dentine.

Histopathology of caries

Histology is the study of the microscopic appearance of tissues and histopathology is the study of the microscopic appearance of a disease process within the tissues – in this case the study of progression of caries through enamel and dentine.

Caries of enamel

Experimental studies have shown that it takes about 4 weeks for the white spot lesion to become visible. Increasing significance is being attached to the early carious lesion of enamel because, at that stage, caries is a reversible condition. Histologically these early lesions have a conical appearance (Fig. 10.4), with the base of the cone at the tooth surface and its apex towards the enamel-dentine junction, with four distinct layers (Table 10.2).

Fissure caries

The histological appearance of fissure caries is similar to smooth surface caries. The lesions start at the sides of the fissure and eventually coalesce at the base of the fissure. The lesion then progresses towards the enamel-dentine junction guided by the orientation of the enamel prisms. At this stage it has the appearance of a cone but with its base towards the enamel-dentine junction. This shape explains why a small enamel lesion at the surface grows larger as the dentine is approached.

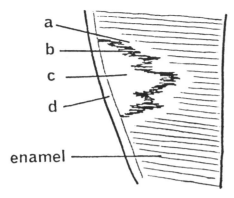

Fig. 10.4 Diagrammatic representation of the early smooth surface carious lesion showing the four zones: **d** the intact surface layer, **c** the body of the lesion, **b** the dark zone and **a** the translucent zone.

The carious lesions of the enamel of primary teeth develop in a similar same way to those in permanent teeth, but the enamel is thinner so is breached more readily. As the pulp of a primary tooth is quite large it becomes quickly compromised by caries (Fig 10.5).

> The essential aspects of the pathology of enamel caries are
> - Experimentally it takes about 4 weeks for a white spot lesion to develop.
> - Histologically the four layers of enamel caries are the surface layer, the body of lesion, the dark zone and the translucent zone.

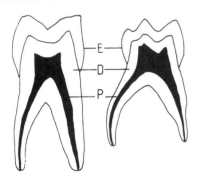

Fig. 10.5 Comparison of primary and permanent molar teeth. The primary molar has thinner enamel (E) and dentine (D) but a larger pulp chamber (P)

Caries of dentine

A similar examination of dentine caries will reveal a roughly conical lesion, with its base towards the surface of the tooth and its apex pointing inwards towards the pulp. Five different zones can be distinguished which, taking the outermost first and the innermost last, have the features shown in Table 10.3.

Table 10.3 Dentine caries

The zones of dentine caries are

- **Zone 1**: an area of totally decomposed dentine.
- **Zone 2**: a zone of decalcified dentine which has been invaded by bacteria.
- **Zone 3**: a narrow band of decalcified dentine which has not yet been invaded by bacteria.
- **Zone 4**: a zone of translucent dentine.
- **Zone 5**: an area in which the dentine is normal but the odontoblastic processes show signs of early degeneration.

Reactions of dentine and pulp to caries

Responses to the progression of dentinal caries can be seen using a microscope. Essentially three reactions can be observed.

- Sclerosis of the dentinal tubules or translucent sclerosis.
- Production of irregular secondary dentine at the dentine pulp interface.
- An increasing inflammation in the pulp as the carious process moves towards it.

Tubular sclerosis

Sclerosis of the dentinal tubules begins in the lumen of each tubule and is due to mineral deposition. This reaction is produced by vital odontoblasts that lie at the periphery of the carious lesion. Dentine tubules that show this change often appears as translucent and this area is referred to as the *translucent zone* – not to be confused with the translucent zone seen in enamel caries.

Irregular secondary dentine

This is the dentine which forms at the dentine/pulp interface and is due to the pulp trying to insulate itself from the advancing carious lesion. This *reactionary* dentine must be distinguished from primary dentine that forms during tooth development and secondary dentine which forms throughout life.

Dental caries
Five zones can be identified in dentine caries.
Three responses occur in dentine and pulp
- tubular sclerosis
- irregular secondary dentine
- pulpal inflammation.

Aetiology of dental caries

Over the years, three principal hypotheses of cariogenesis have been suggested. W. D. Miller is probably the best known of the early researchers into dental caries, having published several papers on the subject in the late 19th and early 20th century. His well known papers were the basis of modern thoughts on cariogenesis: the acidogenic hypothesis. This will be discussed in some detail. Other hypotheses, the proteolytic and the proteolysis-chelation will be discussed first. Although they may also play a part in cariogenesis, the main emphasis is now on the acidogenic hypothesis.

Proteolytic hypothesis

This proposed that the organic portion of enamel or dentine is first destroyed in caries by the proteolytic enzymes produced by plaque bacteria. It was then thought that the unprotected calcified portion was subsequently destroyed, probably by acids. This possibility would seem to apply more in caries of cementum or dentine, where the organic portion is moderately high. It is difficult to imagine that it could be particularly relevant to caries of enamel, where the mineralized portion makes up some 96% of the total.

Proteolysis–chelation hypothesis

Chelation is a complicated chemical process whereby metallic ions are lost because they are attracted to complex molecules. The molecule removing the metallic ion is termed a chelator and it is known that amino acids can act in this way. Chelation does not depend on acidity and can take place at neutral or even alkaline pH. According to the proteolysis–chelation hypothesis, the protein element of the tooth is first broken down into amino acids by the proteolytic enzymes of plaque. The amino acids then form chelates with the calcium ions of hydroxyapatite, gradually decalcifying the tooth substance. Chelating agents are used in dental practice, where they are used to widen root canals in endodontic therapy.

Acidogenic hypothesis

Neither of the two previous hypotheses can adequately explain some important observations in relation to caries. For example, the caries rate in the UK was reduced during the Second World War, when sugar was strictly rationed, and there were low caries rates amongst Inuit populations before the introduction of refined carbohydrates to their diet. The role of both plaque and sugar in cariogenesis is undeniable, and the acidogenic hypothesis still appears to tie them together in the most satisfactory manner. This theory suggests that sugars in the diet are converted into acids, such as lactic and pyruvic acids, by the action of the plaque bacteria. These acids then subsequently destroy the mineral component of the tooth.

Bacteria and dental caries

In the 1950s a series of animal experiments conducted by Orland and Keyes demonstrated that bacteria were essential for the production of a carious lesion. They found that in germ-

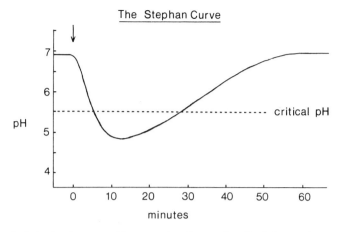

Fig. 10.6 The Stephan curve illustrates the effect on the pH of plaque when a sucrose solution is used as a mouth rinse at the point indicated by the arrow.

free animals who were fed highly cariogenic diets, dental caries did not develop. Conversely, when bacteria were introduced to these animals dental caries did develop. In a further experiment, conducted by Keyes in 1960, germ-free animals were infected with different strains of streptococci which then transferred to uninfected litter mates, who subsequently developed dental caries. Various strains of oral bacteria have been shown to convert sugars into acids, but the micro-organism which has received most recent attention is *Streptococcus mutans*. Early attention was focused on *Lactobacillus acidophilus* and a close correlation was observed between an individual's susceptibility to caries and its concentration in saliva. However, this correlation would appear to be due to *L. acidophilus* thriving in the caries environment. It is now accepted that a broad spectrum of plaque bacteria might be involved, including *S. sanguis* and *S. salivarius*, but that *S. mutans* is by far the most significant.

Sugars and dental caries

The relationship between sugar consumption and caries is well established. The average individual's intake of sugar in the UK is reported as being 58 kg per annum, and this might explain the particularly high caries rate in this country. It has been fashionable in the past to blame refined carbohydrates rather than sugars. High molecular weight carbohydrates such as starches are not that important but low molecular weight carbohydrates such as sucrose are very important. Sucrose is found in both food and many soft drinks. Intermeal 'snacking' with sucrose rich foods or soft drinks allows plaque pH to stay low and demineralize tooth substance. The diet of lower socioeconomic groups in the UK tends to be sucrose rich and this is one of the reasons why caries incidence in this section of the population is high. Unfortunately, this section of the population is very resistant to health promotion efforts and so presents a major challenge to those involved in promoting the importance of good oral health.

Acids and dental caries

A number of organic acids are produced by the action of plaque bacteria on sugars, but probably the most significant is lactic acid. This production of acid is very rapid and immediately after sugar is eaten the pH of plaque begins to drop. Plaque has a resting pH which is fractionally on the acidic side of neutral (pH approximately 6.8), and roughly 10 minutes after exposure to sugar it reaches its lowest pH (in the region of pH 5) before slowly returning to normal over a period of 30–60 minutes. The graph of this change in pH is called the Stephan curve and it is illustrated in Figure 10.6. It is estimated that calcium hydroxyapatite will begin to dissolve when the pH is 5.5 or less and this is referred to as the critical pH.

Dental caries may be explained by the
- Proteolytic hypothesis.
- Proteolytsis-chelation hypothesis.
- The acidogenic hypothesis which emphasizes the importance of bacteria, sugar and acid formation. This is the most supported explanation for caries development.

Secondary factors

Secondary aetiological factors are those not directly involved in causing a disease, but which influence the disease to a greater or lesser extent. These are numerous and it is easier to understand them if they are considered under various headings.

Poor oral hygiene

It is an obvious feature that caries tends to be more prevalent in plaque-infested mouths than clean ones. Plaque is only one factor in caries aetiology and so the caries rate is not related to plaque levels alone. However, the more plaque that is allowed to accumulate on the teeth, the more chance there is for acids to be produced and attack the tooth surface. Furthermore, toothbrushing may remove particulate foodstuffs lodged between the teeth, thus preventing them from releasing sugar into the saliva over a long period of time.

In Chapter 9 it was explained that as soon as plaque is removed from the tooth surface it begins to reform. In a short time plaque organisms are again present on the tooth surface to convert sugars into acids. It is not surprising, therefore, that good oral hygiene alone will not prevent caries, and it must be combined with other preventive measures to be effective.

Diet

The diet has been shown to affect the caries rate in various ways.

Composition

The quantity of sugar consumed at any one time has less effect than the type of sugar consumed. As already noted, sucrose is parti-

cularly harmful. The depth to which the Stephan curve will drop is greatly affected by the type of carbohydrate consumed, but not by the quantity consumed. Other contents of the diet can affect the caries rate. On the positive side, the presence of fluoride in tooth substance can halve the caries rate, as will be described in Chapter 20.

Consistency

Soft sticky foodstuffs will cling to the teeth and remain in the mouth for longer periods than others. They are then able to release sugars over a long period. The dental hygienist should be aware of the evidence which exists to show that fibrous foods do not remove plaque from the teeth to any significant extent and, although they may be preferable to sweet sticky foods, they are no substitute for toothbrushing. Not only do apples not clean the teeth, but their sugar content may have an adverse effect on plaque pH and they have a naturally low pH.

Frequency

As already noted, the acidity in plaque increases immediately after consumption of sugar and then gradually returns to normal (Fig. 10.6). Therefore, the more frequently sugar is consumed, the greater is the period during which acid is available to attack the tooth (Fig. 10.7). Whereas it is accepted that the frequency of eating sugar is more significant than the quantity eaten, the hygienist should avoid the temptation to instruct patients to eat all the sweet things at once! This would run contrary to advice being given by other health educators, and the advice should be to avoid or reduce sweet snacks to the minimum.

One of the most significant pieces of research carried out in relation to diet and caries was the Vipeholm Study conducted in a Swedish mental hospital from 1945 to 1951 (Gustaffson et al., 1954). This work established many of the points discussed above. It was shown that sugar in the diet was needed to produce caries, and that it was more cariogenic if given in sticky form and at frequent intervals: that is, the worst effect was caused by sweet, sticky snacks.

Saliva

A clinical observation is that some families

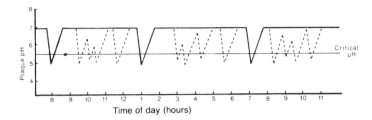

Fig. 10.7 A graph showing the effect of diet on plaque pH. The solid line illustrates the drop in pH resulting from three meals, breakfast, lunch and dinner. The dotted line shows the additional effect of between-meal snacks.

appear to be more prone to caries than others, and that some individuals inherit a greater or lesser susceptibility to caries. This may be explained by dietary and oral hygiene habits acquired from parents, but some of the secondary factors, including saliva, are genetically influenced.

The quantity and flow of saliva may also affect the production of caries. The rate of saliva flow varies throughout the day and is minimal during sleep. This is the reason for stressing the importance of cleaning the teeth before going to bed. Patients who suffer from xerostomia (a pathologically dry mouth which may occur after radiotherapy in the region of the salivary glands or when taking certain medicines) have an increased risk of caries. This is related to the reduced flow and the decreased buffering capacity. The bicarbonate buffering system together with the ammonia and urea components of saliva, can neutralize and buffer acid production in plaque. The buffering action of saliva is a very important natural function of saliva in combating caries.

Saliva also contains protective immunoglobulins which protect against dental caries and these are described in Chapter 7.

The viscosity of saliva may well lead to difficulties with oral hygiene. Some patients can rinse with a single mouthful of water and clear away all the toothpaste from their teeth, whereas others are unable to do this, even after rinsing several times. This ability is referred to as oral clearance which varies greatly between patients.

The teeth and dental caries

There are several ways in which the teeth themselves can influence the caries rate.

Form

Teeth with deep developmental pits and fissures are more likely to be prone to caries. An obvious example of this is the palatal pit often observed near the cingulum of upper permanent laterals. This is a common site for caries. The fissures of teeth narrow to an extent where they cannot be made plaque-free by toothbrushing. This is another reason why toothbrushing alone is inadequate in preventing caries. It can also be a reason for recommending the application of fissure sealants.

Position

Crowding and malalignment make plaque removal more difficult. This will tend to cause an increase in both periodontal disease and caries later in life, which is a good reason for considering orthodontic treatment.

Structure

Areas of hypocalcification may be more prone to caries and teeth with a reasonable fluoride content are less susceptible to caries. The critical pH of calcium hydroxyapatite is approximately 5.5. However, if fluoride is present in the tooth structure, crystals of calcium fluorapatite form and these are less soluble in acid than those of hydroxyapatite. Also fluoride released after acid dissolution will encourage remineralization. The critical pH of calcium fluorapatite is 4.5.

Iatrogenic factors in dental caries

Iatrogenic means caused by human action, and covers the various dental procedures which might increase the caries rate. Even well designed dentures and orthodontic appliances increase the risk, but those appliances and restorations which are poorly made greatly increase the risk of both caries and periodontal disease. Poorly fitting crowns or incorrectly condensed restorations may have voids that will fill with plaque and allow caries to develop. The margins adjacent to the best restorations are liable to secondary caries and, for this reason, the principle of extensively cutting away all fissures before inserting restorations is now considered to be undesirable. Minimal cavities are indicated to preserve sound tooth substance, because it is now recognized that no dental filling material is as durable as healthy enamel and dentine and small fillings are less likely to break down.

Pregnancy and dental caries

It is certainly true that the old adage 'a tooth for a baby', so widely accepted in the past, is completely incorrect. Surveys have shown that caries rates are similar in groups of pregnant and non-pregnant women. It may be more pertinent in relation to chronic periodontal disease, as the gingiva during pregnancy are more permeable to the toxins produced in plaque, and inflammation is more easily provoked. It must be borne in mind that there is no way that calcium from enamel can be absorbed into the blood stream once the tooth had erupted. Therefore, the skeleton of the fetus cannot develop at the expense of the mother's teeth.

> Secondary factors to consider in caries development
> - Saliva.
> - Teeth including, morphology, position and fluoride levels.
> - Quality of dentistry.
> - Oral hygiene.
> - Dietary habits.

Treatment of dental caries

The treatment of caries usually involves its elimination, either by conservative means, such as dental restorations with or without endodontic treatment, or by extraction of the tooth. Urgent treatment may be required if a patient is in pain, and the type of treatment given will

depend on the symptoms. If the patient complains of pain with heat or cold, the exposed dentine can be covered with a temporary filling material such as zinc oxide/eugenol or calcium hydroxide. If the pain is due to irreversible pulpitis or a periapical abscess, the throbbing will only be relieved by drainage. This is done by opening into the pulp chamber.

The dental hygienist is very involved in the management of the very early carious (white spot) lesion. It is well recognized that this early lesion is reversible with the application of fluorides, and a more conservative attitude to this type of lesion is being adopted. The decision as to the treatment of choice for any particular lesion rests with the dentist, but the dental hygienist may be called on to apply topical fluorides repeatedly in an attempt at reversal. Fluoride rinsing may also be recommended for patients who demonstrate multiple white spot lesions.

Prevention of dental caries

The prevention of dental disease, including caries, is of such importance to the dental hygienist that a separate chapter has been allocated to discussing it (Chapter 20).

> Treatment of dental caries may involve
> - Restoration, root filling or extraction of a tooth.
> - A temporary restoration may be needed initially to calm an inflamed pulp.
> - Irreversible pulpitis may require the pulp to be extirpated or the tooth extracted.

Further reading

Cawson R. A. (1984) *Essentials of Dental Surgery and Pathology.* 4th edition. Edinburgh: Churchill Livingstone.

Gustaffson B. E., Quensel C. E., Lanke L. S., Lundquist C., Grahnen I., Bonow B. E., Krasse B. (1954) The Vipeholm dental caries study. *Acta Odont Scand.* 11, 232–364.

Newbrun E. (1989) *Cariology.* 3rd edition. Baltimore: Williams & Wilkins.

Silverstone L. M., Johnson N. W., Hardie J. M., Williams R. A. D. (1981) *Dental Caries: Aetiology, Pathology, Prevention.* London: Macmillan.

11

Inflammatory periodontal diseases

Introduction

Between 10 and 20% of the world's population is highly susceptible to some form of destructive periodontal disease while 40% are likely to suffer from milder forms of plaque-induced periodontal diseases. These vary from early forms of gingivitis, frequently seen in children and adolescents, to advanced periodontitis, more prevalent in the fourth and fifth decades of life. Gingivitis and chronic periodontitis are often considered as two stages of the same disease process, although not all patients suffering from gingivitis will progress to periodontitis. For many years it was believed that the development and progression of periodontal disease was slow, affecting the whole dentition and leading inexorably to the loss of all the teeth. Recently this concept has been challenged and a 'bursts' theory has been described in which destructive episodes occur at particular sites in the mouth; these may be followed by longer periods of remission during which the disease is virtually static. Observation of patients with gingivitis over several years has also shown that very few progress to periodontitis, giving rise to the concept of 'contained gingivitis' and casting doubt on the idea that gingivitis and periodontitis are different stages of the same disease process.

A very small number of sites in patients with periodontitis have been shown to reverse and enter a healing phase whilst others may remain static over a long period of time, although the criteria used to measure periodontitis have such poor reliability that great caution must be used when interpreting these results.

Pathology of inflammatory periodontal diseases

Research has shown that inflammatory periodontal diseases progress through a series of continuous steps from early gingivitis to advanced periodontitis. These stages are described below.

The initial lesion

Within 2–4 days of plaque being allowed to accumulate on the tooth surface, changes occur in the connective tissues underneath the junctional epithelium. Here, in the small blood vessels, the vascular changes of early inflammation are seen. The blood flow slows and, after margination, neutrophilic leukocytes and monocytes migrate from the vessels into the tissues. This is combined with exudation of serum proteins. Many of the neutrophils migrate through the junctional epithelium and into the gingival crevice where, assisted by tissue fluid, termed crevicular fluid, they help to prevent invasion of the junctional epithelium plaque organisms. This initial stage of chronic inflammatory periodontal disease is shown in Figure 11.1. The hygienist would not be able to detect this stage by the use of clinical methods.

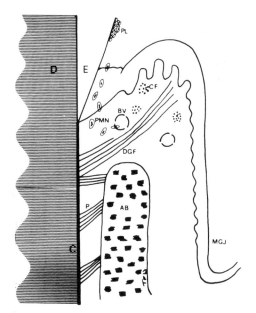

Fig. 11.1 Diagram of the initial lesion: AB alveolar bone, BV blood vessels, C cementum, CF circular fibres, D dentine, DGF dentogingival fibres, E enamel, MGJ mucogingival junction, PL microbial plaque, PMN polymorphonuclear leukocytes.

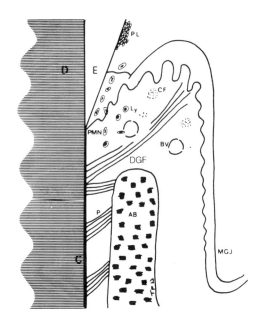

Fig. 11.2 Diagram of the early lesion: Ly lymphocytes, other abbreviations as Fig. 11.1.

The early lesion

After 7–14 days of undisturbed plaque accumulation the features of the early lesion can be detected histologically. The vascular changes are more pronounced, as is the accumulation of extravascular neutrophils (Fig. 11.2). Numerous lymphocytes can also be found located immediately below the junctional epithelium. The predominant immune cell identified at this stage is the T lymphocyte (see Chapter 7). Pathological changes can be seen in the fibroblasts and the collagen content of the gingival connective tissue is markedly reduced.

Changes can also be seen in the basal cell layer of the junctional epithelium. This proliferates into the underlying connective tissue and hyperplastic ridges are formed extending into the infiltrated tissue beneath. Clinically this stage presents as early chronic gingivitis, and is often achieved during experimental gingivitis studies.

The established lesion

Long-term exposure to plaque leads to the development of an established lesion. The main histological feature of this stage is the presence of large numbers of plasma cells. The inflammatory infiltrate now extends laterally towards the oral gingiva so that the inflammation becomes more clinically noticeable. In the inflamed tissue can be detected both T and B lymphocytes as well as immunoglobulins and the other protein components of the immune system (see Chapter 7). The hyperplastic junctional epithelium is often ulcerated and has a continual infiltration by masses of neutrophils passing into the crevice. The crevice itself is deepened and migration of the deeper cells of the junctional epithelium down on to cementum may occur. The deepened crevice forms an ideal site for plaque colonization, which now lies subgingivally (Fig. 11.3).

Clinically this stage may present as either chronic marginal gingivitis or early chronic periodontitis, depending upon whether or not true pockets can be detected.

The advanced lesion

A number of epidemiological studies have shown that not all established lesions will progress to the advanced lesion stage. Identifying the trigger for this change is one of the most tantalizing challenges facing the periodontal researcher.

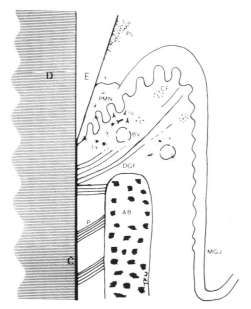

Fig. 11.3 Diagram of the established lesion: Ig immuno-globulins, other abbreviations as Fig. 11.1.

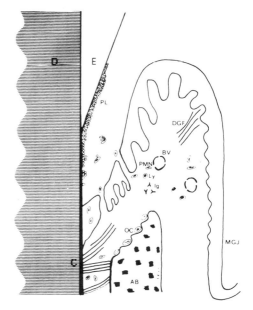

Fig. 11.4 Diagram of the advanced lesion: OC osteoclasts, other abbreviations as Fig. 11.1.

In this stage of the disease the junctional epithelium migrates down the root surface to form periodontal pockets which are colonized by plaque microbes. The lesion extends into the periodontal ligament and alveolar bone (Fig. 11.4) with loss of collagen adjacent to the pocket and fibrosis at more remote sites. Loss of alveolar bone is the result of osteoclastic action. However, periods of quiescence and exacerbation also occur with partial repair being achieved during the quiescent phases.

A number of studies have shown that invasion of the infiltrated tissues by microbes often occurs in advanced lesions and this would account for the prevalence of periodontal abscesses in this stage of the disease. Subgingival plaque organisms frequently become mineralized by calcium and other salts present in the crevicular fluid of the pocket, forming calculus which is firmly attached to the root surface.

Clinically this stage presents as periodontitis.

Pathological stages of inflammatory periodontal diseases
- Initial lesion (subclinical gingivitis).
- The early lesion (early gingivitis).
- The established lesion (chronic marginal gingivitis).
- The advanced lesion (periodontitis).

Gingivitis

Gingivitis is characterized by superficial inflammation of the gingival tissues, shown by the classic signs of redness, swelling and loss of stippling. There is no loss of attachment, significant bone loss or mobility. Any pocketing is of the 'false' variety, caused by gingival swelling, which may be oedematous or fibrous in nature.

Clinical features of chronic gingivitis

The severity of chronic gingivitis may vary from a slight change in texture and colour of the gingival margin, to a severe erythema with a tendency to spontaneous bleeding after minor trauma. Hyperplastic swelling of the gingiva may also be a feature of the disorder. Although the underlying disease is usually a chronic inflammatory process, acute exacerbations are common.

Chronic gingivitis is largely symptomless and most people suffering from it are totally unaware of the fact. On occasions, however, one of the following may be noted.

Bleeding

The gums may bleed with toothbrushing but this is such a common observation that often it is mistakenly thought to be normal. In more severe cases gingival bleeding may occur more readily, perhaps even when masticating. Bleeding is one of the earliest signs of gingivitis and when it occurs on gentle probing is usually a sign that the disease is present. Indeed, this is the basis of the Bleeding Index which is sometimes used in epidemiological studies of periodontal diseases.

Colour

Varying degrees of redness, depending on the severity, replace the healthy salmon or coral pink colour of the gingiva. Initially, there may only be a slight halo of mild redness, not very apparent on first examination.

Texture

A loss of gingival stippling, resulting in a glossy appearance, is one of the earliest signs of chronic gingivitis.

Consistency

In many cases the gingiva lose their firmness and become soft and spongy.

Form

The knife-edge gingival margins and pointed interdental papillae become rounded and blunt, with some degree of gingival swelling. If swelling is severe, pockets may form between the gingiva and the teeth. Because these pockets are limited to the gingiva and there has been no destruction of the periodontal ligament, the terms gingival pocketing or false pocketing are used to differentiate them from the true periodontal pockets described later. Figure 11.5 illustrates the difference between gingival and periodontal pockets. Gingival swelling is usually the result of oedema produced by the inflammatory fluid exudate but on occasions it may be the result of hyperplasia. The term

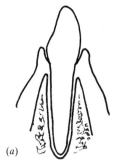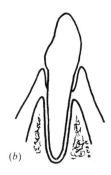

Fig. 11.5 Diagrammatic representation of: (a) false or gingival pocketing, (b) true or periodontal pocketing.

'hyperplasia' was also introduced in Chapter 8 and means the enlargement as a result of an increase in the number of the component cells in a tissue. The repair process involved in the chronic inflammatory response seems to be excessive in these cases. Gingival hyperplasia may be of an oedematous nature, with spongy gingiva which bleed easily, or it may be fibrous in nature, with firm, pink, excessively stippled gingiva. These differences are of significance in relation to both the aetiology and management of gingival hyperplasia.

Halitosis

Halitosis or bad breath is often caused by inflammatory periodontal diseases. However, unless it is particularly severe, the patient tends to be unaware of it, although others may find it all too obvious.

Aetiology of gingivitis

Gingivitis has been shown by epidemiological, clinical and research investigations to be initiated and maintained by the presence of mature plaque deposits around the teeth. Dental plaque has been shown to develop a complex Gram-negative anaerobic flora as it matures. The organisms release a variety of irritant metabolites, destructive enzymes and antigens which stimulate the inflammatory and immune systems. These cause local damage in the gingival tissues which bring about breakdown and the classic signs of gingivitis.

Clinical characteristics of gingivitis
- Gingival inflammation
redness
swelling
bleeding on minor trauma.
- Loss of stippling.
- False pocketing.
- No bone loss.
- No mobility.
- No loss of attachment.
- No true pocketing.
- No recession.

Management of chronic gingivitis

Early gingivitis may be completely reversed by an improvement in the standard of home care, provided that there are no factors present, such as deficient restorations or calculus, that make plaque removal difficult. Later stages may present more complex problems such as gingival hyperplasia, which will sometimes need surgical removal. This section will only deal with the management of chronic gingivitis, the acute forms being described later.

The key factor in the management of all types of periodontal disease is effective home care of the mouth. However it is insufficient to merely instruct a patient on how to brush and clean interdentally and there are a number of obstacles that have to be successfully negotiated before one can achieve the restoration of gingival health.

The encouragement of motivation

The most effective way of triggering motivation is to demonstrate disease in the patient's mouth. The recognition of periodontal pockets and bleeding, especially if there are healthy sites for comparison, will often trigger interest in the measures needed to restore health.

Linking the disease to the cause

Demonstrating dental plaque in diseased sites in the patient's own mouth may be helpful. The use of disclosing agents may assist in this part of the process.

Providing information

Patients may need information on the methods that can be adopted to remove plaque and restore health.

Physical instruction

It may be necessary to teach the patient appropriate methods of oral hygiene.

Setting realistic targets

The use of appropriate indices for the plaque level and gingival inflammation will be of great assistance in this phase of the treatment.

This is only a broad outline of some appropriate methods of oral hygiene. Further information can be found in the section on dental health education.

In addition to the advice on oral hygiene, it is also helpful to undertake a professional prophylaxis for patients with gingivitis. This removes most of the mature plaque deposits, leaves the mouth clean, starts the healing process, and has the effect of reinforcing the patient's home care. The removal of calculus and overhanging margins of restorations makes oral hygiene more effective, and the removal of plaque and stains motivates patients to keep the teeth clean. It will be necessary to follow up the patient to monitor the effect of this therapy, provide feedback and reinforce the motivation. Figures 11.6 and 11.7 illustrate the improvement that may be obtained in these patients.

Key factors in the management of oral hygiene advice
- Encouragement of motivation.
- Linking the disease to the cause.
- Providing information.
- Physically instructing.
- Setting realistic targets.

Types of gingivitis

There are a number of different types of gingivitis including both acute and chronic forms which are shown in the key points box. The chronic types are very prevalent and affect most of the population in one form or another; indeed some epidemiologists claim that most are 'normal' physiological defence responses to dental plaque, although many of the more dramatic manifestations must be considered

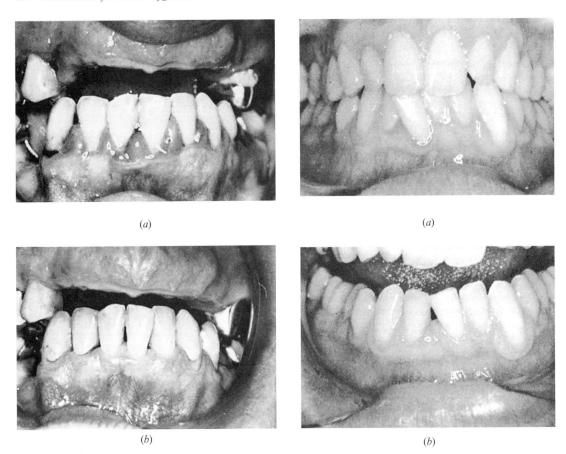

(a)   (a)

(b)   (b)

Fig. 11.6 Clinical photograph of anterior teeth: (a) gingivitis with marked oedematous hyperplasia of interdental papilla, (b) the improvement following effective oral hygiene measures.

Fig. 11.7 Clinical photograph of anterior teeth: (a) pronounced gingivitis with 41 tilted and malaligned, (b) the improvement following effective oral hygiene measures and removal of 41.

pathological. The acute types are relatively rare and often outside the remit of the hygienist to manage.

Acute non-specific gingivitis

This is an acute exacerbation of pre-existing chronic gingivitis and may be latent acute necrotizing ulcerative gingivitis (ANUG). The predisposing factors are those lowering tissue resistance, including systemic diseases such as an upper respiratory tract infection, smoking, stress, lack of lip seal. The treatment is to improve oral hygiene and use chemical anti-microbials if the gingiva are too sore to brush. Scaling and polishing must be undertaken if necessary.

Acute traumatic gingivitis

This usually manifests itself as a localized area of gingival soreness caused by trauma such as aggressive toothbrushing, picking at the gingiva (gingivitis artefacta) or chemical damage as may be caused by chemicals used in dental treatment. The treatment depends upon the cause.

Toothbrush damage

The patient should avoid the area or use chlorhexidine mouthwash instead of brushing until healed. More severe trauma may require the use of lignocaine ointment to numb the area or a periodontal dressing to protect until healing occurs.

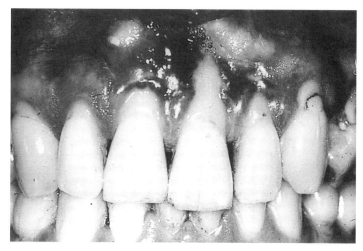

Fig. 11.8 Gingivitis artefacta: acute traumatic gingivitis and recession caused by a finger-picking habit.

Gingivitis artefacta

This is gingival damage caused by self inflicted trauma such as scratching with a finger nail or other object as shown in Figure 11.8. It will appear as an ulcerated area surrounded by hyperkeratosis. It is important to obtain the patient's co-operation in treatment. The use of a vinyl guard to protect the area may be helpful.

Chemical trauma

This may be such as caused by aspirin, toothache tinctures (active ingredient phenol with volatile substances) or acid etchants. It is usually self limiting and the area may be helped by the use of a chlorhexidine mouthrinse which will reduce secondary infection. More damaged areas can be protected with a dressing.

Thermal trauma

Burns to gingiva from hot food (e.g. melted cheese or baked potato) may be treated in a similar manner to chemical damage.

Causes of acute traumatic gingivitis
- Toothbrush damage.
- Gingivitis artefacta.
- Chemical trauma.
- Thermal trauma.

Acute necrotizing ulcerative gingivitis

Acute necrotizing ulcerative gingivitis (ANUG) (Fig. 11.9) is known by a variety of other names, including acute ulcerative gingivitis (AUG), acute ulceromembranous gingivitis, acute fusospirochaetal gingivitis, Vincent's disease and trench mouth. It occurs mainly in young adults, between the ages of 13 and 25 years and is evenly distributed between males and females. Predisposing factors include poor oral hygiene, smoking, stress, and immune suppression.

Clinical features

ANUG produces very marked signs and symptoms which make diagnosis relatively easy. It is a disease of sudden onset. The gingiva become acutely inflamed: they are very red, painful and bleed easily.

Ulceration is the most characteristic feature of the disease. The ulcers have a ragged outline and are extremely painful – a fact which limits the extent of the treatment which can be given at the initial visit. Classically, they form first on the interdental papilla and, with increasing severity, spread to involve the gingival margin, the attached gingiva and, in very severe cases, other areas of the oral mucosa. ANUG of this severity is seldom seen in the UK these days, since it is so painful and the acute symptoms are easily treated. The ulcers are covered with a grey slough, the so-called pseudomembrane,

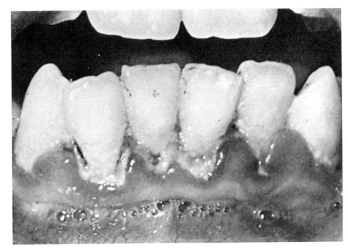

Fig. 11.9 Acute necrotizing ulcerative gingivitis (ANUG) affecting the lower anterior gingiva.

which consists of infected necrotic material which can be wiped off, leaving a raw, bleeding painful area. They are very destructive, eating into the papilla and producing the typical 'punched-out' papilla. The damage caused by the ulcers is so characteristic that many years after they have healed it is often still possible to tell by the gingival appearance that the patient has had ANUG.

When severe, ANUG produces halitosis with a marked characteristic foetid odour, but this is absent in mild cases. Patients may also complain of an unpleasant metallic taste.

Systemic effects

There is usually a degree of lymphadenitis affecting the submental, submandibular and even cervical lymph glands. In severe cases, there may be a degree of malaise and pyrexia, but systemic disturbance, if present at all, is usually mild.

Aetiology

The cause of ANUG is still debated, but there is evidence to suggest that various micro-organisms are involved, together with a lowering of the resistance of the tissues. The typical microscopic picture of scraping taken from the ulcers is of a massive overgrowth of the fusospirochaetal complex: fusiform bacilli, spirochetes (*Borrelia vincenti* or *Treponema vincenti*), and vibrios (Fig. 11.10).

However, the fact that these micro-organisms are invariably present on the ulcers does not mean that they cause ANUG and all attempts to transmit the condition from one person to another, by injecting the bacteria into the tissues, have failed. The typical ANUG microbes may also be found in small numbers in mouths showing no clinical signs of ANUG and close contact with established cases does not seem to cause it to spread. Nevertheless, the fact that ANUG responds so well to antimicrobials does support the idea that specific bacteria are involved.

Mental and physical stress

To overcome the apparent contradiction described above, it has been suggested that the micro-organisms causing ANUG can only have an effect on the gingiva if the gingival resistance has been undermined by either physical or mental stress. This idea gains support from the observation that ANUG spread widely amongst the soldiers fighting in the trenches during the First World War, where physical conditions were appalling and mental stress common.

Systemic disease

ANUG is more common in patients with systemic conditions which lower resistance, especially immunocompromising disorders such as HIV infection.

Local stagnation areas

ANUG frequently appears first in an area of localized stagnation, such as an operculum lying over a partially erupted lower wisdom tooth, or gingiva which has recently been traumatized. Such an area, of course, might well be less resistant to bacteria than other areas and its inaccessibility favours the growth of micro-organisms.

Smoking

Numerous surveys have shown that ANUG is much more common amongst smokers than non-smokers. This may be due to the lower standard of oral hygiene amongst smokers, or the fact that smoking reduces the gingival resistance, by having a constrictive effect on the micro-circulation and damaging crevicular polymorphs.

Characteristics of acute necrotizing ulcerative gingivitis

Predisposing factors
- Poor oral hygiene, smoking, stress, immune suppression.

Clinical features
- Age range: usually 13–25.
- Sore and tender gingiva.
- Bleeding.
- Bad taste and characteristic halitosis.
- Ulceration of interdental papillae sometimes extending to adjacent soft tissue.
- Ulcers covered by grey/yellow slough.
- Sometimes submandibular lymphadenitis.
- Occasionally raised temperature.

The treatment of ANUG depends on its severity. For simplicity, it can be considered under three headings: systemic treatment, localized treatment and follow-up.

Systemic treatment

If adequate local treatment of the ulcers is carried out, systemic treatment may be unnecessary. However, it should be remembered that ANUG is a very destructive condition and rapid resolution is desirable to prevent such damage. Consequently, there would seem little point in withholding antibacterial therapy:

Metronidazole

This is the systemic drug of choice and is administered orally in tablet form. The usual regimen is 200 mg three times daily, for three days, although this dosage may be doubled and the period of time can be extended in severe cases. Metronidazole is a remarkably safe drug with few contraindications. It should not be prescribed for patients who cannot or will not refrain from taking alcohol since it may interact with alcohol to cause headaches, nausea and vomiting. It is also recommended that it should be prescribed with caution in pregnancy, especially during the first trimester. It does not, however, share the same disadvantages as penicillin in causing hypersensitivity reactions in certain patients or producing resistant strains of bacteria.

Penicillin

Penicillin is as effective as metronidazole in treating ANUG but, because of the disadvantages mentioned above, is reserved for those cases in which metronidazole is contraindicated. When used to treat ANUG, penicillin is normally given in doses of 250 mg four times daily for 5 days. However, the use of systemic drugs in the treatment of ANUG without adequate local treatment of the condition is to be deplored since it will frequently lead to recurrence.

Localized treatment

Localized treatment involves the following.

Debridement

It is essential to get the teeth thoroughly cleaned, but, when severe, the pain prevents thorough scaling and the cleaning must be done in stages. Initially it may only be possible to wipe the debris and slough from the gingiva using a cotton wool pledget soaked in an appropriate solution such as hydrogen peroxide. Hydrogen peroxide may have a two fold action: the effervescence mechanically cleans the area and the released oxygen may be toxic to the anaerobic bacteria. Debridement is the term applied to this type of treatment. During the early stages of treatment, the use of an

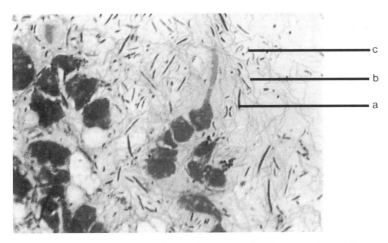

Fig. 11.10 The microscopic picture of a smear taken from a patient with acute necrotizing ulcerative gingivitis (ANUG): **a** fusiform bacilli, **b** spirochaetes, **c** vibrios.

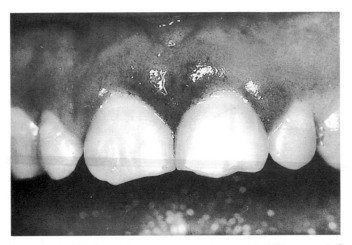

Fig. 11.11 Allergic reaction to toothpaste; the acute gingivitis occurred after changing to a new toothpaste and resolved after discontinuing use.

ultrasonic scaler is often beneficial, with appropriate precautions to avoid inhaling the microbial aerosol. Several visits may be necessary before complete scaling and polishing of the dentition can be carried out. The visits should be arranged within a few days of each other, so that some time is allowed for tissue resolution, but not enough time for the condition to regress.

Oral hygiene
Careful oral hygiene measures must be instigated and maintained. Initially the use of a soft toothbrush may be necessary, but a normal type of brushing should be re-established as soon as possible. Interdental brushes can be beneficial in treating ANUG since the interdental papillae are often destroyed and the resulting space can be gently cleaned without causing pain.

Follow-up treatment

Patients who have suffered from ANUG should be frequently reviewed to ensure that they are keeping their teeth properly cleaned. Because of the gingival damage caused by the ulcers, adequate oral hygiene standards may be more

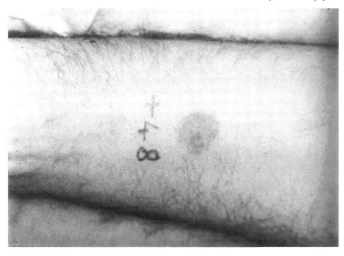

Fig. 11.12 Allergic reaction to toothpaste; positive patch test after 48 h. Same patient as in Fig. 11.11.

difficult to maintain and regular scaling and polishing should be carried out. It may also be necessary for the dentist to perform some periodontal surgery on the affected areas, to restore a reasonable gingival contour.

Management of acute necrotizing ulcerative gingivitis
- Eliminate acute inflammation.
- Debridement and instruction in home care.
- Advise to stop smoking.
- Metronidazole 200 mg 3× a day for a minimum of 3 days.
- Avoid in pregnancy: use penicillin instead. Avoid alcohol.
- Scaling and polishing.
- Maintenance therapy.
- Further more complex treatment such as surgery if indicated.

Acute allergic gingivitis

Hypersensitivity reactions to the constituents of toothpastes and cosmetics are occasionally seen as an allergic gingivitis. The commonest cause is a patient changing to a toothpaste that has not been used before. A similar reaction may occur with items applied to lips, such as cosmetics or lip salve. A typical example may be seen in Figure 11.11. The aetiology may be confirmed by a patch test, as shown in Figure 11.12.

Clinical features

The symptoms reported may vary considerably but common features are a widespread diffuse granular gingivitis involving the full width of the attached gingiva (Fig. 11.11). Other features may include oral ulceration, glossitis and cheilitis. The commonest reported hypersensitivity reaction is to the cinnamonaldehyde constituent of toothpastes. This flavouring is currently used in tartar control toothpastes to hide the unpleasant taste of the pyrophosphate active agent.

Treatment

The condition will resolve with removal of the allergen, but many of these patients will have varying degrees of pre-existing gingivitis and this will require correction.

HIV-associated gingivitis

Acute forms of gingivitis have been described in sufferers from acquired immune deficiency syndrome (AIDS) and have been categorized as definitive forms of periodontal diseases.

Aetiology

It is most probable that these conditions are only an exaggerated or unusual response to dental plaque due to the immune deficits that occur in these patients.

Clinical features

In human immunodeficiency virus (HIV)-associated gingivitis the commonest symptom is an intense marginal gingivitis in a patient who has been diagnosed as infected with HIV. In the more severe cases, there may be ulceration similar to that seen in ANUG. This is a late manifestation in sufferers with HIV infection often occurring just before the onset of full blown AIDS.

Treatment

The primary treatment in these patients is directed towards treating the HIV infection. The oral lesions should always be reported to the consulting physician as they may indicate the arrival of a fully developed AIDS related complex in an HIV carrier. The oral lesions should be sampled with a smear for candidal infection, as this is often present, and may cause an acute form of gingivitis. Assuming that no unusual organisms are found then reinforcing the oral hygiene, together with chemical plaque control by using a 0.2% chlorhexidine gluconate mouthrinse, will help to control the problem. Antibiotics may be required in severe cases.

Types of gingivitis
- Chronic marginal gingivitis.
- Desquamative gingivitis.
- Acute non-specific gingivitis.
- Acute necrotizing ulcerative gingivitis.
- Acute traumatic gingivitis.
- Acute allergic gingivitis.
- HIV-associated gingivitis.

Periodontitis

Unlike gingivitis, where the inflammation is confined to the superficial gingival tissues, periodontitis affects all of the periodontal tissues especially the ligament or membrane. It may be accompanied by a variable amount of gingivitis, which may differ not only from patient to patient, but also from one site to another in the mouth. The characteristics of periodontitis are loss of attachment caused by the apical migration of the junctional epithe-

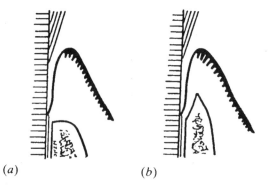

(a)   (b)

Fig. 11.13 Diagrammatic illustration of: (a) suprabony pocket; (b) infrabony pocket.

lium, which may present as pocketing and/or recession, together with bone loss. In the later stages of the disease mobility and drifting of the affected teeth may occur. Other symptoms may include halitosis and pus formation in walls of the pockets, some of which progress to lateral periodontal abscesses.

The bone loss in periodontitis may follow one of two patterns. It may be evenly distributed throughout the mouth, progressing relatively slowly, or there may be localized areas of more severe and rapid destruction. Depending on their relation to the bone loss, the periodontal pockets are termed either suprabony pockets, which are wholly above the crest of the alveolar bone, or infrabony pockets, which are partially contained within the bone (i.e. the base of the pocket lies below the crest of the bone). These two different types are more important in relation to the surgical treatment of chronic periodontitis and are illustrated in Figure 11.13.

Types of periodontitis
Several types of periodontitis are recognized
- Adult periodontitis.
- Prepubertal periodontitis.
- Juvenile periodontitis.
- Adult periodontitis.
- Rapidly progressive periodontitis.
- Refractory periodontitis.
- Acute necrotizing ulcerative periodontitis.
- HIV-associated periodontitis.

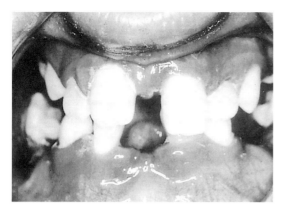

Fig. 11.14 A young patient with prepubertal periodontitis. The incisors are very mobile and have drifted.

Prepubertal periodontitis

As its name indicates, prepubertal periodontitis occurs in young patients before adolescence (Fig. 11.14).

The highest incidence occurs during the eruption of the permanent dentition, although it may be seen involving the primary teeth. The occurrence of true pocketing in children is rare and when it occurs is often a sign of systemic disease, although in some children no underlying predisposing problem can be demonstrated. The diseases that have been identified in sufferers of prepubertal periodontitis include insulin dependent diabetes, leukaemia and neutropenia.

The characteristics of this disease are not well known, although the gingival inflammation is usually extremely acute and granulation or proliferation from the active sites may occur, giving rise to gingival epulides of the pyogenic variety. There is often very a rapid destruction of alveolar bone and sometimes gingival recession. Immune system defects, including functional defects of peripheral blood leukocytes and monocytes, may be found in these patients.

Management of prepubertal periodontitis

It is important that the dentist refers the patient to a physician who should undertake systemic screening. Although in many patients the results may prove negative, the identification of a serious defect in even a small number of these young patients justifies such an approach. The techniques of these investigations and their follow-up is outside the scope of this text, but should include a whole blood and differential white cell counts.

Periodontal therapy, although secondary to the medical treatment, often proves to be difficult as patients of this age are challenging. As a general rule these patients will require regular visits of short duration. The most effective therapies are thorough prophylaxis of the active sites with a low abrasive fluoride-containing paste, together with flushing of the pockets with an ultrasonic scaler, making use of the cavitation effect. Oral hygiene should be kept simple and the guardian must be involved in supervision and monitoring. Scrub brushing will give some subgingival cleaning. Interdental tape, perhaps with a floss holder, must be used in the affected area. The guardian may also be shown how to flush the lesion with a subgingival irrigator filled with an anti-plaque chemical such as chlorhexidine.

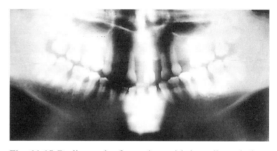

Fig. 11.15 Radiograph of a patient with juvenile periodontitis with bone loss evident around molars and incisors.

Juvenile periodontitis

Juvenile periodontitis is an rare form of periodontitis which occurs around the permanent teeth of adolescents. In localized juvenile periodontitis (LJP) the lesions occur around the first molars and the incisors classically in teenagers (Figs 11.15 and 16) although, as with prepubertal periodontitis, generalized forms have been described. The disease has its onset at puberty, although it may present at any time between eleven and thirteen.

The prevalence is equal in both boys and girls. The amount of gingival inflammation seen in these patients is frequently low and the oral hygiene may vary from excellent to appalling. In all patients, however, the degree of breakdown is excessive for the amount of local irritants. There is some evidence that this

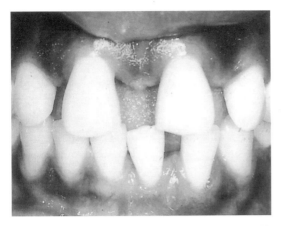

Fig. 11.16 Clinical photograph of a 16-year-old patient with juvenile periodontitis showing drifting of teeth and good oral hygiene.

disease may be subject to remission or burn-out.

The defects occur in siblings and the familial distribution is consistent with an autosomal recessive genetic trait. It is thought that all affected individuals probably have functional defects of neutrophils or monocytes. The microbiology has been studied in some depth and two endotoxin producing organisms *Actinobacillus actinomycetemcomitans* and *Capnocytophaga* have been identified in a large number of these patients. Interestingly the toxins produced by these organisms inhibit phagocytic cell function, which may account for the defects seen in the neutrophil and monocyte function.

Management of juvenile periodontitis

Although the treatment of these patients follows the general principles laid down for adult type periodontitis, the rapid progression of this condition makes the monitoring much more critical. There are two areas, however, in which management does differ radically. It is now widely accepted that these patients should be prescribed tetracycline by the dentist to eradicate the associated organisms. It is a matter of clinical judgement whether the antibiotic is given immediately that the condition is diagnosed, or with mechanical root surface treatment. There is some evidence that this condition does not respond well to root planing, and the most optimal result is obtained from a combination of early surgery and tetracycline.

Rapidly progressive periodontitis

Typically sufferers with rapidly progressive periodontitis have severe and rapidly advancing lesions (Fig. 11.17). which occur between the ages of 25 and 35 years. The lesions are frequently generalized with all the teeth affected to a greater or lesser degree, without any consistent pattern of destruction. The microbiology is uncertain but two organisms are often found: *Porphyromonas gingivalis* and *Actinobacillus actinomycetemcomitans*. During the active phases of rapidly progressive periodontitis the lesions are acutely inflamed and may proliferate to give rise to granulomatous gingival epulides. There is a higher prevalence in individuals with systemic disorders.

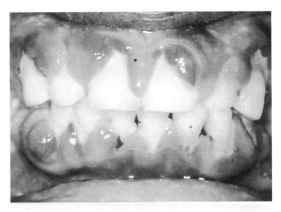

Fig. 11.17 Clinical photograph of a patient with rapidly progressive periodontitis. Note the granulomatous reaction of the gingiva to plaque.

Management of rapidly progressive periodontitis

The general principles of the treatment of periodontitis apply to these patients. Adjunctive treatment with tetracycline, metronidazole or a combination of metronidazole and amoxycillin has been advocated, with variable results. The use of a subgingival irrigation with chlorhexidine is often helpful.

Adult periodontitis

The commonest type of periodontitis is adult periodontitis (Fig. 11.18). This usually occurs in older patients whose tissues respond well to plaque-induced damage and break down slowly over a long period of time. Although there may be periods of rapid breakdown, as with any

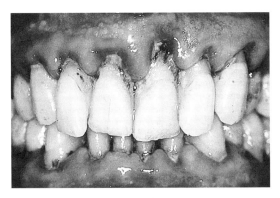

Fig. 11.18 A patient with adult periodontitis showing large amounts of dental plaque deposits but a low grade inflammatory response.

type of inflammatory disease, generally the increase in probing depths is slow. There may be a large amount of reparative fibrosis in the inflamed gingiva.

Management of adult periodontitis

Adult type periodontitis is, after chronic gingivitis, the commonest of the inflammatory periodontal diseases. The management of all forms of periodontitis is necessarily complex and time consuming and the main principles are the following.

- Assessment and diagnosis of the disease.
- Discussion of the findings with the patient.
- Decision on treatment strategy.
- Provision of advice on appropriate plaque control.
- Removal of plaque retention factors.
- The use of chemical adjuncts.
- Allowing a healing period.

Assessment and diagnosis of the disease
It is the responsibility of the dental surgeon to carry out the necessary screening of patients under their care, to undertake an assessment and to arrive at an appropriate treatment plan.

Discussion of the findings with the patient
This is to determine the patient's attitudes and expectations. At this stage relief of pain, if present, may be carried out. Decisions on any teeth of hopeless prognosis (i.e. those with little supporting bone) should be made at this stage, to avoid any misunderstanding about what might be achieved with therapy.

Decision on treatment strategy
Any decision on the type of treatment must be made in conjunction with the patient and with their full informed consent.

Providing advice on appropriate plaque control
This will include advice on home care measures combined with the removal of plaque retention factors such as calculus. Home care would usually involve a subgingival brushing technique, interdental cleansing and, for many patients, the use of disclosing agents where supragingival plaque control measures are suspect.

Removal of plaque retention factors
This will include the removal of calculus and the improvement of restorations and dental prostheses. This part of treatment together with the home care advice is often called the *hygiene phase* or *cause related* therapy and the dental hygienist should be an expert in its application, especially to the patient with adult periodontitis.

The use of chemical adjuncts
In some patients the use of chemical adjuncts to plaque control may be indicated and this is discussed later in this chapter.

Allowing a healing period
After this phase of treatment, a period of time, often 6 to 12 weeks, is allowed for healing before the tissue response is reassessed and a decision is made on the need for further treatment.

The treatment after the hygiene phase will depend upon the healing response (Fig. 11.19). It may include one or more of the following.

- When good healing has been achieved, or if there are signs that healing is occurring, the patient is monitored and treated if indicated to ensure that the tissues return to maintainable health.
- If a healing response is not occurring and the home care is inadequate then the cause should be sought and further advice on oral hygiene provided.
- Where the lack of healing is accompanied by an adequate level of home care, then root planing would be carried out as described on pages 203 and 204.

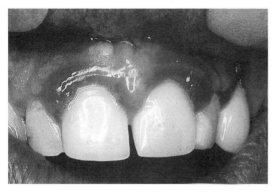

(a)

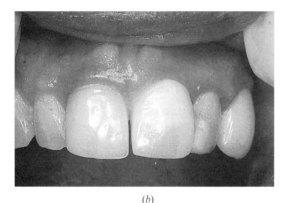

(b)

Fig. 11.19 A patient with adult periodontitis: (a) before periodontal therapy, (b) the patient after non-surgical periodontal therapy.

- For the small group of patients who do not respond to the above regimes it may be necessary for periodontal surgery to be undertaken.

Refractory periodontitis

In a small number of sites in some patients the periodontal lesion will remain active, as shown by continued signs of inflammation, pus formation or pocket deepening despite active treatment (Fig. 11.20).

Before attempting to retreat and stabilize this type of lesion, it is necessary to stop and consider the reasons for the failure of the site to heal. The more frequent reasons are, in order of probability.

- Inadequate oral hygiene.
- Persistence of root surface deposits.

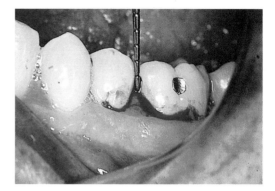

Fig. 11.20 Clinical photograph of a patient with refractory periodontitis. Note the severe inflammation despite previous root planing.

- Root surface defects.
- Inadequate host response.
- Unidentified systemic factor.

Inadequate oral hygiene

This is a level of supragingival dental plaque which is incompatible with marginal periodontal health, which will vary from patient to patient. The level of residual plaque should be sufficiently low as to permit the marginal gingival tissues to be free of visible inflammation. If marginal inflammation persists, then a complex subgingival flora will soon re-establish and pocket activity will again occur.

Root surface deposits

Some deposits are always left after treatment but usually the host response is able to cope with a low level of retained irritants, such as dental plaque, calculus and cementum-bound endotoxin. However, it is not always possible to debride the root surface adequately due to difficulties with access, visibility or root contour as shown in Figure 11.21. In general, anterior, single rooted teeth are usually amenable to instrumentation, whilst posterior, multiple rooted teeth with furcation involvement are least likely to be successfully treated.

Root surface defects

Defects such as grooves, flutes, gingival pits or enamel projections are seen in some sites with refractory inflammation (Fig. 11.22). The root

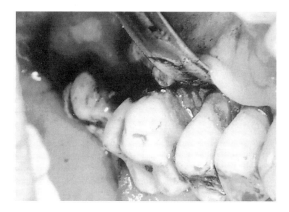

Fig. 11.21 Thin plates of subgingival calculus located deep within periodontal pockets. A flap has been raised to reveal deposits which would have been difficult to detect without direct vision.

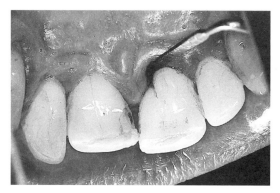

Fig. 11.22 Clinical photograph of a patient with a palatal root groove associated with severe pocketing.

surface defects prevent complete debridement and inflammation therefore persists.

Inadequate host response

This is seen in a small number of individuals. These defects are difficult to detect and impossible to treat. The only factor that can be changed in these unfortunate patients, is to reduce the level of plaque deposits even further.

Unidentified systemic factors

Factors such as anaemia, diabetes or other similar problems occur in a very small number of patients. Although it is not appropriate to screen all patients with refractory lesions, if multiple sites are active, the tissues highly inflamed and the plaque levels low, it is worthwhile for the dentist to arrange for the patient to have a haematological screening including whole blood count, film and serum chemistry.

Management of refractory periodontitis

There are a number of actions that can be taken to stabilize refractory lesions.

Recheck the home care

Firstly check that the patient is using a *subgingival* brushing method. It is important to note that although many methods of brushing, such as the Roll technique, are quite

adequate for the healthy patient, they will not cope with the presence of pocketing or gingival swelling. Also ensure that the patient is using a disclosing agent after brushing to monitor residual plaque levels.

The necessity for good daily interdental cleansing must be stressed and insisted upon. Finally, ensure that the environment in which oral hygiene is undertaken is adequate. Good lighting, a mirror preferably a magnifying one and a comfortable seat are essential.

Subgingival irrigation

Some studies have shown that the introduction of a chemical antiseptic such as 0.2% chlorhexidine digluconate into the pocket will have an additional depressant effect on the subgingival flora. There are two main ways of introducing the chemical subgingivally – the use of a pulsed water irrigator or by using a syringe with a large blunt needle. The irrigation should be undertaken on a daily basis until the lesion is under control.

Repetition of root surface cleaning

It is worthwhile repeating the root planing on a tooth adjacent to an active site, on at least two occasions, with a period of at least 3–6 months in between. It must be remembered that it may take up to 6 months for the full effects of root planing to be achieved. Root surface cleaning should include the use of an ultrasonic or sonic scaler, as the flushing effect will reduce both the level of subgingival microbes and cementum-bound endotoxin.

The root planing may be combined with the use of a topical subgingival antimicrobial such as 2% minocycline, 25% metronidazole or tetracycline cord, which are described later in this chapter.

Use of systemic anti-microbials

The use of systemic agents such as amoxycillin, tetracycline, minocycline or metronidazole may in some cases produce dramatic improvements, provided they are combined with mechanical root surface treatment in the form of root planing or flap surgery.

Undertake periodontal flap surgery

For those sites which persist despite the previous treatment and when the home care is considered adequate, then the dentist may raise a periodontal flap to permit access to the root surface for instrumentation. The commonest procedure undertaken is the replaced flap, often called the modified Widman procedure.

Prolonged professional debridement

Sometimes, when the lesions will not stabilize it is necessary to undertake repeated professional debridement of the active pockets, especially with the sonic or ultrasonic scaler. This will be sufficient in many patients to prevent extension of the lesions with the problems of further loss of attachment.

HIV-associated periodontitis

Periodontitis associated with patients whose immune systems are compromised by HIV infection may show unusual features. The marginal gingivitis may be intense and sometimes the overlying soft tissue will be necrotic exposing marginal bone around the tooth. Pocketing, when present, will be deeper than expected. There is often an associated candidal infection.

The main manifestations of HIV periodontitis are as follows.

- HIV-associated gingivitis.
- Acute necrotizing ulcerative gingivitis.
- Acute necrotizing ulcerative periodontitis.
- Aggressive periodontitis.
- Acute necrotizing stomatitis.
- Gingival ulceration.

Management of HIV-associated periodontitis

It is essential that any treatment undertaken for these patients involves close liaison with the physician managing the HIV infection. The most important benefit that the hygienist can give to the patient is to institute excellent plaque control measures. This should include the regular use of chlorhexidine mouthrinse. The mouth must be monitored on a regular basis and checked carefully for signs of pathological change.

When HIV-associated periodontitis does occur then it should be treated with a regime of scaling, root planing and the use of anti-microbials. If in addition there is a candidal infection in the mouth this needs treatment with antifungals. The periodontitis should be managed conservatively and surgery avoided if at all possible in view of the poor healing potential of these patients. If bone denudation occurs then it should be covered with a dressing and antibiotics prescribed in conjunction with the physician responsible for the medical care.

Clinical characteristics of periodontitis
- Variable degree of gingivitis.
- Loss of attachment
  pocketing
  recession.
- Pocket activity
  bleeding on deep probing
  suppuration
  loss of attachment.
- Bone loss.
- Mobility and/or drifting.

Anti-microbials in the management of inflammatory periodontal diseases

Mouthrinses

A number of mouthrinses have been successfully used in the treatment of inflammatory periodontal diseases despite the risk that the superficial signs of disease (e.g. redness, bleeding from the marginal gingiva) may lessen, but the pocket activity may extend, leading to insidious progression of periodontitis over a period of time.

The most successful antiplaque chemical used in mouthrinses to date is the bis-biguanide salt, chlorhexidine gluconate, which has a broad anti-microbial spectrum and is active against both Gram-positive and Gram-negative bacteria. Chlorhexidine has been shown in long-term studies to reduce plaque and gingivitis by an average of 55% and 45% respectively; 30% of a chlorhexidine rinse is retained in the mouth, and elevated levels are found in saliva after 24 hours.

Another anti-microbial is Triclosan which is approximately 65% as effective as chlorhexidine, especially when combined with a copolymer or zinc salt to improve oral retention. It is slowly released from oral surfaces to give a level in saliva capable of inhibiting bacterial growth and hence plaque accumulation, for extended periods between applications; 25–35% is retained and an elevated level remains in plaque and saliva for 8 hours, and for 3 hours on mucosal surfaces.

The other chemical mouthrinse in addition to chlorhexidine which has been approved by the Council of Dental Therapeutics of the American Dental Association, is Listerine, a phenolic antiplaque compound with anti-inflammatory properties. This has a moderate clinical efficacy in the reduction of plaque and gingivitis with average reductions of 35% in both parameters. There are no data on the oral retention for Listerine.

Other mouthrinses containing cetylpyridinium chloride, sanguinaria, stannous fluoride, hydrogen peroxide and perborates have relatively poor clinical efficacy. Cetylpyridinium chloride is a quaternary ammonium compound used in many mouthrinses available over the counter. Although similar *in vitro* activity to chlorhexidine has been reported, little or no plaque inhibiting activity exists *in vivo* after mouthrinsing. Short-term studies show an average of 35% plaque reduction, but a six months study reported only 14% reduction in plaque although a there was a 24% reduction in gingivitis.

Sanguinaria, a plant alkaloid, has a high affinity for plaque, but binds too tightly for anti-microbial activity to be manifest *in vivo*. Short-term studies have shown some plaque and calculus reduction, but long-term studies show no significant reduction in plaque or gingivitis. When used as a mouthrinse and dentifrice, significant reductions in plaque and gingivitis in the 15–50% range have been reported.

Short-term studies on stannous fluoride have reported promising results on plaque and gingivitis reduction, but long-term studies showed minimal beneficial effects.

Hydrogen peroxide and perborates are oxygenating agents which, when acted upon by tissue- and bacterial- derived enzymes, release oxygen with an effervescence. These have anti-inflammatory properties and therefore less gingivitis is observed. However, the bacteria producing the inflammation have not been shown to be reduced. Contradictory findings in short-term and unimpressive long-term findings have been reported. Increased tissue injury, which may delay wound healing has also been suggested with these substances.

In summary it can be concluded that although plaque control is best accomplished by brushing and flossing, some patients could benefit from the use of mouthrinses having an antiplaque action, as an adjunct to mechanical methods. These include patients having poor plaque-removal habits due to physical and/or cognitive impairment, patients with poor motivation and patients having local 'plaque retentive' factors such as malposed teeth, malocclusion, crowns, bridgework and/or partial dentures, or orthodontic bands. The most effective time to use a mouthrinse is after root surface treatment such as root planing. This slows down recolonization of the pockets and improves healing after non-surgical periodontal therapy.

Subgingival anti-microbials

Most types of inflammatory periodontal disease can be healed or stabilized by conventional non-surgical management methods which include the following.

- Oral hygiene (home care) advice.
- Correction of plaque retention factors.
- Root surface treatment
    root planing
    root cleaning
    root debridement.
- Re-evaluation.

However, 10–30% of inflammatory periodontal sites do not respond to conventional mechanical treatment. To date there have been two options for the management of these refractory sites: keep on repeating the initial therapy or undertake periodontal surgery. The advent of subgingival anti-microbials has given a third option or at least another step before proceeding to irreversible periodontal surgery.

Subgingival anti-microbial delivery systems have a number of advantages in the management of diseased periodontal sites including site specific delivery, effective concentration at the inflamed site, the potential for prolonged action as well as a decreased risk of side effects or interactions. The techniques are not dependent upon patient compliance.

Characteristics of subgingival anti-microbials

- Site specific delivery of therapeutic agents.
- Effective concentration profiles at the inflamed site.
- Potential for prolonged action.
- Decreased risk of side effects or interactions.
- No dependence upon patient compliance.

Subgingival anti-microbial delivery may be used in the management of periodontitis, as an adjunct to mechanical subgingival debridement, in order to overcome the problem of ensuring the entry of anti-microbials into periodontal pockets. Local delivery may be achieved in the following ways.

Pulsed oral irrigation

Studies have shown that pulsed oral irrigation after scaling and root planing may further reduce plaque levels, bleeding index and pocket depths. With regard to the most efficacious chemical for use with such a system, chlorhexidine appears to be the agent of choice although there is no agreement as to the most appropriate concentration. Indeed there is considerable disagreement as to the activity of chlorhexidine in periodontal pockets. There is general agreement in the literature that pulsed oral irrigation reduces gingivitis and improves the efficiency of antimicrobial chemicals. However, when the efficacy of scaling and root planing is compared with subgingival irrigation, the former is the most effective. Therefore, pulsed irrigation is only useful as an adjunct to standard therapy in some patients.

Topical anti-microbials

A number of products have been developed to deliver an anti-microbial subgingivally in an active site as an adjunct to mechanical treatment. In the UK the following sustained release systems are available at present:

2% Minocycline gel (Dentomycin®) requires 3 or 4 applications each at 2 weekly intervals with no repetition within 6 months. It inhibits most periodontal pathogens but is rapidly cleared from pocket.

25% metronidazole gel (Elyzol®) is applied twice at one-week intervals. This product has a slow release base (biodegradable monoglycerid gel rich in mono-olein with sesame oil).

25% tetracycline hydrochloride in ethylene vinyl acetate copolymer monofilament (Actisite®). This elastic cord is packed into the pocket and left for a 12 day period. Despite being very time consuming to insert this product has long retention and sustained release. The cord requires subsequent removal and is very bulky in the pocket and this causes a degree of discomfort, both during insertion and the following period.

55% Chlorhexidine gluconate in a hydrolysed gelatine chip (Periochip®). This is based on a sustained release device, which a method of delivering the anti-microbial subgingivally over a prolonged period of time. Unlike other subgingival products Periochip is not based on an antibiotic and therefore has few side effects. It is very easy and quick to insert with minimum discomfort to the patient. As the product is biodegradable there is no need to remove and it has been shown to have effective activity over a 10 day period

It may be concluded that the local delivery of anti-microbials has a part to play in the management of inflammatory periodontitis. The appropriate therapeutic strategy is to use them as an adjunctive treatment after adequate mechanical therapy and they would appear to be most effective when used in local persistent pockets.

Further Reading

Ciancio S. G. (1988) Use of mouthrinses for professional indications. *Journal of Clinical Periodontology* **15**, 520–523.

Coventry J. F., Newman H. N. (1982) Experimental use of a slow release device employing chlorhexidine gluconate in areas of acute periodontal inflammation. *Journal of Clinical Periodontology* **9**, 129–133.

Consumers Association (1994) Antibiotic gels for periodontal disease. *Drugs and Therapeutic Bulletin* **32** (6), 43–44.

Mandel I. D. (1988) Chemotherapeutic agents for controlling plaque and gingivitis. *Journal of Clinical Periodontology* **15**, 488–498.

Rawlinson A., Walsh T. F. (1993) Rationale and techniques of non-surgical pocket management in periodontal therapy. *British Dental Journal* **174**, 161–166.

Walsh T. F., Glenwright H. D., Hull P.S. (1992) Clinical effects of pulsed oral irrigation with 0.2% chlorhexidine digluconate in patients with adult periodontitis. *Journal of Clinical Periodontology* **19**, 245–248.

12

Epidemiology of dental diseases

Introduction

Epidemiology is concerned with the presence of disease in a community or country. It may be required to know the amount, severity, spread and origin of a particular disease. Therefore the epidemiologist deals with disease in groups of people, compared to the clinician who deals with disease in the individual. From this information decisions may be made on the allocation or targeting of resources, or whether to increase the number dental auxiliaries, such as dental hygienists.

Periodontal indices

The hygienist may be working in a community or research study to determine the amount of periodontal disease in a population. It is necessary, if comparisons are going to be made, to reduce the findings to precise mathematically expressed terms. It would be impossible to say which was worse: 100 'fairly deep pockets' or 150 'rather loose teeth'. A number of indices have been used express in figures our observations. The hygienist may have the important task of making the measurements required from each examination, as very often many hundreds of subjects have to be examined and the data recorded. It is necessary to devise systems which are simple and not time-consuming. Indices have been devised for the measurement of caries and these have been described previously, plaque levels and gingivitis and periodontitis, including the following.

Indices of plaque levels

Plaque indices are also used by many clinicians on an individual patient basis, to provide a numerical record of the amount of plaque present on the teeth at each visit. Not only can this be a useful clinical record, it can also be used to motivate the patient by providing a clear goal for which to aim: an agreed plaque score. Numerous indices of this type have been developed, but the two most popular are the oral hygiene index and the plaque index.

Oral hygiene index (OHI)

This was developed by Greene and Vermillion (1960) and in its original form was a combination of two indices: a calculus index and a debris index.

Calculus index
Scores of 0–3 are awarded to each test site on the basis of the following criteria.

  0 No calculus present.
  1 Supragingival calculus covering less than one-third of the tooth surface.
  2 Supragingival calculus covering between one- and two-thirds of the tooth surface or odd flecks of subgingival calculus.
  3 Supragingival calculus covering more than two-thirds of the tooth surface or continuous bands of subgingival calculus.

Debris index
The initial suggestion of debris is now usually interpreted as plaque and this part of the index

is now often used on its own. The criteria for scoring are as follows.

0   No debris or extrinsic staining.
1   Debris covering less than one-third of the tooth surface, or any degree of extrinsic staining.
2   Debris covering between one- and two-thirds of the tooth surface.
3   Debris covering more than two-thirds of the tooth surface.

The mean of the separate scores for each surface tested is taken as the score for each index. The two scores may then be recorded separately or the mean of the two taken as the overall OHI score.

Simplified oral hygiene index (OHI-S)

It is important that any index used should not be too time-consuming, in view of the large number of the subjects which may have to be studied. For this reason Greene and Vermillion simplified their index. The principle of the calculus and debris indices remains the same, as do the criteria for awarding the scores. However, six tooth surfaces are selected as being representative of the whole mouth.

- The buccal surface of the first standing upper molar on each side.
- The lingual surface of the first standing lower molar on each side.
- The labial surface of tooth 41 and 21 or, if either is missing, tooth 31 and 11.

Plaque index

This was developed by Silness and Loe (1964) and was designed for use with their gingival index. The level of plaque present on each tooth surface tested is scored using the following criteria.

Code 0   no plaque present.
Code 1   a film of plaque, visible only by removal on a probe or by disclosing.
Code 2   moderate accumulations of plaque within the pockets or on the margins which can be seen with the naked eye.
Code 3   heavy accumulations of soft material filling the niche between the gingival margin and tooth surface. The interdental area is filled with debris.

All sites can be tested, or six selected teeth may be taken as representative of the whole mouth. These are teeth 16, 12, 24 and 36, 32, 44. In each case the mesial, distal, buccal and lingual surfaces are separately assessed and the final plaque index score is the mean of all these scores.

Modified plaque index

One variation of the plaque index that is often used is to record presence or absence (1 or 0), usually after staining with a disclosing agent. This method has a number of advantages, including being quicker to undertake, having less variation within and between examiners, and being easier to analyse than the multiple codes of the other indices.

Code 0   no clinical plaque deposits visible in the gingival area.
Code 1   plaque deposits visible after disclosing in the gingival area.

Gingival indices

Gingival indices are used to assess the level of inflammation and therefore the degree of activity of the periodontal lesions. To increase the reliability of the assessment they are always combined with other observations before making a clinical decision about the activity of the lesion.

PMA index

This was the first index to be developed. The abbreviations stand for papilla (P), marginal gingiva (M) and attached gingiva (A) and each of these areas is examined and scored from 0 to 4, depending on the severity of the inflammation. Numerous variations of this index exist which was primarily used in surveys of acute gingivitis and is now of largely historic interest.

Gingival index

This was developed by Loe and Silness in 1963. The mesial, facial, distal and lingual of each tooth to be assessed is examined and graded according to the following codes.

Code 0   normal gingiva.
Code 1   mild inflammation, slight change in

colour, slight oedema, no bleeding on probing.

Code 2 moderate inflammation, redness, oedema and glazing. Bleeding on probing.

Code 3 severe inflammation, marked redness and oedema or ulceration. Tendency to spontaneous haemorrhage.

The codes may be totalled to give a gross score or divided by the number of points and teeth to give a mean. Alternatively, the number of readings of each code may be noted separately, to give a more statistically meaningful result.

Bleeding index

Developed by Cowell *et al.* in 1975, this index uses the most reliable sign of gingival inflammation, bleeding from the pocket after gentle probing.

Grade 0 no bleeding on gentle probing with a blunt probe.

Grade 1 bleeding on gentle probing up to 30 s later.

Grade 2 immediate bleeding on gentle probing.

Grade 3 spontaneous bleeding.

Gingival bleeding index

This variation of the bleeding index described by Ainamo and Bay in 1975 has the distinct advantage of using presence or absence of bleeding as its criterion. This improves the reliability of the recording.

Code 0 no bleeding after gentle probing with a blunt probe.

Code 1 bleeding within 10 s after gentle probing with a blunt probe.

Periodontal indices

All indices to determine the severity of periodontitis are compound assessments which incorporate a number of different criteria. Some years ago indices such as the periodontal index (Russell, 1956) were used to measure the severity of disease, an impossible task. Now the community periodontal index of treatment needs (CPITN) has largely replaced the previous indices. One variation of this, the basic periodontal examination (BPE) has been developed as a chair side screening index and will be described below.

Periodontal index (PI)

Russell (1956) developed this index, in which the gingiva of all standing teeth are examined and scored as follows.

0 No periodontal disease, mild gingivitis.
2 Marked gingivitis, but no pocketing.
6 Gingivitis with pocketing.
8 Advanced destruction with loosening of the teeth.

The individual's score is calculated by dividing the total score by the number of units assessed.

Basic periodontal examination (BPE)

The screening system described here is based on the community periodontal index of treatment needs (CPITN), as amended by the working party of the British Society of Periodontology and first produced in their policy statement *'Periodontology in General Dental Practice in the United Kingdom,'* and is reproduced with their kind permission. The authors have made some minor changes from the BSP document and these are indicated by italics.

For the periodontal examination the dentition is divided into six sextants. The use of a periodontal probe is mandatory. The recommended probe is the *World Health Organization probe which has a ball end 0.5 mm diameter. A colour coded area extends from 3.5 mm to 5.5 mm. A newer version of the WHO probe has a second dark band running from 8.5 mm to 11.5 mm to assist in estimating the depth of very deep pockets* (Fig. 12.1). Probing force should not exceed 20–25 g.

The probe tip is gently inserted into the gingival pocket and the depth of insertion read against the colour coding. The total extent of the pocket should be explored, conveniently by 'walking' the probe around the pocket. At least six points on each tooth should be examined: mesiobuccal, midbuccal, distobuccal and the corresponding lingual sites.

For each sextant the highest score *together with an * if appropriate* is recorded. A sextant

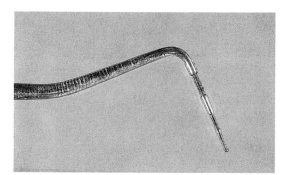

Fig. 12.1 The C version of the WHO probe.

with only one tooth is recorded as missing and the score is included in the adjacent sextant. A simple box is used to record the scores for each sextant as shown in Fig. 12.2. *The following codes are used.*

Code 4: coloured area of probe disappears into the pocket indicating probing depths of at least 6 mm.

Code 3: coloured area of probe remains partly visible in the deepest pocket in the sextant.

Code 2: coloured area of probe remains completely visible in the deepest pocket in the sextant. Supra- or subgingival calculus is detected or the defective margin of a filling or crown.

Code 1: coloured area of probe remains completely visible in the deepest pocket in the sextant. No calculus or defective margins are detected. There is bleeding after gentle probing.

Code 0: healthy gingival tissues with no bleeding after gentle probing.

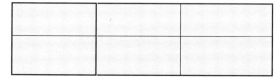

Fig. 12.2 The basic periodontal examination recording box.

*In addition to these scores the authors recommend that the symbol * be added to the sextant score whenever there is a furcation involvement or there is total attachment loss of 7 mm or more at any site within that sextant. It should be noted that this advice differs from the BSP policy.*

The management of patients according to their sextant scores is suggested below.

Code 0: no treatment.

Code 1: oral hygiene instruction.

Code 2: OHI plus removal of calculus and correction of plaque retentive margins or fillings or crowns. Patients whose CPITN *(BPE)* score for all sextants are CODES 0, 1, 2 should be screened again after an interval of one year.

Code 3: as Code 2 but a longer time will be required for treatment. Plaque and bleeding scores are collected at the start and finish of treatment. Pocket probing depths in the sextants scoring Code 3 should be taken at the finish of treatment. Subsequently these records should be taken at intervals of not more than one year, along with BPE/CPITN screening of other sextants.

Code 4: a full probing depth chart is required together with recordings of gingival recession, furcation involvement and any other relevant clinical details. Individual intra-oral radiographs will be taken of teeth which show furcation involvement or loss of attachment of 7 mm or more at any site.

Code * treatment will include oral hygiene instruction, removal of calculus and overhangs and root planing. Re-examination is then required to assess the results of treatment to date and the need for further treatment which may include periodontal surgery.

Practitioners may wish to refer patients with scores of 4 or * for specialist care.

It should be noted that this screening system is not intended to be used for monitoring purposes during treatment. Readers are referred to the BSP policy document for recording and monitoring methods suited to this purpose.

Mobility index

This is a very useful index which may be used to assess whether mobility is increasing over a period of time (Grace and Smales, 1989).

Grade 0 No apparent mobility.
Grade 1 Perceptible mobility but less than 1 mm buccolingually.
Grade 2 Definite mobility between 1–2 mm buccolingually.
Grade 3 Gross mobility exceeding 2 mm buccolingually and/or vertical mobility.

It should be noted that in order to distinguish mobility grades from pocket depths, they are usually recorded in Roman numerals on periodontal charts, e.g.: I, II, III.

Indices of special interest to the dental hygienist
- Plaque index (Silness and Loe, 1964).
- Gingival index (Loe and Silness, 1963).
- Gingival bleeding index (Ainamo and Bay, 1975).
- Basic periodontal examination (BPE) or amended community periodontal index of treatment needs (CPITN) (British Society of Periodontology, 1984).

Periodontal probing

Despite arguments as to the significance of periodontal probing depths in the progression of periodontitis, they do represent an accurate picture of the disease to date and are one of the most important prognosticators of the likely life of the tooth. The measurement of probing depth depends upon the following factors.

- The probing force used.
- The depth of the pocket.
- The amount of inflammation in the area.
- The access to the pocket.
- The presence of features which will impede the probe such as calculus or the presence of restorations, or root surface features such as furcations.

The probing force used determines the penetration of the probe into the junctional epithelium. The latest recommendations are that a very light force should be used, in the order of 15–25 g. This force, if applied to a periodontal probe placed under the fingernail, would not cause any discomfort.

The depth of the pocket and the amount of inflammation present will also determine the probing depth achieved. The greater the degree of inflammation in a pocket, the further the probe penetrates into the junctional epithelium. For this reason the probing depths should always be reassessed after initial therapy has reduced inflammation.

The access to the pocket and the presence of root surface deposits will determine the ease with which the pocket can be entered by the probe. The classic example is furcation pocketing where, because of the morphology of the root, the full extent of the lesion cannot be explored. This should be borne in mind when examining periodontal pockets.

Probing sites

Probing depths may be measured at two, four or six sites around the tooth. The more sites assessed, the more accurate the information gained and the fewer the periodontal lesions that will be missed. At the simplest level, measuring mesial and distal sites on each tooth will identify the great majority of problems, as it is unlikely that a tooth with, for example, a mid facial lesion, will not also have a mesial or distal lesion. A more accurate method is to measure the mesial, distal, facial and lingual pockets. The most accurate method is to measure the probing depths on the mesial, distal and mid facial or lingual aspect on each side of the tooth, giving six readings per tooth.

Factors influencing chronic periodontal diseases
Age

A large number of surveys have confirmed the common clinical impression that the severity of periodontal disease increases throughout life. It has already been mentioned that this observation is so common that it has given rise to the erroneous impression that periodontal breakdown is an inevitable physiological age change, rather than a pathological condition which can be prevented by adequate plaque control. Gingivitis is common in the deciduous dentition and is so common in the early teens that the term 'puberty gingivitis' is often used. Periodontitis, on the other hand, is uncommon under 13 years of age, but becomes more common in the later teens. One survey on late teenagers in the UK by Sheiham (1969) showed that one-quarter of them were affected by periodontal breakdown to some extent. The increase in severity progresses steadily throughout life, and whereas caries is the main cause of tooth loss in the first three decades of life, over 30 chronic periodontal disease is by far the commonest reason for extractions. It is estimated that taken over a whole life span, caries and periodontal disease each cause 40% of all extractions, with the remaining 20% being extracted for miscellaneous other reasons such as crowding, impaction, trauma, etc.

Gender

The influence that the gender of a person has on periodontal disease is confusing, with many surveys indicating that the periodontal condition of females is better than males and others suggesting the opposite. When groups of equal oral hygiene standards are compared, no difference is found and it would appear that the gender of the subjects makes no difference, but that in many countries the condition of females is better than that of males simply because women care more for their appearance, including their oral hygiene. However, the periodontal health of pregnant women has been shown to be poorer than that of males and non-pregnant women and the recent increase in smoking amongst young females will inevitably lead to a worsening of the periodontal health of females.

Ethnic group

A marked difference in periodontal health has been observed between various ethnic groups. For example, Asian and African populations have, on average, more severe periodontal disease than Europeans or Americans. However, this has been shown to be the result of differences in oral hygiene habits, education and nutrition, rather than race itself. However, some specific disorders such as juvenile periodontitis do have an ethnic distribution as described in Chapter 11.

Systemic diseases

Many systemic diseases increase the progression of inflammatory periodontal diseases. Amongst these are human immunodeficiency disease (HIV), diabetes, inflammatory bowel disorders, including ulcerative colitis and Crohn's disease, leukaemias and neutropenia. A number of types of medication including phenytoin, calcium antagonists and cyclosporin are associated with gingival hyperplasia. The reader is referred to specialist texts for information.

Epidemiology of dental caries

The most common technique used in epidemiological surveys of caries is the DMF method. D, M and F stand for decayed, missing and filled and by counting the number of DMF teeth it is possible to assess the extent of the caries. If the DMF tooth surfaces (DMF-S) are counted the technique becomes more sensitive. With the DMF index a tooth with an occlusal filling would score the same as a tooth with an MOD filling and an additional buccal filling. With the DMF-S, the tooth with the occlusal filling would score 1, but the tooth with the MOD and buccal fillings would score 4, reflecting the greater severity of disease. A tooth extracted because of caries would score 5 with the DMF-S; that is, all five surfaces missing. In the case of children a very similar caries index is used with the letters def(t) or def(s) where e stands for extracted teeth rather than those exfoliated in the normal way.

Age

It is a common clinical impression, supported by several surveys, that caries affects children and adolescents more than adults. Since the DMF scores are cumulative and show the total caries experience throughout life they must, by definition, increase with age. However, the increase is very rapid between tooth eruption and the second decade of life, after which it begins to slow down.

In the UK the first survey undertaken on children's teeth was undertaken in 1973 and published by Todd in 1975. It revealed the following facts.

- 63% of 5-year-olds had active caries on some of their deciduous teeth.
- 57% of 15-year-olds had active caries on some of their permanent teeth.
- 88% of 15-year-olds had some of their permanent teeth filled.
- 33% of 15-year-olds had had one or more extractions for caries.

More recently, reductions in the incidence of caries have been reported in the 1993 survey published by O'Brien in 1995. The caries incidence figures for the national surveys undertaken 1973, 1983 and 1993 were compared. Amongst the information published is the following.

- In 1973, 71% of 5-year-olds had experienced caries, but this had dropped to 48% in 1983. In 1993 similar rates of decay were noted.
- In 1973 the average 5-year-old child had had caries affecting 3.4 teeth, by 1983 this figure had dropped to 1.7. Similar rates were reported in the 1993 survey.
- In 1973 the average 15-year-old had had caries affecting 8.4 teeth, but by 1983 this figure was only 5.7. In the 1993 survey this figure had dropped to 2.2.

Other data from the 1993 survey indicate that the incidence of dental caries in the UK is in decline although it does highlight the plight of children in social groups IV and V which includes many living in cities, amongst whom it is rising. This perhaps is where dental promotional campaigns need to be concentrated in the future.

An area of concern for members of the dental team which has been highlighted by the 1993 child dental health survey is the rise in dental erosion seen in children's teeth. This is due to the rapid rise in the consumption of carbonated drinks and colas which frequently have quite a low pH. Dental hygienists must warn parents of this danger when they advise on the mouth care of children. This is covered in Chapter 13.

Gender

Surveys have suggested the following.
- In the deciduous dentition, caries is slightly more prevalent in boys than girls.
- In the permanent dentition, caries is at first slightly more prevalent in girls than boys, but evens out in later life.

However, both these differences are small and neither is of any real significance. Several well conducted surveys have failed to support the popular belief that caries is more prevalent during pregnancy.

Geographical distribution

Although there is evidence of caries in the human skulls of the Neolithic period (between 12 000 and 3000 years BC) it is essentially a disease of modern civilization and diet. A survey of the teeth of Alaskan Inuits in 1936 showed that those living in remote villages had 0.1% carious teeth, whereas those living near trading posts selling processed foods had 13% carious teeth. Another survey, in 1923, showed that among the indigenous population of Southern Rhodesia caries was present as follows.

- 5% of those who had only recently come in contact with European food.
- 20% of those who had been in contact with it for longer periods.
- 50% of those who had been in contact with it for most of their lives.

Other racial and geographical differences in caries incidence have been reported but, in general, these could be explained by variations in diet and oral hygiene standards. Fortunately, the incidence of dental caries in all developed or industrial countries like the UK and the USA is falling and this is thought to be due to improved dental awareness and the ubiquitous use of fluoride containing toothpastes. However, in disadvantaged sections of society in these countries the incidence is not falling but rising and this presents the challenge for dental professionals in the next decade or so.

Distribution within the mouth

Numerous studies have shown that the right and left halves of the dental arches are equally affected by caries, but roughly 60% of all caries occurs in the maxillary arch and 40% in the mandibular arch. There is a very marked variation in the susceptibility of individual teeth to caries, from an incidence of 95% in the first molars to 3% in the lower incisors. It is important to recognize which teeth are the more likely to become carious. The table of incidence reported by Brekhus (1931), following a survey in the USA in 1931, is given for reference purposes (Table 12.1).

The different surfaces of the teeth also vary considerably in their susceptibility to caries, and almost half of all carious lesions involve the occlusal surface. Of the remainder, more occur on the mesial and distal surfaces than on the lingual and buccal.

Table 12.1 Caries incidence of individual teeth

Teeth	Incidence of caries
First molars	95%
Second molars	75%
Upper second premolars	45%
Upper first premolars and lower second premolar	35%
Upper incisors	30%
Upper canines and lower first premolars	10%
Lower incisors and canines	3%

These figures were reported by P.I. Brekhus in 1931, based on a survey of 3711 students of the University of Minnesota.

Epidemiology is the study of disease prevalence within a population

- The DMF-S is a useful index in the measurement of caries in a given population.
- Caries incidence in the developed world is falling in all sections of society except the poorest where it is rising.
- With more refined diets, the chances of developing caries increase.
- The teeth which are least susceptible to develop dental caries are the lower incisors and canines.
- The most susceptible teeth are the first permanent molars.

Further reading

Brekhus P. J. (1931) A report of dental caries in 10,445 university students. *J. Am. Dent. Assoc.,* **18**, 13–50.

Grace A. M., Smales F. C. (1989) *Periodontal Control. An Effective System for Diagnosis, Selection, Control and Treatment Planning in General Practice.* London: Quintessence.

Mendieta C., Reeve C. M. (1993). Periodontal manifestations of systemic disease and management of patients with systemic disease. *Current Opinions in Periodontology,* 18–27.

O'Brien M. (1995) *Children's Dental Health in the United Kingdom.* London: HMSO.

Silness J., Loe H. (1964). Periodontal disease in pregnancy. 2: Correlation between oral hygiene and periodontal condition. *Acta Odont. Scand.,* **22**, 121–135.

Todd J. E. (1975) *Children's Dental Health in England and Wales, 1973.* London: HMSO.

Todd J. E., Dodd T. (1983) *Children's Dental Health in the United Kingdom, 1983.* London: HMSO.

13

Oral medicine

Introduction

Oral medicine is that aspect of dentistry that deals with the diagnosis and treatment of conditions that affect the oral mucosa and of oral manifestations of systemic disease together with the treatment of those patients who suffer from various types of facial pain.

The oral cavity cannot be treated in total isolation from the rest of the body. Just as certain oral conditions can have an effect on the whole body, so can general medical conditions affect the oral cavity in various ways. For this reason it is important to take a careful medical history before treatment (Table 13.1).

Table 13.1 The history

A detailed history can be of relevance to the dental hygienist in the following ways

- There are local conditions which produce oral signs, such as oral ulceration or white patches.
- There are systemic conditions such as iron deficiency anaemia and its associated glossitis which produce oral signs. Certain types of medication will induce changes that are seen in the mouth such as drug induced gingival hyperplasia.
- There are conditions which will affect the treatment which may be given, such as those requiring prophylactic antibiotic cover.
- There are conditions which may put the health of the dental hygienist at risk, such as hepatitis B.

The dental hygienist needs to be aware of those conditions which may present in the mouth because any treatment given might need to be modified. Indeed the hygienist might spot a suspicious lesion in the mouth which has developed since the dentist last examined the patient, in which case the dentist should be consulted again as to the most appropriate treatment for this lesion. It is most convenient to cover the various types of lesion that can present in the mouth under the following headings.

Oral ulceration

The most common disorder to affect oral mucosa is ulceration, although the reason for the ulceration may not always be immediately apparent. An ulcer may be defined as a break in the surface continuity of epithelium. When a patient presents with an ulcer it is necessary to find out how long it has been present, if there has been any trauma to the area and if they suffer from mouth ulcers on a regular basis. The ulcer is then examined and its size and position noted, together with the type of margin it presents. An ulcer with a raised, rolled and everted margin frequently proves to be malignant. It is the responsibility of the dental hygienist to inform the dentist of any suspicious ulcer found in the mouth so that it can be examined and a decision made on treatment. There are two reasons for this approach: the first is to exclude malignancy and the second is

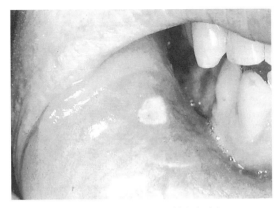

Fig. 13.1 A minor aphthous ulcer which had been present for about 5 days.

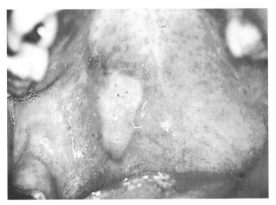

Fig. 13.2 A major aphthous ulcer on the soft palate which had been present for 3 weeks.

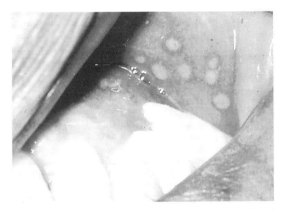

Fig. 13.3 Herptiform aphthae adjacent to a periodontal dressing.

to provide effective treatment and to quickly ease any pain. The presence of an oral ulcer may have two local effects; its presence will

limit efficient cleaning in the area, so this will lead to a local increase in plaque levels. This may then lead to increasing secondary bacterial contamination of the ulcer. Some of the more common types of oral ulceration will now be described.

Recurrent aphthous ulceration (RAU)

This is a common form of oral ulceration in which the ulcers recur frequently. It affects predominately young people of 10–30 years and is seen more commonly in females. The ulcers can vary in size from a few millimetres to over a centimetre in diameter and are most commonly found on non-keratinized mucosa (Figs 13.1–13.3). The hygienist should be careful to avoid any trauma to the mucosa in these patients as this may predispose to the formation of an ulcer. There are three types recognized (Table 13.2).

Table 13.2 Aphthous ulceration

Different types of recurrent aphthous ulceration are

- **Minor**: account for 80% of cases and last for about 10 days: Fig. 13.1.
- **Major**: account for 10% of cases, tend to be large and very painful and can last for several weeks: Fig. 13.2.
- **Herpetiform**: account for 10% of cases and last for about 10 days and are more common in females: Fig. 13.3.

Traumatic ulceration

This can be produced as a result of physical, chemical or thermal injury. Biting the mucosa of the cheek would be an example of physical injury. The once-common habit of placing an aspirin tablet next to a painful tooth would produce a chemical burn of the mucosa and a thermal burn can arise from hot sticky food, such as pizza, being eaten. Benzydamine mouthwash (Difflam) may help to reduce the discomfort in such cases.

Viral ulceration

Two groups are responsible for the majority of viral conditions that present to the dental clinician; the Herpes and Coxsackie viruses.

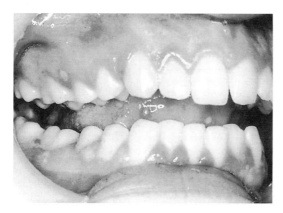

Fig. 13.4 Primary herpetic gingivostomatitis with characteristic ulcers throughout the mouth together with acute gingivitis.

Herpes simplex virus is responsible for primary (or acute) herpetic gingivostomatitis. Initial infection may be mild and produce very few symptoms or it may be severe with general widespread oral ulceration, causing extreme difficulty in eating, talking or cleaning the teeth. It is more commonly seen in children but can occasionally occur in adults. When the condition is severe the patient will feel ill, as though they have flu except that instead of a blocked nose and wheezy chest they will have a sore mouth and throat. In common with flu they will feel weak and will require lots of rest. The oral lesions of herpes start as multiple small vesicles (blisters) which rupture to form ulcers and can present on keratinized or non-keratinized mucosa (Fig. 13.4). These can last for up to 2 weeks. Acyclovir may be prescribed by the doctor or dentist and this helps to reduce the duration of the acute phase of the condition. Gentle rinsing of the mouth with Corsodyl® mouthwash will help to reduce plaque levels and secondary infection of the ulcers.

The other viral conditions which can affect oral mucosa are less common or severe. Herpangina is seen in children and affects the posterior part of the mouth and throat. It is caused by a Coxsackie virus but it is only a mild infection. Hand, foot and mouth disease is also seen in childhood and should not be confused with the foot and mouth disease that affects farm animals. Hand, foot and mouth disease produces oral ulcers together with red spots on the hands and feet. It can occur as an outbreak in primary schools and is very infectious. It is not particularly severe and requires only oral

swabbing with Corsodyl® to reduce plaque contamination of the oral ulcers. Both of these conditions should resolve in about a week.

Bullous conditions affecting the oral mucosa

A bulla is a large fluid filled vesicle that forms in epithelium or in the superficial connective tissues. These conditions are rare. Pemphigus vulgaris is an example of an intraepithelial bullous condition and benign mucous membrane pemphigoid a subepithelial bullous condition. The bullae often rupture to leave ulcers. The hygienist treating these patients will need to be very careful not to traumatize the oral mucosa as for example using cotton rolls in the sulcus can stimulate a bulla to form. The oral mucosa in these patients is often very fragile.

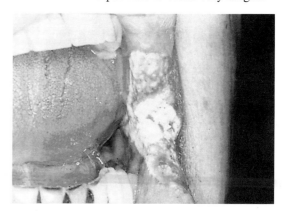

Fig. 13.5 Chronic hyperplastic candidosis affecting the left commissure of the lip.

White patches

The majority of white patches seen in the mouth are benign, but certain conditions may be premalignant or malignant. Unfortunately, it is difficult to decide which white patches are benign and therefore it is best to biopsy all white patches.

When a white patch (or keratosis) is seen it is advisable to see if a traumatic cause could be responsible such as cheek biting or placing an aspirin tablet next to the tooth. However, in someone who is a heavy smoker, smokers keratosis must be considered. This may be premalignant and so biopsy is mandatory. Infection with candidal organisms is another cause of white patches and in this case thrush, also known as acute pseudomembranous candidiasis, may be present and this occurs in patients taking broad spectrum antibiotics or using steroid inhalers to control asthma. Thrush may involve the soft palate in those who use a steroid inhaler. HIV infection in its late stages can be a further cause for oral thrush developing in young adult patients. Another infection seen in the mouth is chronic hyperplastic candidiasis and this is more common in the elderly patient (usually a denture wearer) and affecting the mucosa of both corners of the mouth (Fig. 13.5).

Premalignant and malignant conditions

There are about 2000 cases of oral cancer diagnosed each year in the UK. It is for this reason that patients over the age of 50 years should be screened regularly by a dentist, particularly if they are exposed to known risk factors such as smoking or excessive alcohol consumption. Often the first sign of neoplastic (malignant) change in the oral mucosa is a white patch. This is sometimes referred to as 'leukoplakia'. Widespread use of this term has resulted in it being associated with oral malignant change. However, the word leukoplakia means literally a 'white patch'. The most significant aetiological factors associated with leukoplakia, which subsequently develops into oral cancer, include tobacco usage, excessive alcohol consumption, nutritional deficiency and candidal infection. Microscopically the early histological changes are referred to as epithelial dysplasia and may be classified by the pathologist as mild, moderate or severe. Once the basal cell layer in the epithelium has been breached by malignant cells, the diagnosis of early squamous cell carcinoma can be made.

Squamous cell carcinoma

This is the commonest of all oral cancers and accounts for 1% of malignancies found in the body. It is more commonly found in lower socioeconomic groups and, as in the case of dental caries, is another reason for directing oral health promotional resources to this sector of the population. Dental team members must be vigilant when examining the mouth and look for any suspicious lesions that may need a

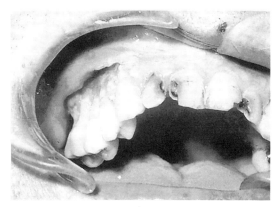

Fig. 13.6 Primary squamous cell carcinoma involving the gingiva of 16, 15 and 14.

biopsy to confirm the diagnosis. If a dental hygienist spots such a lesion then the advice of the dentist must be sought to decide the most appropriate next step in treatment (Fig. 13.6).

Once the diagnosis of squamous cell carcinoma has been confirmed by biopsy, various forms of treatment are available including surgery, radiotherapy, laser therapy and chemotherapy. These would all be provided in a hospital environment.

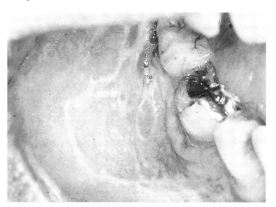

Fig. 13.7 Typical 'lace' pattern seen in lichen planus.

Lichen planus

Oral lichen planus is a condition of unknown aetiology which principally affects the buccal mucosa, but the tongue, lips and attached gingiva can also be affected. When it is seen on the buccal mucosa it appears commonly as an interlacing network of white striae (Fig. 13.7). When it affects the gingivae, they become very red or erythematous even when plaque control is excellent. As the aetiology is un-known, effective treatment can be elusive but it always includes oral hygiene therapy and sometimes steroid treatment. Some medication may produce a lichenoid reaction in the mouth and when this occurs it may be necessary to change this, after discussion of the case by the dentist with the doctor.

> Oral ulcers can be due to
> - Trauma.
> - Recurrent aphthlous ulceration including minor, major, herpetiform.
> - An acute viral condition (e.g. herpes simplex).
> - A bullous condition (e.g. pemphigus vulgaris).
> - Malignant change (e.g. squamous cell carcinoma).
>
> Any suspicious lesion must be seen by the dentist at the earliest opportunity. White patches must always be considered suspicious.

Systemic conditions presenting in the mouth

Many systemic conditions may have oral presentations. One of the more common conditions presenting oral signs and symptoms is anaemia; both iron deficiency and pernicious anaemia. The oral aspects of anaemias include a sore and burning sensation in the tongue which otherwise appears normal. Alternatively the tongue may become smooth and red, losing its papillae and is referred to as atrophic glossitis. Atrophic glossitis is seen in patients with severe anaemia and is now rarer than in the past. Candidiasis can aggravate anaemia and may be a presenting feature in these patients. There are many and varied presentations of systemic disease in the mouth and the dental hygienist who works with medically compromised patients can glean a greater insight into the oral manifestations of systemic disease from one of the standard textbooks written about this subject and reference to one of them is recommended.

Conditions affecting the gingiva

Various systemic and local conditions can affect the gingiva. The systemic ones which most frequently affect the gingiva do so by altering the host response to dental plaque which results in an exaggerated tissue response. A good example of this is seen in acute leukaemia where the gingival tissues may become swollen, pseudopockets form and the tissues may bleed spontaneously, this haemorrhage often being difficult to arrest. This condition is rare as the prognosis of acute leukaemia is generally poor. In diabetes mellitus, a condition where the regulation of glucose in the body is defective, there is also an increased incidence of periodontal pocketing. This is due to a defect in the function of polymorphonuclear leukocytes, specifically impaired chemotaxis and phagocytosis. Where there is a systemic condition present the resolution of the oral symptoms will be closely dependent on its successful treatment. However, the dental hygienist can often help the patient by giving advice on oral hygiene including using careful brushing and flossing techniques. The use of antiplaque mouthrinses such as chlorhexidine gluconate may also aid the patient with their mouth care.

The local conditions which produce gingival problems include localized gingival swellings (referred to as an epulis), overhangs from restorations and acute diseases which can involve the gingiva. These are acute (or primary) herpetic gingivostomatitis and acute necrotizing ulcerative gingivitis (both are covered in Chapter 11). A granulomatous epulis (also called the pyogenic granuloma) usually forms in response to some localized irritation of the gingiva such as calculus or an overhanging

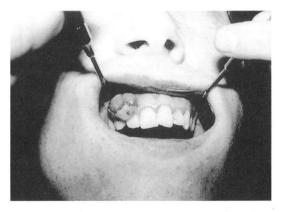

Fig. 13.8 Pregnancy epulis or pyogenic granuloma in a pregnant patient. The exacerbation of the pre-existing gingivitis is also noticeable.

restoration and is seen most commonly in pregnant women who have poor oral hygiene. For this reason it is referred to as a pregnancy epulis (Fig. 13.8). Treatment includes advising on good oral hygiene and removal of overhangs and calculus. If surgical removal is necessary this is best done by using electrosurgery to reduce the chances of excessive bleeding after excision.

There are other gingival swellings that can present which range from periapical granulomas on non-vital tooth to various cysts which can develop in the jaws. Nevertheless, any gingival swelling could be malignant in nature and the dentist should always be consulted when in doubt.

Drug induced gingival changes

Several types of medication can produce effects on the gingival tissues. The most well known is the gingival hyperplasia seen in patients taking phenytoin, an anti-epileptic medication (Fig. 13.9). A second group of drugs, the calcium channel blockers also produce gingival overgrowth, the commonest being nifedipine (Fig. 13.10). These drugs are used to control hypertension and angina. Cyclosporin may also produce gingival overgrowth (Fig. 13.11). This is taken to prevent rejection in transplant patients.

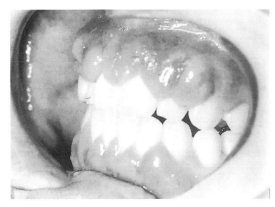
Fig. 13.10 Gingival hyperplasia seen in a patient taking nifedipine.

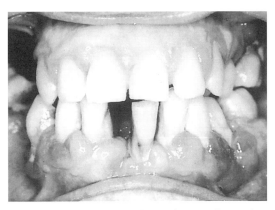
Fig. 13.11 Gingival hyperplasia seen in a renal transplant patient taking cyclosporin to prevent organ rejection.

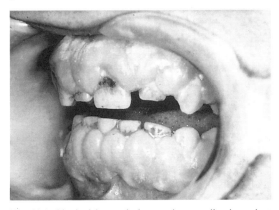
Fig. 13.9 Gingival hyperplasia seen in an epileptic patient taking phenytoin.

Once severe hyperplasia has occurred, the hygienist's role is to minimize plaque levels and improve home mouth care so that the dentist will be able to perform a gingivoplasty. After any gingival surgery the hygienists should supervise a good level of home mouth care to prevent the hyperplasia returning.

Conditions influencing hygienist treatment

There are a number of conditions that may alter the way that the hygienist carries out the treatment.

Rheumatic fever

Rheumatic fever is a condition that has been mentioned previously in this book. It is caused by a bacterial infection of the throat with *Streptococcus haemolyticus*. This organism produces an exotoxin which circulates in the blood stream and attaches itself to the synovial lining of the joints. This induces an autoimmune response leading to inflammation of the joints. In some cases the lining of the heart may be similarly involved and the heart valves may be permanently damaged. This is termed rheumatic heart disease and the damaged valves can be detected by the cardiac murmur which they cause.

Should a subsequent bacterial infection of the blood stream occur (i.e. a bacteraemia), particularly if this involves *Streptococcus viridans*, a common oral micro-organism, further damage to the valves may result. This is known as infective endocarditis and is a serious condition which can be fatal. It has been shown that various dental procedures, such as tooth extraction and scaling, can result in *Strep. viridans* from the oral cavity entering the blood stream and, for this reason, patients who have had rheumatic heart disease are given antibiotic prophylaxis before extractions, scalings, or treatment likely to cause a bacteraemia. The antibiotic prophylaxis required is discussed in more detail in Chapter 22.

Obviously it is a very serious matter to give a patient repeated antibiotics throughout life and so prophylactic cover should only be given where necessary: for example for scaling and not for other procedures such as fissure sealing or polishing.

Certain other types of patients may also require antibiotic cover: those who have functional heart murmurs or congenital heart defects and those who have had valvular surgery. There is an ever-increasing number of patients with artificial joint replacements and the current advice in the British National Formulary is that they do not require antibiotic prophylaxis but not all orthopaedic surgeons agree. On these matters, the dental hygienist must be guided by the dentist under whose direction they are working. The dentist, in turn, may well ask for the advice of the patient's general medical practitioner or hospital consultant.

Pregnancy

Pregnancy can affect the treatment given by the dental hygienist in several ways.

- **Chair position**: consideration should be given to the patient's comfort, especially during the final trimester. Being treated in a horizontal position is often uncomfortable at this stage. It may also be necessary to reduce the length of the appointments.
- **Scaling and polishing**: the condition of the patient's gingiva may be such that more numerous and more frequent appointments will be necessary throughout the pregnancy.
- **Medication**: it is recommended that metronidazole should not be used during pregnancy and tetracycline, which would stain the infant's primary teeth, should be avoided.

Pregnancy can cause a marked gingivitis to occur. This is referred to as 'pregnancy gingivitis' and it tends to become more florid as the patient progresses towards full term. The gingival tissues become inflamed and bleed more on brushing (Fig. 13.8). It is thought to be due to the gingival tissues becoming more permeable to the harmful effects of dental plaque, due to the hormonal changes that occur during pregnancy. The way to control it is to improve oral hygiene and it is helpful to reassure the patient that good plaque control will help it to resolve the condition.

Drug induced gingival hyperplasia can be caused by

- **Phenytoin**: a medication used to control seizures in epileptic patients.
- **Nifedipine**: a medication used to control hypertension and regulate cardiac function.
- **Cyclosporin**: a medication used to prevent rejection in transplant patients.

Antibiotic prophylaxis is needed for certain categories of patients.

Various factors need to be considered when treating pregnant patients.

- Chair position.
- More frequent scaling and polishing.
- Metronidazole and tetracyclines are contraindicated in pregnancy.
- Pregnancy gingivitis may occur in some women.

Bleeding disorders

Severe bleeding disorders, such as haemophilia

(which is due to a deficiency of the clotting factor VIII: also known as antihaemophilic globulin) or Christmas disease (which is due to a deficiency of clotting factor IX, also known as Christmas factor) would normally contraindicate treatment outside special units. The responsibility of caring for such patients rests with specialists in their field, but any dental hygienist called on to treat such patients must ensure that the scaling technique is as atraumatic as possible.

Patients with minor bleeding disorders may well be treated in dental practice, but in all cases the supervising dentist would give guidance, having where necessary discussed treatment with the medical practitioner. This also applies to the growing group of patients who are taking anticoagulants after a recent heart attack or stroke: a careful atraumatic technique is essential.

Some patients who have had a stroke or heart attack are prescribed aspirin on a daily basis. This helps to 'thin the blood' by affecting the function of platelets so that clots are less likely to form. This may increase gingival bleeding slightly after scaling but the usual local measures will arrest it.

Other conditions influencing treatment

There are many other conditions which cause treatment procedures being altered or adapted, some of them in a very minor way. Such conditions include infection by human immunodeficiency viruses, mental and physical disability, old age and general ill health. A further condition of particular significance to the dental hygienist is the presence of an artificial cardiac pacemaker. This is being fitted to an ever-increasing number of patients who have had a heart attack resulting in cardiac arrhythmias. It is recommended that the ultrasonic scaler should not be used on such patients because of the risk of upsetting the rhythm of the pacemaker. In addition those patients wearing a hearing aid may not tolerate use of the ultrasonic scaler.

Care should be taken with patients who are receiving or have received steroids in the past year. They will often be less able to withstand stressful situations such as dental treatment without additional steroid support. Steroids are anti-inflammatory drugs used to control conditions such as rheumatoid arthritis and asthma and since they reduce the inflammatory response, they reduce the tissue resistance to infection. The supervising dentist will probably seek direction or assistance from the patient's medical practitioner before treating these patients.

Conditions which might put the dental hygienist's health at risk

Dental hygienists must be vigilant when treating patients who have a condition which could be transmitted to the clinician.

Hepatitis

This may be caused by a number of viruses, of which hepatitis B and C are the most important. Further details are given in Chapter 7.

Human immunodeficiency viruses

Two viruses have been identified to date and the reader is referred to Chapter 7 for more details of these and the appropriate precautions.

Other conditions

The dental hygienist works in close proximity to patients and so the risks of contacting any infective condition tend to be greater than for anyone else. For this reason, all hygienists wear protective facemasks and spectacles, especially when using the ultrasonic scaler (Table 13.3).

- Patients with haemophilia and Christmas disease will probably require dental treatment, including scaling, in hospital.
- Patients with pacemakers and hearing aids should not be exposed to the ultrasonic scaler.
- Hygienists must wear facemasks and protective spectacles at all times when scaling and polishing.

Table 13.3 Infective conditions

Infective conditions which carry risk for the hygienist include

- Those which are relatively minor in their effects, such as the common cold and influenza. It is useful to remember that nasal secretions have been shown to be positive for hepatitis B and hepatitis C in carriers of these viruses. The dental hygienist must ensure that universal precautions for infection control are observed.
- Those more major conditions for which preventive measures exist, such as tuberculosis. In view of the working environment, the hygienist really ought to take advantage of all available immunization procedures. Tuberculosis incidence is on the increase particularly amongst the destitute and in people from certain ethnic groups. There is also a strain of tuberculosis which is now resistant to most drugs and this presents a very worrying development for all health care workers.
- Those other conditions for which no adequate preventive measures exist, such as syphilis. Fortunately normal careful surgery hygiene should provide adequate protection from most of these conditions. However, if any unusual ulcers or other lesions are observed in the oral cavity the advice of the supervising dentist should be sought.

Further reading

British National Formulary, published by the British Medical Association every six months.

Lamey P. J., Lewis M. A. O. (1997) *A Clinical Guide to Oral Medicine*. Basingstoke: BDJ Books.

Scully S., Cawson, R. A. (1993) *Medical Problems in Dentistry*. 3rd edition. Oxford: Wright.

14

Abnormalities of the teeth

Introduction

In this chapter, abnormalities of the teeth (other than caries) are discussed. It is usually sufficient for the dental hygienist only to recognize the condition and understand the terminology, but those conditions which are felt to be of clinical relevance are discussed in greater detail.

Tooth surface wear

The use of the term 'tooth surface wear' has become popular in the last few years and it is used to describe tooth tissue loss due to erosion, attrition and abrasion. It does not replace these terms but is used before a definitive diagnosis can be made, usually at the patient's first visit.

Erosion

Erosion is the removal of tooth substance by chemical means, usually by acids. Erosion is almost always caused by acid from one of three sources: hydrochloric acid regurgitated from the stomach, acids from the diet, or from acid atmospheric pollution in the workplace. Regurgitation is not unusual in the elderly where chronic indigestion and hiatus hernia may be present, but it is also seen in anorexia nervosa and this may be reason for abnormal tooth wear in a young person. The affected surfaces appear smooth and highly polished. They

gradually lose their individual distinguishing features and may eventually develop shallow depressions (Fig. 14.1).

Erosion is most commonly associated with the frequent consumption of acidic foodstuffs: the habitual drinking of carbonated drinks or regular sucking of citrus fruits. It used to be a relatively common hazard in industries in which acids were used (such as plating, galvanizing, pickling, engraving, battery manufacturing and crystal glassworks) due to the inhalation of acidic fumes. However, industrial health regulations have eliminated most of these problems in the UK.

An increasing cause of erosion in modern times is chronic vomiting, where gastric hydrochloric acid comes into contact with the teeth, particularly the palatal surfaces of the upper teeth (Fig. 14.2). A form of anorexia nervosa, called bulimia, in which vomiting is self-induced after meals in an effort to achieve weight loss without curbing the appetite, is becoming more prevalent in modern society. Erosion is also seen in patients suffering from hiatus hernia with reflux of gastric contents into the mouth. Those with this problem may present with marked palatal erosion.

Dental erosion may also be seen in older people suffering from dry mouth because the flow of saliva is much reduced. Patients who might at one time have eaten several items of fruit per day with no ill effects now suffer from erosion due to the loss of the protective functions of saliva. Chronic alcoholism may also allow regurgitation to occur although the

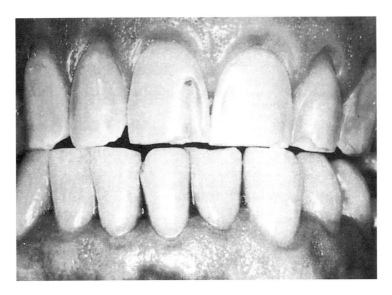

Fig. 14.1 Erosion of the anterior teeth caused by frequent eating of citrus fruits.

individual may be unaware of it. The popular image of the chronic alcoholic being a derelict is true for a small minority who would very rarely seek dental treatment, the discrete middle class alcoholic is much more likely to seek dental advice for the problems of tooth wear.

Attrition

This is wear caused by tooth-to-tooth contact. It may be seen if the diet has a very abrasive component or if the teeth are used for masticating very tough food such as natural Inuit or aborigine populations. It is commonly seen in developed countries or when clenching or tooth grinding habits are taking place (Fig. 14.3). These habits are very complex in nature and 'bruxism' is a combination of dental, emotional, occupational and systemic factors. Attrition is commonly seen as wear facets which are small polished areas on enamel surfaces where heavy tooth contact is occurring. Once dentine is exposed, and especially if acid erosion is also present, then 'cupping' will occur as dentine is worn away more quickly.

Primary teeth, being relatively softer than permanent teeth, are more susceptible to attrition and are often quite markedly worn by the time they are shed.

Variations in the severity of attrition may be related to differing dietary habits or even to certain occupations (such as mining) where

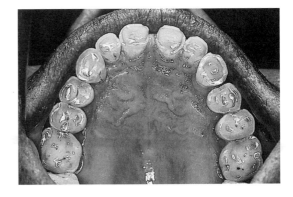

Fig. 14.2 Marked erosion in a patient who suffers from gastric acid reflux. Typically the upper palatal surfaces are more effected than the buccal.

abrasive dust may become mixed in the saliva. Men usually show a greater degree of attrition than women.

Occasionally, with advancing age, attrition may result in the loss of the full thickness of enamel, with exposure of dentine, which often becomes stained. In some cases this exposed dentine may be sensitive, but more usually the attrition progresses so slowly that the formation of secondary or sclerotic dentine prevents sensitivity from developing.

Attrition may be increased greatly by parafunctional habits such as tooth grinding.

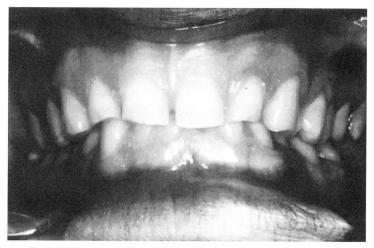

Fig. 14.3 Marked attrition of the anterior teeth resulting from bruxism.

Abrasion

This is the progressive loss of hard tooth substance caused by mechanical factors other than mastication or tooth-to-tooth contacts (Table 14.1). Examples of this include destructive toothbrushing techniques (Fig. 14.4) and habits such as pipe smoking, where the pipe is continually held in the mouth. Abrasion due to working in a dust polluted environment is less commonly seen now as a result of improved working conditions. Such conditions may still be found in coal mines or brick works and may be seen in employees who fail to wear protective masks.

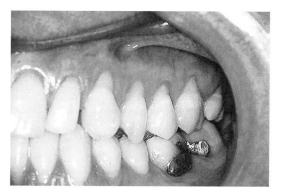

Fig. 14.4 Marked abrasion caused by aggressive toothbrushing.

Types of tooth wear

- Erosion: the removal of tooth substance by chemicals usually acids.
- Attrition: wear as a result of tooth-to-tooth contact.
- Abrasion: loss of hard tooth substance caused by mechanical factors.

Management of tooth wear

The management of a patient who presents with tooth wear has two phases. The first is to monitor the progression of wear using serial study models and clinical photographs and during this time take all steps possible to prevent further deterioration. Secondly, active intervention if the wear is found to be progressing to the extent that any further tissue loss is going to be difficult to restore. After careful treatment planning and, if possible, correction of aetiological factors, reconstruction of the worn dentition should be considered.

Parafunctional activity may vary from bruxism to digit-sucking or the chewing of pens and pencils. Bruxism is the term for the abnormal grinding of the teeth and can often be detected in patients who are unaware of the habit, by the degree of wear seen (Fig. 14.3). Bruxism may be related to stress and often happens only during sleep. Parafunctional habits usually result in attrition but when wear is caused by foreign objects, such as the holding of tacks between the teeth, then abrasion will occur (Table 14.2).

Table 14.1 Tooth abrasion

The main causes of tooth abrasion are

- **Toothbrush abrasion:** the aggressive use of a toothbrush, particularly if used with an unnecessarily abrasive paste and a horizontal scrubbing action, can result in cervical abrasion. The enamel of the tooth, being harder, tends to be little affected, but any exposed dentine at the cervical margin can become rapidly worn, with a smooth, shiny, horizontal furrow developing. If this is observed, the patient's toothbrushing habits must be examined and altered as necessary.
- **Foreign objects:** teeth may be abraded by objects such as pipes which may wear teeth where they rest, chiefly on occlusal surfaces. The holding of pens, tacks, nails and pins will lead to characteristic notching.

Table 14.2 Parafunction

Parafunction means altered or abnormal function. It may be classified in three ways according to the cause

---

- Tooth-to-tooth function.
- Tooth to soft tissue.
- Tooth to foreign object.

Developmental abnormalities

Tooth size

The terms 'microdontia' and 'macrodontia' are used to describe teeth which are respectively abnormally small or abnormally large. Generalized microdontia or macrodontia are quite unusual conditions but on occasions the teeth may be of normal size and yet appear to be small or large in relation to abnormally sized jaws. Microdontia of individual teeth is a common condition: the teeth most commonly affected are the third molars and the upper permanent laterals. When the laterals are affected they often have small conically shaped crowns and are referred to as peg laterals.

Tooth number

Although not common, it is by no means rare to find additional teeth present in the dentition. These are termed supernumerary teeth. Usually, supernumeraries are smaller than normal and they may be abnormally formed. The commonest site for such teeth is the midline of the maxillary arch between the permanent central incisors. This type of supernumerary is called a mesiodens (Fig. 14.5). Many of these teeth do not erupt.

The failure of teeth to develop is called anodontia. Complete anodontia is extremely rare and only occurs in conjunction with other severe hereditary defects. However, hypodontia or partial anodontia which implies the absence of one or two teeth, is common. The teeth most often found to be missing are the third molars, upper permanent laterals and second premolars, in that order.

Tooth shape

It is usually enough for the dental hygienist to recognize the various terms applied to abnormalities of tooth form.

Dilaceration

This indicates a sharp, abnormal bend or curve in the root or crown of a tooth and is a relatively common abnormality.

Gemination

This results from the attempted division of a single tooth germ into two teeth and usually presents as two crowns, partially or completely separated, with a single root. It is not common.

Fusion

This is the reverse of gemination in which two normally separate teeth become joined together. The degree of union depends on the stage of development at the time of union. It is also uncommon.

Concrescence

This is a form of fusion which occurs after the roots of the teeth have fully formed. The teeth

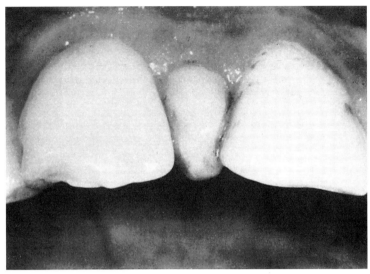

Fig. 14.5 A mesiodens which has erupted between the central incisors.

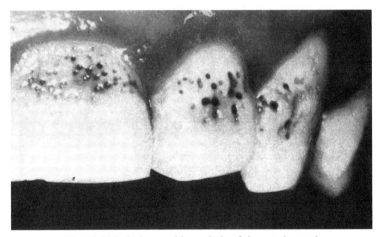

Fig. 14.6 Marked enamel hypoplasia of the anterior teeth.

become joined by cementum only.

Odontomes

This is a term applied to the irregularity of teeth which may vary from an unusually shaped tooth to a totally unrecognizable calcified mass (which does not usually erupt). A compound odontome contains rudimentary teeth or denticles and a complex odontome consists of a disorganized mass of dental tissue.

Tooth structure

Hypoplasia (or incomplete formation) of the tooth may affect either enamel (enamel hypoplasia) or dentine (dentine hypoplasia) or both. Usually this condition is relatively mild, with a few small pits and grooves, often stained, on the surface of one or two teeth (Fig. 14.6). There is a very rare condition in which generalized severe hypoplasia occurs, termed amelogenesis imperfecta.

The cause of dental hypoplasia is usually obscure, but several possibilities exist. It has been suggested that hypoplasia of individual teeth may result from infection of the developing tooth, for example from an abscess affecting its deciduous predecessor, or from trauma, as might result from extraction of the deciduous predecessor. Systemic conditions such as the childhood fevers (measles, chickenpox, etc.) have also been incriminated and this type of cause would be supported by the observations that, when several teeth are affected, the parts of the various teeth affected are those which would all be developing at any one time. The antibiotic tetracycline, if given at the time of development of the crowns, may also cause enamel hypoplasia.

Of particular interest to the dental hygienist is the hypomineralization which is seen in fluorosis. In mild fluorosis, such as is seen in areas with approximately two parts per million fluoride in drinking water (2 p.p.m.), mottling of the teeth is seen. This is mild and usually not disfiguring. Where the fluoride level is higher (5 p.p.m. and above) the enamel may be grossly affected with pitting and brown staining giving rise to severe enamel hypoplasia.

Abnormalities of tooth formation

- Tooth size: microdontia or macrodontia.
- Tooth number: supernumaries or hypodontia.
- Tooth shape: dilaceration, gemination, fusion, concrescence, odontomes.
- Tooth structure: hypoplasia.

Further reading

Ash, M. M. (1992) *Oral pathology: an introduction to general and oral pathology for hygienists.* 6th edition. Philadelphia: Lea Febiger.

Ibsen O. A. C., Phelan J. A. (1992) *Oral pathology for the dental hygienist.* 2nd edition. Philadelphia: Saunders.

Miller R. L. (1995) *General and oral pathology for the dental hygienist.* London: Mosby.

Scully C. M. (1994) *Color atlas of oral diseases in children and adolescents.* London: Wolfe Medical Publications.

Tyldesley W. R., Field E. A. (1995) *Oral Medicine.* Oxford: Oxford Medical Publications.

15

Dentine sensitivity

Introduction

The term 'dentine hypersensitivity' is often used to describe the condition in which pain is felt when mild stimuli are applied to apparently normal dentine exposed at the cervical margin of the tooth. While it is true that exposed dentine can be exquisitely sensitive, it is common to find areas of gingival recession, sometimes quite extensive, which are entirely symptomless. In Chapter 6, the fact that dentine is a naturally highly sensitive tissue was discussed; a fact which would be all too obvious to anyone who had a tooth drilled without local analgesic cover! For this reason, many of those involved in this field feel that the term 'dentine sensitivity' is to be preferred to 'dentine hypersensitivity'.

Clinical features of dentine sensitivity

Dentine sensitivity is no new phenomenon. As long ago as 1884, P. Calvo wrote in 'Dental Cosmos': *'There is a great need of a medicament, which while lessening the sensibility of dentine, will not impair the vitality of the pulp'*.

It has been estimated that the incidence of dentine sensitivity in the dentate population can be a high as 30% (Table 15.1).

Stimuli

Patients may complain of pain being caused by a wide variety of everyday stimuli: hot or cold foodstuffs, sweet substances, toothbrushing and even light touch. Cold is the most frequently implicated factor, with as many as 75% of patients suffering from this condition complaining that cold, either alone or in combination with other stimuli is the principal cause. In contrast, few patients complain of pain resulting from hot stimuli alone.

Pain

Classically, the pain induced in sensitive dentine is sharp, severe and of short duration. It develops immediately the stimulus is applied and ceases when this stimulus is removed. The quality of the pain is the same, whether caused by cold, touch or sweet foodstuffs. Only heat elicits a different quality of pain; developing more slowly and lasting for a time after heat is removed.

By definition, dentine has to be exposed to the oral environment for dentine sensitivity to occur. However, the term is only applied to situations where no pathology (such as dental caries) exists. Sensitivity of dentine associated with abrasion and erosion is becoming more prevalent, but the commonest site for such sensitivity remains the cervical margin of the tooth. Gingival recession must have occurred to expose part of the root surface, but the degree of recession is not related to the incidence of sensitivity. Severe symptoms commonly occur where minimal gingival recession has occurred and commonly quite extensive areas of exposed root are entirely symptomless.

Table 15.1 Dentine sensitivity

The clinical significance of dentine sensitivity

- **Quality of life.** For some individuals, the discomfort can significantly reduce the pleasure gained from certain foods and drinks and may even restrict outdoor activities in cold weather.
- **Oral hygiene.** Cervical sensitivity can impair plaque control, with the risk of development of periodontal disease. This in turn might lead to progressive gingival recession, with further exposure of dentine. There is also evidence that plaque accumulation on exposed dentine is liable to make the sensitivity worse.
- **Dental treatment.** No one who has worked as a dental hygienist needs reminding that root sensitivity can preclude thorough scaling and polishing, without the use of local analgesia.

Distribution

Most investigations report that cervical sensitivity is almost exclusively found on the buccal and labial surfaces. It is also more common in the canine and premolar regions than elsewhere and it has been suggested that this distribution might be linked to the possibility of excessive toothbrushing in these areas.

The level of sensitivity in any given site varies a good deal with time; at times severe and at other times absent. Although occasionally an individual site may be particularly troublesome, the commonest picture is of pain which moves from site to site and which varies in severity.

Sensitive dentine can be found in patients of any age from mid-teens onwards. It is, however, most prevalent in young adults; particularly between the ages of 15 and 35 years. There is a tendency for the problem to be more common amongst women than men.

Clinical significance of dentine sensitivity
- reduced quality of life
- interference with oral hygiene
- need for local analgesia for dental treatment.

Types of causative stimuli: cold, touch chemical and heat.

Quality of pain
- with cold, touch or chemical stimulation a sudden, sharp pain of brief duration
- with heat, a gradually increasing throbbing pain, lasting longer than the stimulus.

Distribution
- commonest on buccal surfaces of canine and premolar teeth
- most prevalent between ages of 15 and 35 years
- more common amongst women than men.

Aetiology

Undoubtedly, the pain felt by those suffering from dentine sensitivity is due to stimulation of the nerves of the pulp of the tooth with transmission from the pulpal nerves to the brain. How the pulpal nerves are excited by the various stimuli applied to the outer surface of the dentine remains something of an enigma. In Chapter 6 possible mechanisms of transmission through the dentine are suggested. The hydrodynamic hypothesis is currently the most plausible.

Despite the fact that Sir John Tomes wrote in 1856: '*The Dentinal Tubules are constantly filled by fluid, pressure made upon the fluid at the exposed end of the tubes is felt by the pulp at their inner extremities*', it was not until the 1960s that Brannstromm showed that stimuli which cause pain when applied to the dentine also produce movement of the fluid through dentine.

When the outer surface of dentine is exposed to the oral cavity, there is a slow, steady outward flow of pulpal fluid through the tubules into the oral cavity. It is suggested that, when the rate of flow of the fluid changes, stimulation of the pulpal nerve endings might occur. It has been demonstrated that some of the pulpal nerve endings projects a short distance into the dentinal tubules, where they are closely associated with the odontoblastic processes. A sudden increase in the rate of flow of fluid could, it is suggested, 'suck' the odontoblast against the inner opening of the tubule, making it impinge on the trapped nerve ending.

Support is given to this theory by the fact that all of the main stimuli, cold, sweet solutions and probing can dramatically increase the rate of outward flow of the fluid in the tubules as the following points confirm.

- **The application of cold** causes contraction of the fluid in the outer parts of the tubules, which in turn draws further fluid from the pulp.
- **Sweet solutions** have the same effect through osmosis; i.e. the attraction of water from a dilute solution into a more concentrated one with a view to equating their strengths.
- **Touch**, for example, by placing a dental probe on the root surface, sets up surface tension, thus sucking fluid out of the microscopic tubules.

Since the ultimate response to these three totally different types of stimuli is the same, this might explain why they all produce identical types of pain.

As noted already, heat is the one stimulus which appears to produce a different quality of pain from the others. When heat is applied to the root surface, it will cause expansion of the fluid. The flow of fluid initially slows, then stops and eventually reverses direction. Once again, this conveniently matches the observation that the pain caused by heat is slower to develop and slower to revert to normality when the heat is removed.

Since dentine is a naturally sensitive tissue, yet not all exposed dentine is sensitive, it might be more valuable to investigate why such areas are not sensitive, rather than why others are. Electron microscopy has shown that where dentine is sensitive there are always patent tubules opening onto the outer surface, whereas in other areas the tubules are frequently occluded by sclerotic dentine, irregular secondary dentine, calculus, or a smear layer. Such findings further support the hydrodynamic theory since blockage of the tubules would prevent fluid flow.

Aetiology of dentine sensitivity

The details of the hydrodynamic theory.
The effects of various stimuli
- cold (contraction of the fluid within the dentinal tubules)
- touch (surface tension)
- sweet solutions (osmotic pressure)
- heat (expansion of the fluid within the dentinal tubules).

Treatment of dentine sensitivity

In 1908, GV Black observed that *'obtundants have been tried by hundreds of dentists and then faded out of the memory of men. Such has been the fate of every obtundant for sensitive dentine that has come forward during 70 or more years of dental practice.'* Despite the large amount of research aimed at improving the clinical management of dentine sensitivity, the treatment is still largely empirical, poorly understood and ill defined. A large number of substances have been recommended for topical application to the dentine surface; including arsenic (for which there might be difficulty obtaining a product licence in modern times) and phenol (which might well have had its effect by killing the pulp). For the sake of discussion, treatment methods can be divided into three main headings: surface barriers, topical agents and dentifrices.

Surface barriers

Various adhesives and resins have been applied to the dentine surface as protective barriers.

Fluoride varnishes

Varnishes such as Duraphat® and Cervitek® appear to have a beneficial effect. Whether this is due to the varnish itself or the fluoride content is unclear. It is often necessary to repeat the application from time to time if the effectiveness wears off.

Siloxane esters

Substances such as Tresiolan, have been used in the past. They polymerize on moist surfaces, but they too are quickly abraded and tend to leave the surface as sensitive as it was before.

Glass ionomer cements and resins

When bonded on to the tooth surface these are more robust materials and undoubtedly have a place in the management of localized, severe, persistent dentine sensitivity. Unfortunately, they are difficult to apply in areas of minimal gingival recession. In cases where the recession is more extensive, further gingival recession after the application of the material may well result in recurrence of the sensitivity. Furthermore, such treatment is less suited to the management of more widespread and transient dentine sensitivity.

Topical applications

As noted already, a wide range of obtundants, including phenol, zinc chloride, silver nitrate and arsenic have been used in the past. Since these agents, in general, tend to cause unacceptable damage to the pulp and gingivae, their use cannot now be recommended.

Salts containing calcium or strontium ions have been applied to the dentine surface in an attempt at plugging the patent openings of the dentinal tubules. Such salts have been applied as pastes or burnished onto the tooth surface with reported benefits, although their long-term effectiveness is doubtful. In addition, the burnishing procedure can be very uncomfortable and may even contraindicate this approach.

Dentifrices

Probably more research has been devoted to dentifrices than to any other form of desensitizing treatment. The use of dentifrices has three distinct advantages (Table 15.2).

- Repeated application of agents with a short-term effectiveness can be achieved.
- Repeated applications of some agents is reported to have a cumulative effect.
- The abrasive or filler of the dentifrice may block the patent tubules for a time after each brushing session.

Table 15.2 Desensitizing agents

Desensitizing agents found in dentifrices

- 10% strontium chloride.
- 5% potassium nitrate.
- 5.53% potassium citrate.
- 2% sodium citrate.
- various fluoride salts.

Strontium

The principal behind using strontium ions is similar to that referred to under the heading of 'Topical applications'. Strontium ions will replace calcium in the crystalline structure of the dentine and it is suggested that, in so doing, they gradually occlude the dentinal tubules. A single application of strontium chloride is clinically ineffective and the purpose of incorporating it in a dentifrice is to achieve a long-term cumulative benefits.

Potassium

The theory behind the addition of potassium ions to toothpaste is that potassium blocks nerve transmission. A problem associated with this theory is that the outward flow of fluid in the dentinal tubules would tend to act as a barrier to the potassium ion reaching the nerve endings at the pulpal end of the tubule. Recent work has suggested that the potassium ions might have a direct effect on the odontoblastic process causing the release of nitric oxide at the pulpal surface of the dentine; this in turn would have an analgesic effect on the nerve endings.

Fluoride

The addition of fluoride to desensitizing dentifrices is important from the point of view of caries prevention in relation to exposed root surfaces. However, there is evidence that the fluoride itself contributes to a reduction in dentine sensitivity.

Formalin

Until relatively recently desensitizing dentifrices containing formalin were available. The inclusion of formalin in toothpaste was designed to reduce the vitality and activity of the odontoblastic processes by mummifying them. However, the suggestion that these processes conduct painful stimuli has been largely discounted. Furthermore, a number of patients reported problems with allergic reactions to the formalin, which resulted in the withdrawal of such products.

Research into the effectiveness of the various agents used to manage dentine sensitivity has been complicated by a number of factors, including the variability of the discomfort in any given site, the difficulty in standardizing the different stimuli used to excite discomfort and the wide range of stimuli involved. Perhaps the greatest complication, however, is the placebo effect which is so noticeable in the management of dentine sensitivity. Even water, when used under test conditions can produce a reduction in sensitivity of up to 25%!

What is clear is that further research is required to discover an agent which has no undesirable effects and which is consistently effective over a long period of time, either by blocking the dentinal tubules or by producing a favourable defensive reaction within the pulp. GV Black's 1908 statement is as valid today as it was when he made it; '*But the relief of suffering is an ever present duty and the search for this very desirable thing should continue*'.

Treatment of dentine sensitivity
Surface barrier agents.
- fluoride varnishes
- siloxane esters
- glass ionomer cements and resins.
Topical applications.
- Dentifrices
- active ingredients: strontium, potassium, fluoride, formalin.

Further reading

Addy M., West N. (1994) Etiology, mechanisms and management of dentine hypersensitivity. *Current Opinion in Periodontology*, 71–77.

Orchardson R., Gangarosa, L. P. (1994) Hypersensitive dentine: biological basis of therapy. *Arch Oral Biol* (Supplement), 1S–153S.

16

Emergencies in the dental surgery

Responsibilities of the dental hygienist in an emergency

Although in the UK dental hygienists are permitted only to carry out specified dental work under the direction of a dental surgeon who has previously examined the patient, this regulation cannot be taken to limit the responsibility of a dental hygienist in an emergency, nor to excuse being inadequately trained and prepared to handle an emergency situation, should one arise. When working under the direct supervision of a dentist, the dental hygienist's duties in an emergency are clear:

- recognition of an emergency and summoning assistance,
- immediate first-aid treatment of that emergency,
- assisting with subsequent treatment.

However, in a situation in which the supervising dentist is not immediately on hand the hygienist must be prepared to take charge of the situation and be responsible for the management of the patient.

Emergencies and their management

Fainting

Fainting, or syncope, is the commonest cause of loss of consciousness that occurs in the dental surgery. It is estimated that as many as 1 patient in 200 faints or feels faint whilst attending the dental clinic. Clearly the dental hygienist must recognize the early signs of fainting and take appropriate action and in order to do this a knowledge of the cause of the condition is needed.

Clinical features

Initially the patient becomes pale, sweaty and distressed and may complain of dizziness, confusion, nausea and weakness. The pulse will become thin and rapid. This should be tested in the neck rather than the wrist since the carotid pulse is the stronger and will be more easily detected in the collapsed patient. Gradually consciousness may be lost and there may be muscle twitching or even convulsions.

Aetiology

The cause of fainting is a lack of oxygen and nutrients reaching the brain because of a reduced blood supply to the head. In Chapter 3, when discussing the sympathetic nervous system and the secretion of adrenaline from the adrenal glands, the so-called 'fight-or-flight' reaction was discussed. If sympathetic stimulation or adrenaline secretion is strong enough, then fainting will occur. Because of the increased distribution of blood to the peripheral circulation (e.g. to skeletal muscle) the supply to the brain becomes inadequate. Various factors may increase the likelihood of a patient fainting in the dental chair, including fear, pain, hunger, stuffiness of the room and posture, although modern dental chairs are better in this respect than their earlier counterparts.

Treatment

The first action, when a patient feels faint or has actually fainted, is to adjust the chair so that they are lying flat with the feet raised slightly higher than the head. This is the single most important action and alone is usually sufficient to revive the patient. In situations where this is not possible, such as in a theatre or church, it is common to place the individual with the head down between the legs. This is a poor substitute and is not recommended in the dental surgery. Tight clothing around the neck should be loosened and a window opened to ventilate the room. As the patient recovers, reassurance may be needed and giving the patient a sweet drink will speed recovery. Finally, the patient should not be allowed to leave without the dentist being informed of what has happened, since they are ultimately responsible.

Fainting or syncope

Clinical picture
- pallor, sweating, nausea, confusion
- thin rapid pulse, twitching
- gradual loss of consciousness.

Aetiology
- reduced flow of blood to the brain
- fear, pain, hunger and stuffy atmosphere.

Management
- adjust the chair so that patient is lying flat with feet slightly raised
- loosen tight clothing around patient's neck.
- room ventilation
- reassurance
- assistance with recovery (sweetened drink and gradually move the chair into a more upright position)
- report and record the incident.

Cardiac arrest

Cardiac arrest is the cessation of the beating of the heart, either completely or by fibrillation, when there is no effective output of blood. It can occur for a number of reasons, including respiratory failure or obstruction, adverse drug reactions or coronary thrombosis.

The signs are sudden collapse, absence of a pulse (this is best checked at the carotid pulse in the neck) and pallor. A late sign is dilatation of the pupils of the eyes. Immediate treatment is necessary as lack of oxygenated blood to the brain will cause irreversible brain damage within 3 minutes.

A cardiac arrest is invariably followed by respiratory failure, so the dental hygienist should be familiar with cardiopulmonary resuscitation.

Cardiac arrest
- Possible causes: respiratory obstruction, adverse drug reaction, coronary thrombosis.
- Signs: sudden collapse, no pulse, pallor, dilatation of pupils.
- First aid treatment: immediate cardiopulmonary resuscitation; brain damage within 3 minutes.

Cardiopulmonary resuscitation

If a patient is not breathing and the heart has stopped beating, artificially taking over respiration and circulation, termed cardiopulmonary resuscitation (CPR), may save their life.

Table 16.1. The ABC of cardiopulmonary resuscitation

- A: make sure the airway is open.
- B: breathe for the patient by artificial ventilation.
- C: circulate the blood by external chest compressions.

Exhaled air ventilation

Exhaled air contains about 16% oxygen which is more than sufficient to sustain life. One of the more efficient ways of ventilating a patient who has stopped breathing is to transfer air from the operator's own lungs into the patient's, by the mouth or nose. Having checked that the oral cavity is clear and that nothing is blocking the airway, the operator should tilt the patient's head well back, by placing one hand underneath the neck, to prevent the tongue from contacting the posterior wall of the pharynx and blocking the airway. The operator then takes a deep breath and blows into the patient's mouth or nose, whilst blocking off the other with the free hand. An eye should be kept on the chest to ensure that it rises with inflation. When the mouth is removed, the elastic chest wall will recoil and expel the air that has been forced in. After the first two inflations check the pulse to make sure the heart is beating. If the heart is beating normally, continue to repeat the inflations at approximately 15 times a minute (one inflation every 4 seconds) until natural breathing is restored.

External cardiac massage

A non-beating heart can be compressed through the chest to force blood out and around the body. This is achieved by pressing firmly down on the lower half of the sternum. When the pressure is released the chest returns to its normal position and blood flows back along the veins and refills the heart as it expands. External chest compression is always preceded by artificial ventilation and it is most important to establish first that there is no heartbeat by checking the carotid pulse. To be fully effective the casualty must be lying on a firm surface. This is achieved by either placing the dental chair in a fully horizontal position or, preferably with the patient lying flat on their back on the floor. Place the palm of one hand on the centre of the lower half of the sternum with the fingers raised off the ribs. The palm of the second hand is placed over this and the fingers are locked together. Keeping the arms straight, rock forward to apply downward pressure, moving the sternum down about 4–5 cm in an average adult. Rock back to release the pressure and repeat this for 15 compressions, at a rate of approximately one every second.

If alone, the operator should give two exhaled air inflations for every 15 chest compressions and check the pulse at regular intervals. If assistance is available then one person should carry out the ventilation and the second the chest compression, at a ratio of one inflation to five compressions, with the pulse being checked every 3 minutes. Without assistance the procedure can be exhausting and can only be

maintained for a short time. It should, however, be kept up as long as possible, until the patient recovers, or until help arrives. On recovery, the patient should be moved into the recovery position and closely monitored. In the recovery position, the patient is semi-prone; that is lying on the stomach with one knee raised and the head turned to the side. This position prevents the tongue from falling backwards to block the airway and ensures that, if the patient is sick, the vomit will not be inhaled.

The patient should never be left alone during cardiopulmonary resuscitation other than momentarily, when the initial diagnosis of cardiac arrest is made, in order to summon help.

Cardiopulmonary resuscitation
Exhaled air ventilation
- Patient flat on back on floor.
- Mouth to mouth or nose respiration.
- Check for chest movements.
- Repeat at rate of 15 per minute (one every 4 seconds).

External cardiac massage
- Firm pressure to lower half of sternum.
- Repeat once every second.
- Check for carotid pulse at regular intervals.

For two operators
- One performs artificial ventilation, one carry out cardiac massage.
- Use a ratio of 1 ventilation to 5 cardiac compressions.

For solo operator
- Two inflations for every 15 chest compressions.

Coronary thrombosis

Coronary thrombosis is the blockage of the blood supply to the heart muscle and is called a heart attack in lay terms. This may occur suddenly, such as when a blood clot blocks a cardiac blood vessel (a myocardial infarction), or it may be the result of slow blockage of the vessels due to atherosclerosis. The end result in both cases is ischaemia of part of the heart muscle and possible necrosis of that muscle due to lack of oxygenated blood. The condition may rapidly cause a cardiac arrest and sudden loss of consciousness, but commonly the patient remains conscious, becoming distressed and breathless. There is usually severe pain (angina), with the pain radiating from the chest down the left arm. Vomiting may occur and care must be taken that the airway is not obstructed.

The patient should be kept still and warm until medical assistance arrives and be allowed to adopt the most comfortable position, which is often sitting upright. The dental hygienist should be prepared in case a cardiac arrest occurs and cardiopulmonary resuscitation becomes necessary.

Coronary thrombosis

- Caused by a myocardial infarct or atherosclerosis.
- If there is sudden loss of consciousness: cardiopulmonary resuscitation.
- If still conscious the patient will be distressed and breathless and have angina.
- The conscious patient should be made comfortable, kept quiet and supervised until help arrives.

Breakage of an instrument during treatment

Inhalation of a foreign body, such as the broken head of a rubber polishing cup or tip of a scaler is always a possibility during dental hygienist procedures. If, during treatment, part of an instrument should break off and disappear, it could have serious consequences and must not be ignored, even if it causes no distress whatsoever. Initially, the hygienist should examine the oral cavity thoroughly in an attempt to find the missing article, being careful not to aspirate it from the mouth without noticing. If it is not found, it may have taken either of two routes. Most probably it has been swallowed, in which case there is no real problem. If it has been inhaled, this is a very serious matter. The dentist must be informed of what has happened and will probably arrange for the patient to have radiographs taken to find out whether the object is lying in the

stomach or the lungs.

Should the foreign body be seen to be in the stomach or intestines, no further treatment is indicated, but should it be seen to be in the lungs, the patient will require hospitalization for its removal.

Breakage of an instrument during treatment

- Search the oral cavity for the missing part.
- If not found, report incident to dentist immediately.
- Two possible routes
    oesophagus to stomach: no real problem
    trachea to lungs: a serious problem.
- Likely referral to hospital for X-rays and any necessary treatment.

Epileptic fit

The person suffering from epilepsy is more vulnerable to an attack in the dental surgery, due to the stress involved in treatment.

An epileptic patient will usually have a history of the complaint and may also be able to tell when a fit is imminent, enabling the hygienist to take any necessary precautions. An epileptic attack may range from a momentary loss of consciousness, seen in the patient with petit mal epilepsy, to more serious symptoms of involuntary movements, convulsion, salivation, loss of consciousness and cyanosis seen in the grand mal forms.

In the former situation no treatment is necessary. The latter patient should have dentures and spectacles removed immediately and clothing carefully loosened, if this can be done safely. Equipment should be moved out of range to leave a clear space around the patient. No attempt should be made to move, lift or forcibly restrain the casualty unless there is any particular danger. Nor should anything be put into the patient's mouth. On recovering from a grand mal attack, the patient may take some time to return to normal and may be confused for a while.

In all cases, the dentist should be consulted before allowing the patient to leave the surgery. The incident should be recorded on the patient's notes and the patient should not be allowed to leave without a responsible escort.

Table 16.2. Management of the unconscious patient

At some time the hygienist is likely to be faced with an unconscious casualty and must decide upon the cause and the appropriate treatment. In this event the following rules will ensure that the casualty has the greatest chance of survival

---

- **Check the airway**. Look in the mouth to ensure that there is no obstruction and remove any loose dentures or clear the mouth of any blood or vomit. Loosen any tight clothing around the patient's neck and tilt the head firmly backwards to move the tongue off the back of the pharynx and free the airway.
- **Check the patient** for any obvious cause of loss of consciousness. Check for signs of head injury or any bracelets or cards warning of medical problems.
- **If the patient has stopped breathing**; exhaled air ventilation should be undertaken.
- **Check the pulse** at the carotid artery and if this is absent cardiopulmonary resuscitation should be carried out.
- **Send or shout for help**. If essential, leave the patient only momentarily to summon help. Otherwise the patient should never be left alone.
- **Position the patient** correctly. The unconscious patient should be immediately laid flat and on no account left sitting upright in a dental chair. Initially whilst the airway and heartbeat are being checked the patient should be laid flat on their back. However, once breathing and heartbeat are restored, the patient should be moved into the recovery position.
- **Monitor the patient** until consciousness is regained or help arrives.

Epileptic fits
Petit mal
- short period of confusion or loss of concentration
- report the incident to the dentist
- patient to leave surgery only with escort.

Grand mal
- loss of consciousness with convulsions
- move equipment, etc. out of range
- protect but do not attempt to move patient
- possible period of confusion on regaining consciousness
- Report the incident to the dentist
- Ensure patient leaves with escort.

consciousness the patient appears pale, restless, often confused and may feel hungry. Differentiating between the two conditions may be difficult to the inexperienced, but, fortunately, the diabetic person can usually tell what is happening and take appropriate action. In the conscious patient, administering sugar by mouth will bring about the rapid recovery of the hypoglycaemic patient, but will make little difference to the hyperglycaemic patient.

Diabetic crisis
Hyperglycaemia
- due to inadequate insulin dosage or excess sugar consumption
- slow onset of drowsiness, with sweating
- less urgent, but should be reported immediately.

Hypoglycaemia
- due to excess insulin being taken or lack of food
- rapid onset with feeling of hunger
- serious situation requiring immediate medical assistance

If uncertain of diagnosis, in emergency a sweet drink should be given.

Diabetic crises

A diabetic patient may suffer from two forms of crisis: hypoglycaemic, caused by excess insulin or lack of food, and hyperglycaemic, which occurs when the patient has not taken the insulin, or has eaten excess carbohydrate.

The hyperglycaemic crisis is of slow onset, with the patient tending to be drowsy, flushed and sweating. The hypoglycaemic crisis is of sudden onset and is more dangerous as it leads more rapidly to a diabetic coma. Before losing

Temporary dressings

A hygienist will occasionally suffer the misfortune of dislodging a restoration during the process of scaling and as a consequence have to arrange for a temporary restoration to be inserted until the dentist can replace the restoration. This will most commonly occur when scaling around restorations which lie close to the gingival margin. The types of restoration most likely to be dislodged are old amalgams or composites which had not been acid etched originally. At the time of writing this edition, the UK General Dental Council is recommending that a dental hygienist's scope of work be increased to include the placement of a temporary dressing in this situation.

It would be important to inform the patient that a restoration has fractured and that a temporary restoration is to be inserted until the dentist can deal with the situation. Then the dentist must be notified as soon as is convenient and an appointment can be made for the patient to have the tooth permanently restored. It is also worth remembering that the dental hygienist may only place a temporary restoration where the permanent restoration has been dislodged during the process of scaling carried out by the hygienist and under no other circumstance.

The aim of inserting a temporary dressing is to cover exposed dentine, prevent sensitivity and protect the pulp. If the tooth is non-vital the aim is to temporarily fill the cavity to prevent it becoming a food trap and also a source of annoyance to the patient. In Table 16.3 the various materials are listed which can be used as temporary restorations

When placing a temporary restoration it would be preferable to use a material that would be durable for at least a month and ideally one that will have an affinity to tooth substance. It might be appropriate to consider a glass-ionomer (GI) material such as Ketac Fill® or Fuji II® which will form a bond to tooth substance. Alternatively, a non-eugenol material could be used such as Coltisol® or Cavit®, but before using these materials it would be important to check that there is enough retention in the cavity to hold it in place. It would, for example, be difficult to place one of these dressings (which do not bond to teeth) in a cavity that was originally an abrasion cavity, had minimal retention and had been restored with a glass-ionomer or composite. In such cavities the retention depends on the tooth bonding properties of the final restorative material so when inserting a temporary dressing it could be appropriate to use one of the glass-ionomer cements (GIC).

Technique of placement

When a restoration is dislodged it is important to carefully remove any loose bits of remaining filling material using only an excavator. If the tooth is vital and sensitive it may be uncomfortable for the patient if the 3-in-1 syringe is used. Therefore, the tooth might have to be isolated with cotton rolls and the cavity dried with cotton pellets held in tweezers. The material should preferably be mixed by a dental nurse, so that the cavity can be kept dry and then the temporary dressing is carefully inserted using a flat plastic instrument. Any excess is removed from around the margins using either a dental probe or a sickle scaler when it has set enough for it to be trimmed easily.

Temporary dressings

Regulations: dental hygienists may place a temporary restoration only when a permanent restoration is dislodged during treatment.

Purpose
- cover exposed dentine
- prevent sensitivity
- protect the pulp
- prevent food stagnation
- avoid irritation to the patient.

Materials
- retentive cavities: recognized temporary materials such as Coltisol® or Kalzinol®
- non-retentive cavities: glass-ionomer materials.

Placement
- remove any remaining debris
- dry cavity
- mix material to instructions
- place with flat plastic
- remove excess.

Further reading

Colquhoun M., Handley A. J., Evans T. R. (1995) *ABC of*

Table 16.3 Restoration materials

Materials which can be used for temporary restorations

- For small retentive cavities: Coltisol®, Cavit® or zinc oxide, Eugenol®.
- For larger cavities which are retentive: Kalzinol®.
- For larger less retentive cavities: a Polycarboxylate material such as Poly F®.
- Where retention is poor such as a fractured cusp Ketac Fill® of Fuji II®.

Resuscitation. The Resuscitation Council (UK). 3rd edition. London: BMJ Publishing Group.

Marsden A. K., Moffat Sir Cameron, Scott R. (1992) *First Aid Manual: The Authorised Manual of the St John's Ambulance Association and the British Red Cross*. 6th edition. London: Dorling Kindersley.

Skeet M. (editor) (1988) *Emergency Procedures and First Aid for Nurses*. 2nd edition. Oxford: Blackwell Scientific.

17

Patients with special needs

Introduction

For some patients the long-term maintenance of their teeth requires special attention, although it could be argued that all patients require special care. With improved methods of preserving life and with increasing longevity of the population it is likely that greater numbers of patients will attend for treatment with some degree of handicap or disability, whether developmental or acquired. Patients in these categories have special needs and considerable extra efforts are required of us if we are to satisfy those needs adequately. To simplify the approach to this aspect of dental care, modes of treatment for patients with the various types of special need will be described separately.

Motor disabilities

Motor disability may arise from a variety of causes. It may follow physical damage to the spinal cord or brain, e.g. paraplegia and cerebral palsy; be of developmental origin, e.g. spina bifida; or be the result of a disease such as Parkinson's, multiple sclerosis or myasthenia gravis. The significant problems of patients with a motor handicap are now better recognized and more attention is being paid to their solution. Problems may arise at various stages and are particularly acute when a wheelchair is the normal mode of transport.

Good access to the surgery is essential and ideally there should be easy access for a wheelchair. Steps are virtually impossible to negotiate single-handedly in a wheelchair or walking aid and the alternative of a shallow ramp should be provided. Corridors must be at least 1 m wide and all doors at least 80 cm wide. Floor surfaces must be smooth without loose rugs or changes in level. When access is adequate for wheelchairs there will be no problems for less badly handicapped patients.

Once in the surgery a decision has to be made with wheelchair patients whether it is more convenient to treat the patient in the wheelchair or in the dental chair. Most patients can transfer to a dental chair if the wheelchair can be 'parked' alongside. The degree of help needed is best determined by patients themselves who are normally quite adroit at the necessary manoeuvres. Alternatively, experienced companions or relatives can be of great assistance. If transfer to the dental chair is difficult a detachable headrest may be attached to the back of the wheelchair and the wheelchair moved to a site convenient for the light and other equipment. When wheelchair patients are treated frequently in specialized units it may be best to use a special wheelchair lift which tilts the chair into the operating position.

With regard to oral hygiene, the ability of the patient may vary considerably. Some may be able to manage on their own, but many will require some assistance. As a general rule, it is better not to over-assist those who can manage independently, as they will frequently resent the intrusion. It may be helpful to adapt the handle of the brush, or use an automatic brush which

---

Table 17.1 Physical problems

The main physical problems that may be encountered in patients include

---

- **Manual dexterity**: patients with arthritis or those who have suffered from a lack of limb development may have difficulties in holding a toothbrush. The authors have seen one patient with no hands who managed to clean his teeth by having an electric toothbrush fixed to a wall.
- **Postural problems**: many patients, such as those crippled by kyphoscoliosis, will be unable to sit in a normal position in a dental chair.
- **Ability to co-operate**: patients with cerebral palsy often have exaggerated and involuntary contractions of the oral musculature and this will provide a barrier to a dental examination. Sudden closure of the mouth may occur, presenting a danger to both patient and operator.
- **Poor eyesight**: this may make effective oral hygiene difficult to achieve.
- Impaired hearing: this will make communication difficult.

---

may, if necessary, be fixed to a solid surface, for patients with problems involving the hands.

Where the patient must rely on others to assist with or carry out oral hygiene, it is essential to involve the carer in the plaque-control instruction. Ideally, a spouse or close relative may be involved, although for hospital or long-stay patients, the nursing staff may have to assist. The dental hygienist would be unwise to underestimate the problems involved in this. In the first case, the same person may not always be responsible for helping the patient, and secondly, the nurses caring for handicapped individuals may have many other aspects to cope with, and may not see dental care as having a high priority. Much may be achieved, however, by spending time to relate with and motivate such staff adequately.

It is vital that those in the dental field do not try to work in isolation. Communication should be established with other professionals with special skills in the medical sphere. For example, occupational therapists may well be able to advise on the adaptation of a tooth-brush and physiotherapists may help train the patient in the physical action of brushing. Those dental hygienists working in the community dental services should take every opportunity to give dental preventive advice to anyone involved in the care of handicapped individuals (Table 17.1).

During prolonged treatment provision must be made for any necessary 'physiotherapy'. Patients may need to exercise muscles to restore the blood circulation in order to avoid skin problems similar to bed-sores. Handicapped patients can be questioned on this aspect beforehand and a rest from treatment taken at regular intervals. If oral hygiene instruction is to be given frequently to patients in wheel-chairs, a sink at a suitably low level and lever handles on the taps are essential.

Plaque control methods will vary from normal only insofar as the patient lacks normal control of their hands and fingers. In cases where manipulative skills are poor, the tooth-brush can be adapted to give greater security of control. Elastic bands can be permanently attached to give extra support or the handle of the brush can be thickened with cycle handle-bar grips or modified with cold-cure acrylic. Caries control by fluoride rinses is advisable. In severe cases chemical plaque control may be necessary, although regular professional attention will be required to remove the resultant staining.

Cognitive disability

Many patients with a mild degree of mental disability (IQ 50–70) are excellent dental patients. Although forgetful and in need of frequent reminders, they are enthusiastic and with understanding from the operator they come to relish a visit to the surgery. A patient with a greater degree of mental handicap than this finds oral hygiene difficult to perform and presents greater problems. Successful treatment then depends on a thoughtful and often prolonged approach. An added complication is that some forms of mental disability, e.g. Down's syndrome, can be associated with heart lesions and warrant antibiotic prophylaxis for some forms of treatment.

Patients with mental handicaps present a

Table 17.2 Mental handicaps

Mental handicaps that may be encountered in patients include

- **Cognitive deficiency**: low intelligence may mean that communication and co-operation are difficult.
- **Communication deficits**: this may be due to problems with hearing, eyesight, speech or interpretation. The dental hygienist should not assume without supportive evidence that because the patient cannot communicate effectively there is a cognitive deficiency.
- **Inability to concentrate**: some patients, especially those with cerebral dysfunction, may be restless and have an inability to concentrate. Distractions on the periphery of vision may preferentially attract the patient's attention.
- **Apprehension**: in many otherwise healthy patients, apprehension at attending the dentist may be so severe as to be classified as a psychosis. Apprehension may be a particular problem in some children with other handicaps who have been cared for by very protective parents.

large variety of problems. These may vary from a refusal to co-operate or even permit examination, to the severe problems of aggressive periodontitis often seen in sufferers from Down's syndrome.

In order to assess the full extent of the problem, a full history is essential, with the carer being involved in this. As well as providing information for a full assessment, the time involved in this exercise will help in the establishment of a trusting relationship, which is essential if co-operation is to be achieved. If there is one rule that should be followed with these patients, it is to 'make haste slowly'. A considered, friendly, measured approach will save time in the long run. The actual treatment may be relatively simple, but success or failure often depends upon the preliminary attempts at making contact with the patient.

First, whatever the age of the patient, the support of the carer, whether nurse, parent or relative, must be recruited. Without their understanding of methods of achieving oral health and willingness to carry them out on a daily basis little is possible apart from giving dietary advice and recommending topical fluoride application in the form of fluoridated toothpaste. With the help of the carer a full range of oral care is possible.

Next the confidence of the patient must be acquired, a process that can require several visits and involve slow, gradual introduction of the patient to the instruments and techniques of plaque and deposit removal. New items and actions are introduced by a process of show-tell-do and to ensure concentration and avoid discordant sensory stimuli the environment must be distraction-free without intrusive music. Repetition is an essential element of the introductory stage. Obviously threatening equipment must be inconspicuous, slow movements are performed and every attempt must be made to involve the patient in treatment by providing relevant, non-harmful items to take home, e.g. disposable dental mirror heads, oral hygiene leaflets and samples of toothpaste. The nature of the items can be selected according to the mental age of the patient and can be a useful form of home education for both patient and carer.

Finally, while successful progress to home therapy often occurs, oral health will have to be maintained by relatively simple methods. It is advisable to teach the scrub brushing technique and complex manoeuvres with floss silk and interspace brushes will be impossible. Chemical plaque control can be tried when all else fails. Chlorhexidine in the form of rinse or spray is very effective but the strong taste can produce a negative reaction. Cetyl pyridinium chloride and fluoride mouthrinse is a more acceptable but less effective alternative. It has to be acknowledged that extra time and effort must be made when treating patients with mental disability. There is no substitute for frequent maintenance and supervision, and constant reinforcement of the attitudes of patient and carer are essential.

In view of the large range of handicaps that may be encountered, it is also important that the hygienist has a source of reference to go to in order to look up the known facts relating to any problem, and is not too proud to do so (Table 17.2).

The main physical problems include
- Manual dexterity.
- Postural problems.
- Cerebral palsy.
- Poor eyesight.

Some of the mental handicaps are as follows
- Cognitive deficiency.
- Communication deficits.
- Inability to concentrate.
- Apprehension.

The older patient

Elderly patients often suffer from a deterioration in oral hygiene leading to root caries and tooth loss unless efforts are made to bring the disease under control. Several factors contribute to the state of affairs. After retirement and loss of the daily routine that a career brings there is a tendency to eat irregularly, at short intervals, and not at the intervals dictated by work. Fermentable carbohydrate comes into contact with the teeth more frequently and caries follows. Retirement may also bring a reduction in income and cheaper foods are chosen with a greater proportion of refined carbohydrate. If this is also associated with loss of a spouse an apathetic life style may be adopted and snack type foods chosen which require less preparation.

Apathy extends also to oral hygiene habits with plaque remaining in permanent contact with the teeth. Oral hygiene may be made worse if there is a lack of saliva. Hyposalivation is not inevitable with ageing. Although some degeneration of salivary gland tissue takes place the amount is not usually significant enough to cause functional difficulties. Hyposalivation is more usually a side effect of drug therapy, antidepressant drugs being a particular problem in this respect.

Oral hygiene in the elderly is maintained principally by the normal methods of adulthood, although an electric toothbrush can be useful if there is some degree of physical impairment. If there is recession of the gingivae, desensitizing treatment may be required and to avoid root caries a daily fluoride mouthrinse is to be recommended. If hyposalivation is causing a problem an artificial saliva can be prescribed to aid lubrication of the mouth. A fluoride-containing aerosol spray type is best.

The difficulty that must be overcome is lack of enthusiasm. Elderly people are reputed to find learning difficult. This is an oversimplification. The elderly can learn complex tasks to great proficiency and are capable of intense intellectual effort. The problem lies in motivation. For the young person knowledge is of immediate benefit and the advantages of learning are apparent. For the middle-aged, too, learning is necessary to maintain their position in the world. The elderly on the other hand are no longer so pressurized and the techniques of improved oral hygiene and altered dental practices have to be reinforced by frequent repetition and clear identification of the advantages and goals to be achieved.

In the absence of cerebral pathology, much is possible. Once elderly people have been convinced of the need for good oral hygiene and have mastered the necessary techniques, they become model patients. Indeed they often look forward to their review appointment and anticipate the social aspects with pleasure.

For those who find attending the surgery difficult, then a domiciliary visit will be necessary. These will need to be carefully planned and discussed with the supervising clinician. Specific equipment is available and the hygienist is advised to consult a specialist text for further information.

Endocardial disease and orthopaedic prostheses

A medical history which includes an episode of rheumatic fever must be viewed with suspicion. Rheumatic fever can be associated with endocardial disease, and the bacteraemia caused by dental procedures such as extraction, scaling and root planing can result in an increased risk of a bacterial endocarditis; a condition which is frequently fatal even with treatment.

Opinions differ on the need for antibiotic cover for such patients during dental operations, some feeling that in the absence of a clinically detectable heart murmur antibiotic cover is unnecessary. Until the experts concur it is only sensible to provide antibiotic prophylaxis (Table 17.3).

The need for antibiotic prophylaxis for patients with a prosthetic hip or knee joint is

Table 17.3 Infective endocarditis

Recommended antibiotic regimes for patients at risk from infective endocarditis

- For patients who are not allergic to penicillin, the necessary regime is 3 grams of amoxycillin by mouth, under supervision, 1 hour before the operation.
- Children under 10 years have half the adult dose and children under 5 have quarter the adult dose.
- Patients allergic to penicillin are given 600 mg of oral clindamycin 1 hour before the operation. For children under the age of 10 the dose of clindamycin is half the adult does and under 5, one quarter. The same regime is required for patients with patent ductus arteriosus or septal defect.
- Prescription of the regime at intervals of shorter than one month is thought to be inadvisable in view of the possibility that resistant organisms may arise and if present will negate the beneficial effect of antibiotic prophylaxis.
- When a special risk patient (one with a prosthetic valve, previous endocarditis, or a patient who has been prescribed penicillin more than once within the last month) is to be treated under general anaesthetic, the prophylaxis is slightly different. Those with no allergy to penicillin are given amoxycillin 1 gram and gentamicin 120 mg, both intramuscularly, immediately before the operation, and 500 mg of oral amoxycillin 6 hours later.
- With a patient allergic to penicillin the therapy changes to 1 gram of vancomycin intravenously over 60 minutes prior to the operation, followed by gentamicin 1.5 mg/kg body weight i.v. immediately before the operation.

more debatable. In this situation it is best to follow local practice and when the surgeon responsible for the implant wishes to avoid any risk of infection, prophylaxis can be prescribed as for endocardial disease.

Immunocompromised patients

Patients with defects of their immune system are becoming increasingly common. Apart from developmental diseases such as hypogammaglobulinaemia or agranulocytosis, a patient's immune response may be therapeutically diminished after transplantation or treatment of neoplastic disease. Recently HIV infection has become of increasing significant importance.

Such patients are particularly at risk from infections acquired in the surgery and cross-infection procedures should be as those for hepatitis B. The patient is to be especially protected against the risk of infection from the operator, and organisms not normally pathogenic can be the source of severe infections.

Oral hygiene is very important. Patients in this category are liable to infections of the mouth. Oral candidosis, which gives rise to sore red areas, can be a particular problem. Chlor-

hexidine mouthrinses are a useful prophylactic measure but when oral candidosis is present it is often the sign of a more generalized infection and treatment with systemic antifungal drugs is normal. Ketoconazole is the agent of choice at present but the risk of kidney damage must be borne in mind.

Patients with diabetes

Diabetes is a common, incurable disease caused by reduction or lack of insulin production by the pancreas and characterized by high glucose levels in the blood. If occurring for the first time in a patient older than 40 it is often insidious in onset, and the effects mild and controlled by weight reduction and modification of the diet. When diet modification is difficult oral hypoglycaemic drugs are helpful and help stimulate insulin production. In a young patient the disease is usually more sudden and severe, and there is a complete lack of insulin production. To maintain a near-normal blood glucose level rigid control of sugars in the diet is needed and injections of insulin are required.

The significance of diabetes to dentistry lies in the finding that insulin dependent diabetics appear to be more susceptible to periodontal diseases and the periodontal state of some diabetics is characterized by rapid breakdown, a state which appears to be due to an altered host response. Research has shown that there is a defect in neutrophil polymorph function in insulin dependent diabetics.

The goal to be achieved is a high standard of plaque control and along with dietary control must go emphasis on oral hygiene if the teeth are to be preserved. At the same time it is important to eliminate other local irritants such as calculus or overhanging restorations. Generally those diabetics who find it easy to regulate their diet and maintain their blood glucose level also find it easy to accept the habits of regular oral hygiene. As a corollary, those who find difficulty in regulating their blood glucose require constant reinforcement of the need for plaque control.

Diabetics also require consideration with regard to their appointments. Normally they require three main meals each day with intermediate snacks. This means that the times they can attend the surgery may be restricted. Early and late times may coincide with meals, and mid-morning and mid-afternoon appointments may have to be avoided, or if necessary interrupted, to allow food intake.

Complex restorative dentistry

As the population becomes increasingly dentally sophisticated, so the demand for complex restorative procedures increases. Broken down teeth are replaced by crowns and the appearance of discoloured teeth improved by veneers. Weakened teeth can be reinforced by inlays, the mobility of loose teeth can be reduced by the use of interlocking crowns, and lost teeth can be replaced by bridges. Even after loss of all the teeth there is the possibility that dental function can be restored permanently by means of osseointegrated transmucosal implants.

Most forms of complex restorative dentistry merely involve precise replacement of the form of the missing tooth and from the point of view of hygiene, normal methods of plaque control are adequate. Bridges and transmucosal implants require special attention because their shapes diverge from normal dental anatomy and their problems merit individual consideration.

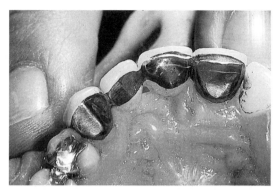

Fig. 17.1 A fixed-fixed bridge requiring special cleaning methods.

Dental bridgework

When applying oral health measures there are two kinds of bridge. Fixed and semi-fixed bridges are attached to the teeth on either side of the missing tooth or teeth and have pontics with relatively inaccessible fitting surfaces (Fig. 17.1). Free-end cantilever or spring cantilever bridges are attached either to a tooth on one side of the missing tooth or teeth, or are attached to a tooth remote from the missing tooth or teeth. These latter types permit easy access to the fitting surface through one or both contact points (Fig. 17. 2).

In general there are few problems in ensuring good oral hygiene and the performance of dilatory patients can be encouraged by discussions of the costs involved if any of the complex restorations have to be replaced. Difficulties arise when the anatomical shape of the restoration is abnormal. Typically this is when the adjacent teeth are joined at the contact point. As mentioned above, this is always the case with fixed and semi-fixed bridges and only free-end cantilever and spring cantilever bridges allow the under surface of the bridge to be cleaned via a contact point. Similar problems occur when united crowns are made or when interlocking inlays are prescribed.

Inaccessible fitting surfaces of bridges or the interproximal surfaces of united crowns necessitate the use of specially designed oral hygiene aids and the use of some form of floss threader must be taught. The simplest form of floss threader is a piece of thin, stiff plastic tape one end of which is formed into a loop (Fig. 17.3). By threading the floss silk onto the loop and passing the free end of the tape between the

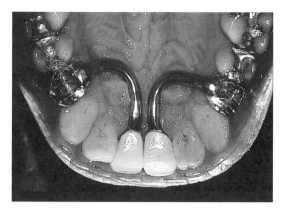

Fig. 17.2 Spring cantilever bridges with extensive bars that require cleaning in addition to the pontics.

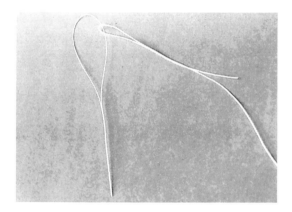

Fig. 17.3 Floss threader and floss.

interproximal surfaces beneath the fused contact point the floss silk is passed from the buccal to the lingual surface and after removal of the thread can be used in the normal way to clean the undersurface of the bridge or contact point. This technique is most easily performed on anterior teeth after a demonstration given with the patient observing by means of a mirror. The method works less well on posterior teeth where access is more difficult and the patient may have to supplement oral hygiene by use of an interproximal brush. An alternative to a floss threader is the use of 'Superfloss' which has an integral threader which has one end stiffened to permit passage through the interproximal spaces. In extreme cases chemical plaque control by means of chlorhexidine mouthrinses may be the only way of maintaining plaque-free fitting and interproximal surfaces. Staining can

then result and may need to be removed at regular intervals.

Osseointegrated implants

Restoration of a functional dentition for the edentulous patient by means of implants has been attempted for many years. Some success was achieved with subperiosteal metal frames but in the long-term, epithelial downgrowth from the oral mucosa encapsulated the implant and rendered it liable to infection and sequestration. Predictable success was first achieved by Branemark using titanium implants placed within surgically created slots in the bone. After ensuring immobilization of the implanted structures, osseointegration occurs between bone and titanium via the molecule-thick layer of titanium oxide on the implant surface. On completion of osseointegration, superstructures are placed over the embedded sections and a complete denture or an implant-supported bridge inserted.

To ensure continued success of osseointegrated implants, the maintenance of plaque-free abutments is vital and the cleanliness of that part which pierces the mucosa has the highest priority. The spaces between the abutments are best kept clean with an interspace brush (Fig. 17.4) and other abutment surfaces can be cleaned with Superfloss. Although careful daily use of these oral hygiene aids should maintain the abutments plaque-free, review of all such patients by a hygienist is advisable at regular 6 month intervals. Any deposit can then be removed and oral hygiene reinforced. Hard deposits are removed with special polymeric based instruments to avoid scratching or contaminating the relatively soft titanium surface by contact with another metal.

Removable dental prostheses

The patient with a removable dental prosthesis has special problems with oral hygiene. Although dentures are designed to be as hygienic as possible inevitably the mouth of a patient without a prosthesis will be more healthy than one with. No matter what the design of the denture there is a biological price to pay. It is the duty of the clinician to keep the price to a minimum. Because the problems with the different types of prosthesis differ, those

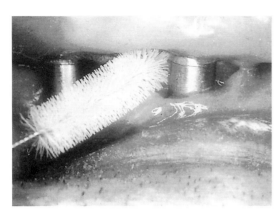

Fig. 17.4 An osseointegrated implant abutment being cleaned with an interdental brush.

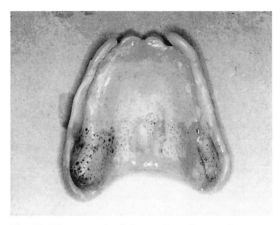

Fig. 17.5 Plaque on the fitting surface of a complete upper denture revealed by disclosing solution.

related to complete dentures, overdentures and partial dentures will be approached separately.

Complete dentures

The proportion of the adult population wearing complete dentures is becoming smaller as standards of oral hygiene improve and the incidence of caries diminishes. In the UK, nevertheless, 19% of adults wear complete dentures and their specialized needs are all too infrequently recognized. Plaque can accumulate on dentures as it can on teeth, and the consequences are staining, calculus formation and bacterial infection. The role of the hygienist is to institute a denture cleansing routine which is effective and acceptable to the patient. The majority of complete denture wearers are elderly and after the insertion of new complete dentures, efforts have to be made to overcome, by enthusiasm and practical help, the problems of learning and decreased manual dexterity so often present in this section of the population.

Denture hygiene instruction should begin before replacement dentures are fitted, by the demonstration of plaque on previous dentures. Disclosing solution is highly effective, and emphasizes the need for a proper denture cleansing routine (Fig. 17.5). For immediate dentures instruction is given at a review stage. Although instructions on the cleansing of dentures will have been given when the dentures were inserted, it is sensible to review procedures and reinforce motivation.

The simplest method of cleansing dentures is with soap and a soft nailbrush or with denture toothpaste and a special denture brush. While having the advantage of cheapness and simplicity, the methods have drawbacks. The denture becomes slippery and the patient must be warned to clean the dentures over a towel or basin of water, either of which will break the fall and prevent fracture if the denture is dropped. The other drawback is that patient's manual dexterity may be diminished and cleaning may be inefficient even when a large, specially designed toothbrush is bought.

An alternative is to use an immersion cleanser. Immersion cleansers come in tablet form and are added to warm water to form a solution in which the denture is immersed for a specific period of time. The most effective immersion cleansers contain detergents or hypochlorite either alone or in combination and a few contain hydrochloric acid. The action may be aided by bleaches (peroxides and borates) and proteolytic enzymes. While hypochlorite is a very effective plaque-removing agent and hydrochloric acid will remove calculus, both cause corrosion of metals and must never be used when the denture has a metal base. Patients should also be warned to follow carefully the instructions for use. Hot water will cause stress relief and distortion of acrylic dentures, and if bleaches are also present whitening of the surface resin occurs.

Partial dentures

On functional grounds, partial dentures may be divided into two extreme types, those supported by the natural teeth and those supported by the soft tissues and bone. An intermediate group

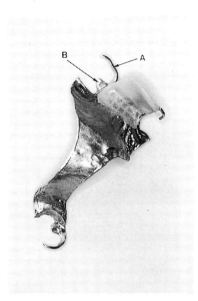

Fig. 17.6 A typical metal-based partial denture. Arrows point to: clasps **A** and rests **B**.

occurs, the denture must very often be replaced. Even greater problems occur if a tooth is lost. Loss of an abutment tooth means that the denture must be replaced, but because many partial dentures depend for their continuing satisfactory support on maintenance of the remaining teeth as parts of an intact arch, unless the denture is of a simple, acrylic-resin base soft tissue supported type, loss of any tooth often means that the denture must be replaced. This may be very inconvenient, because after tooth loss a temporary denture will be required until the initial rapid resorption phase of alveolar bone is over.

The patient with a partial denture needs the help of a hygienist because there will be serious financial consequences if further caries occurs. Instruction in the cleansing of the denture, on the lines described above for complete dentures, is secondary to ensuring that oral hygiene is of a very high standard. Patients must be told not to leave the denture in their mouth when carrying out procedures. When examining the mouth hygienists should also include examination of the partial denture. Special note should be made of any wear of either the denture or abutment teeth, or of loss of retention.

also exists in which support is divided between teeth and bone. Dentures with tooth support must be designed to meet much greater stresses, comparable in magnitude to those resisted by the natural teeth. For this reason they have a metal base, usually cast cobalt/chromium alloy. Those with only soft tissue support usually have an acrylic resin base. Nevertheless, patients often prefer the feel of a thin metal base and for this reason a metal base may be needed. It may also be prescribed if stresses are unusually high, e.g. when the lower incisors contact an upper base due to a complete overbite, or when a prominent palatal torus produces a point of weakness or stress concentration.

The majority of partial dentures depend for their efficient functioning on an integration with the remaining teeth. Resistance to masticatory forces is provided by occlusal rests which fit into slots in either teeth or restorations. Resistance to vertically displacing forces is provided by direct retainers or clasps which fit into undercuts on the axial surfaces of the crowns of teeth (Fig. 17.6). Resistance to lateral displacing forces is countered by contact of the denture base with non-undercut tooth surfaces.

The prevention of any further caries must be a high priority. If caries of a tooth contacting a partial denture occurs, restoration is difficult if the original tooth/base contact is to be re-established. If caries of an abutment tooth

Overdentures

Overdentures are provided primarily when there is fear that if teeth are lost the resulting alveolar bone resorption will compromise denture stability. Consequently, selected tooth roots are preserved after removal of their crowns and the retained root preserves alveolar bone which in turn provides lateral stability for the denture (Fig. 17.7). The exposed root surfaces also serve to provide extra vertical support to the denture and hence overdenture therapy may also be advisable in cases where the face height is to be increased and extra stresses will be imposed on the denture-bearing area.

Inevitably, if root surfaces are to be covered by a denture base there will be the risk of further caries and regular attention by a hygienist will help preserve roots which would be otherwise quickly lost, and patients must be warned to brush root surfaces as well as teeth. Extra precautions include prescription of fluoride mouthrinses (0.05% daily) or use of APF gel (1 drop weekly applied to the fitting surface of the denture over the root surfaces). Alter-

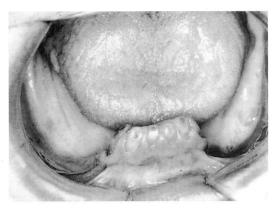

Fig. 17.7 Retained roots acting as abutments for an overdenture. The alveolar bone in this area has been retained by this treatment.

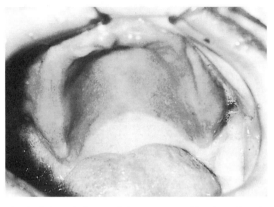

Fig. 17.8 A typical case of denture stomatitis where there is inflammation and papillary hyperplasia of the maxillary denture-bearing surface.

natively, after brushing their teeth, to prolong the period of fluoride treatment the patient can apply a small amount of fluoridated toothpaste to the fitting surface of the denture over the root face.

Denture stomatitis

Denture stomatitis is usually found beneath complete upper dentures but can occur beneath any form of oral prosthesis, including orthodontic appliances. Alternative names for the disease are denture associated candidosis and denture-sore mouth. It is characterized by redness of the denture-bearing area and is often associated with papillary hyperplasia (Fig. 17.8). The cause is proliferation of a fungus (normally *Candida albicans*) in the plaque deposited on the denture and the predilection for an upper denture may be a consequence of its relatively good retention and the consequent fluid stasis beneath it. Its incidence is greatest in the elderly and it has been claimed to occur at some time in one third of the denture-wearing population. While the symptoms are relatively mild, the condition tends to occur in individuals susceptible to infection and apart from the local elimination of disease, treatment is provided to prevent spread to other sites.

Diagnosis is made on clinical grounds and confirmed by swabbing the fitting surface of the upper denture and identifying large amounts of *Candida* in the plaque. Except when trauma is diagnosed, treatment involves improvement of oral hygiene and disclosing solutions are helpful for identifying plaque both in the surgery and at home. The aim of preliminary treatment is a permanent improvement in oral hygiene and methods of cleansing dentures have to be emphasized. If removal of plaque by mechanical means is difficult, immersion in hypochlorite solutions is usually effective. When no improvement can be made by these methods, locally applied antifungals are prescribed. Nystatin pastilles are excellent but have a strong taste which patients object to and a more acceptable choice is miconazole oral gel, a few centimetres of which is squeezed from a tube onto the fitting surface of the denture after each meal. Treatment is carried on for about 6 weeks to ensure that all spores are killed, but relapse is common unless the conditions predisposing to the infection are eliminated.

Some resistant cases are associated with a systemic defect, either anaemia, diabetes or immunocompromising condition. For this reason particularly florid or resistant forms should be regarded with suspicion and the appropriate tests prescribed.

A condition which is frequently associated with denture stomatitis is angular cheilitis where the angles of the mouth are red, cracked and painful (Fig. 17.9). The condition is rationalized as being initially due to a reduction of the height of the lower third of the face due to excessively worn dentures or dentures in which the upper anterior teeth give inadequate lip support. In either case the skin at the corner of the mouth becomes creased and macerated by escaping saliva. Infection from an associated denture stomatitis can then follow.

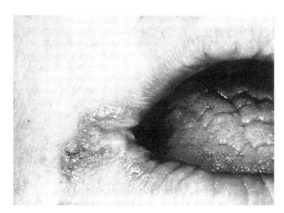

Fig. 17.9 A typical case of angular cheilitis. *Candida albicans* was isolated from the area.

Treatment involves correction of any denture fault and treatment of the infection after identification of the offending organism. Swabs should be taken of the angles of the mouth and the anterior corners of the nose (a likely site for cross contamination). *Candida albicans* and/or staphylococci are the usual organisms found. Fusidic acid ointment will eliminate staphylococci and miconazole ointment is effective against both *Candida albicans* and staphylococci.

Post-surgical maintenance

Periodontal surgery is less frequently practised now but is invaluable in selected cases. After surgery it may be necessary to close the wound and restrain the tissues with sutures. Protection in the immediate post-surgical period may then be afforded by applying a periodontal pack. Maintenance routines depend on the procedures adopted and cannot be overstressed. Many studies have shown that correctly applied maintenance therapy is more important than the type of surgical procedure undertaken.

If sutures and no pack have been used then a chlorhexidine antiseptic mouthrinse is prescribed for use twice a day to keep the area plaque-free. A soft brush may be used on the teeth but interdental cleaning is not advisable in the surgical area.

In the presence of a periodontal dressing or pack, normal plaque control methods are impossible locally and the patient should be advised to avoid sticky foods at the site and to rinse carefully to remove accumulated debris. Normal oral hygiene methods can be used elsewhere.

A week or so later, after removal of pack or sutures, the teeth are polished with a soft rubber cup, prophy point and a fluoride containing prophylaxis paste. It is important to undertake this on a regular basis during the following few months while the periodontal tissues are healing. It has been shown that by preventing mature plaque deposits in this way, subsequent healing is improved. If the patient's level of home care is less than perfect it may also be advisable to prescribe the use of chlorhexidine mouthrinse for up to 2 months after surgery, in any case regular maintenance on a 3 month basis is continued until the area is stable before increasing the interval to 6 and then 12 months.

Immediately after periodontal surgery the soft tissues will shrink and an interdental brush will be more appropriate for use than floss or tape. If exposure of sensitive dentine becomes troublesome, application of a topical desensitizing agent will be needed.

Patients undergoing oral surgery

Many dental hygienists are employed at least part-time in the oral and maxillofacial surgery departments of hospitals. If possible, the patients should be seen preoperatively, so that a scale and polish can be carried out and the oral hygiene problems which the patient is likely to encounter postoperatively can be discussed. Some cases will require to use a soft toothbrush for a while and others, with limited opening, will benefit from small or single-tufted brushes.

Particular problems will be encountered with patients being treated for a fractured mandible or maxilla. Many of these patients will have their upper and lower teeth fixed together with splints for a considerable time. Oral hygiene is very difficult and such patients should be seen at frequent intervals for cleaning of the teeth and splints. In all oral surgery cases the value of chlorhexidine should be borne in mind. Where mechanical plaque removal is not possible, chemical plaque control may be substituted.

Postoperative oral surgery patients may be restricted to a soft or liquid diet and there is a great risk that such a diet will be rich in sugar and, therefore, highly cariogenic. Once again, the patient with dental splints in place for some weeks is a particular worry. The dental hygienist must be able to give appropriate advice to these patients.

It is important to try to see the patients once healing is completed, so that a fine scale and polish can be carried out.

When visiting the patient (and any handicapped or bedridden person) the provision of a portable irrigating spray is important. There are still oral irrigators powered by carbon dioxide capsules or cartridges. We have even used small hand-size garden sprays pressurized by pumping and piston. When using an ultrasonic unit the water source could be a larger garden spray (holding 2 litres) and this can be attached to the water socket of the unit. Mouthwashes should be prescribed and provided and it is important to use one that has a strong distinctive taste because much stagnation occurs in the mouth during the day and the patients often complain of a foul taste. A soft toothbrush is provided, with instructions as to its use in accessible regions.

Orthodontic patients

Orthodontists are making increasing use of dental hygienists in their specialist practices and it is important that hygienists are aware of the current methods of treatment and their own role in the management of patients with orthodontic appliances.

The patient will usually go through the following stages during treatment.

Assessment appointment

This will include a full history and examination, impressions for study casts and radiographic survey. From this information a diagnosis and treatment plan will be decided upon. The hygienist can help at this stage by giving oral hygiene advice and dental health education in relation to the proposed treatment.

Appliance fitment

The procedure with removable appliances consists of fitting and activating the appliance as well as ensuring that the patient can remove and reinsert it. Fixed appliances require a more complicated and time-consuming process. The first stage is preparing the teeth for bonding. The enamel is cleaned with a non-fluoride-containing prophylaxis paste and, after this is washed away, the teeth are isolated and dried before the enamel is etched. To this bonding composite is applied to fix the appropriate brackets to the teeth. After fixation these are connected with wires and/or elastics.

The hygienist can assist not only with appropriate advice on oral hygiene, but in the cleaning and bonding processes, as these are very similar to the procedures used in fissure sealing. Patients with removable appliances need advice in relation to both cleaning of the teeth and the care of the appliance. After every meal or snack the appliance should be removed and carefully brushed clean in soapy water. In patients with fixed appliances, the care is more difficult. Special orthodontic brushes are available, as a brush with a very small head is needed for cleaning the bands, brackets, springs and wires. The value of a chlorhexidine rinse should be remembered.

The possibility of dental caries affecting the teeth with either type of appliance is increased. Therefore these patients should have a closely supervised programme of preventive treatment, including topical fluorides, fissure sealing and dietary advice.

Recall visits

The patient is recalled about every 6 weeks for the appliance to be checked and further activation to be undertaken. The oral hygiene must be checked and patients should be routinely seen by the dental hygienist.

Completion of active treatment

If a removable appliance has been worn it is deactivated or a passive retainer is fitted and worn for about 3 months, after which it is worn at night-time only for a further 3 months. A fixed appliance has to be removed and the bonding composite or cement cleaned from the teeth, after which a fixed or removable retainer is fitted. The hygienist may assist with tooth-cleaning and the subsequent monitoring of the oral health.

Review

The patient will be reviewed every 6 months for 12 months once the retainers are removed. During this period it is important that the oral

Table 17.4 Orthodontic treatment

The objectives of orthodontic treatment are to improve aesthetics, function and oral health. The main methods used are extractions and appliance therapy, whether fixed or removable, and functional.

- Removable appliances may be passive, such as space maintainers or retainers, or active. Active appliances may use forces from wires, springs, elastics or screws to move teeth or utilize muscle forces to cause changes, as with functional appliances. Generally, removable appliances move teeth by tipping actions and rarely can be relied upon to move teeth by a bodily motion.
- Fixed appliances use components which are cemented or bonded on to teeth. The commonest components are bands which are cemented around teeth, or brackets which are held by etch retained composites. Active fixed appliances use forces from wires, elastics or springs to move the teeth. The movements can be very complex and include tipping, bodily movement, torquing, rotation, forced eruption and depression of teeth.
- Either fixed or removable appliance therapy can be helped by the use of extra-oral headgear which, by acting as a secure anchorage, provides extra force and increased control of the movements.

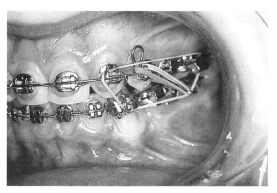

Fig. 17.10 A fixed orthodontic appliance that will need special care in its cleaning.

hygiene is monitored carefully. Any areas of decalcification may require treatment with topical fluorides to encourage remineralization (Fig. 17.10 and Table 17.4).

Patients with cleft palates

Possibly the most important group of patients the hygienist may have to treat are those with cleft palates. It is enormously important that these patients should retain their teeth in a healthy state for two reasons. Firstly, the teeth may be needed for oral orthopaedic treatment: appliances can only be used, for example to widen the dental arch, if adequately healthy teeth are present to support the appliance. Secondly, the congenitally missing teeth must be replaced by a partial denture or bridge. If patients with a cleft palate ever require a full

upper denture, retention of the denture is a very difficult problem.

Unfortunately, patients with clefts are often less well motivated towards retaining their teeth, since the appearance of the teeth before treatment is often poor. Also, by the very nature of their problem, plaque control is often more difficult for them. Nevertheless, it has been showed that the prevention of caries in cleft palate patients is possible, given the intensive preventive care that such patients deserve.

Patients with specific disabilities that will require careful oral hygiene advice and management
- Motor disabilities.
- Cognitive disability.
- The older patient.
- Patients with endocardial disease.
- Immunocompromised patients.
- Patients with diabetes.
- Patients with cleft palates.
- Patients with denture stomatitis.
- Patients undergoing oral surgery.

Dental appliances that will require careful cleaning
- Crown and bridgework.
- Osseointegrated implants.
- Removable dental prostheses.
- Complete dentures.
- Partial dentures.
- Overdentures.
- Orthodontic appliances.

Further reading

Jacob M. C., Plamping D. (1992) *The Practice of Primary Dental Care*. Oxford: Wright, Butterworth-Heinemann.

Manson J. D., Eley B. M. (1995) *Outline of Periodontics*. 3rd edition. Oxford: Wright, Butterworth-Heinemann.

Murray J. J. (1996) *The Prevention of Dental Disease*. 3rd edition. Oxford University Press.

Pine C. (1996) *Community Oral Health*. Oxford: Wright, Butterworth-Heinemann.

18

Instrument care and use

Introduction

The effective debridement of a root surface depends not only upon the use of appropriate techniques, but also on correctly maintained instruments. In 1905 C.V. Black said: '*Nothing in the technical procedures of dental practice is more important than the care of the cutting edges of instruments*'. This statement applies equally to the dental hygienist today who must know how to care for, as well as use, instruments.

Care of instruments

After use, instruments should be thoroughly washed and scrubbed under cold running water to remove all traces of blood and other debris, then dried. They can be further cleaned in an ultrasonic bath. Handpieces and other mechanical items need to be lubricated with a non-oil-based lubricant before sterilization. After sterilization hand instruments should be checked for sharpness and, if found to be blunt, sharpened then resterilized. It is no longer safe to sharpen instruments before sterilization, as this poses a threat to the operator, particularly from blood-borne viruses, and the sharpening equipment would, in time, become heavily contaminated. It is not necessary to sharpen instruments after every use, but the careful worker should undertake this on a regular basis, which will depend upon the patient flow and the use made of the instruments. Obviously

if an instrument is patently blunt it must be sharpened, but maintaining them on a regular schedule will prevent them from becoming totally ineffective.

Instruments must be sharp for effective and efficient scaling and root planing. Sharp instruments will improve your speed and make the procedures easier for both the operator and the patients (Table 18.1). Dull instruments not only increase patient discomfort and therefore operator stress, but may burnish the calculus flat and make it more difficult to detect.

Table 18.1 The principles of sharpening

The following steps should ensure that instruments remain sharp

- Sharpen the lateral sides of instruments, not the face. This ensures that the instrument maintains its most efficient shape.
- Do not overheat the instrument during sharpening. The temper of steel is lost when overheated and its sharpness will not be retained.
- Reduce the entire lateral face. If only one part of the side is reduced, it will not be straight and therefore it will not be possible to keep the cutting edge against the root surface during scaling.
- Make the sharpening stroke by moving the instrument towards not away from you, as this will minimize the formation of a wire edge.
- Lubricate the stone well during sharpening.

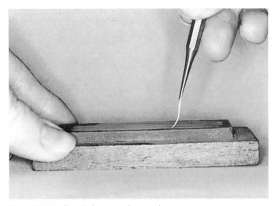

Fig. 18.1 A flat Arkansas sharpening stone.

Testing for sharpness

There are three basic methods of detecting blunt instruments: effectiveness during use, visual inspection and using test sticks. A blunt instrument will not 'bite' on the root surface and the operator will need to apply increased pressure for it to be effective. When visually inspecting the cutting edge of an instrument it is helpful to examine it using a magnifying viewer with about ×5 magnification. The cutting edge should not show any reflection when it is rotated through the light.

The final method of testing the degree of sharpness is to use a series of test strokes. Many operators use the finger- or thumbnail for the assessment. Although, with correct sterilization procedures, this should not pose an infection risk, it is a procedure that must be decried as, if it is undertaken frequently, it must lead to a weakening of the fingernail. A preferable method is to use an acrylic test stick. The instrument is held against the stick, activated and the resulting bite evaluated. Care must be taken that instruments with long cutting edges, such as sickles, are tested along the entire working length.

Sharpening is undertaken using a stone and the type chosen will depend upon the shape of the instrument to be sharpened. Mounted stones are recommended only for the very experienced, as they are difficult to control and can quickly ruin an instrument by taking off too much metal, or generating heat by friction and thus affecting the temper of the instrument. A flat, unmounted hard Arkansas or diamond-coated stone is the best choice for all instruments with straight cutting edges, whilst rounded or cylindrical stones are better for those with rounded cutting edges (Fig.18.1). The Arkansas stone is the one used most commonly for sharpening. It should be wiped clean after use and re-oiled before storage. It can be sterilized in an autoclave but must always be re-oiled before storage. Mechanical motor-driven sharpening honing units are also

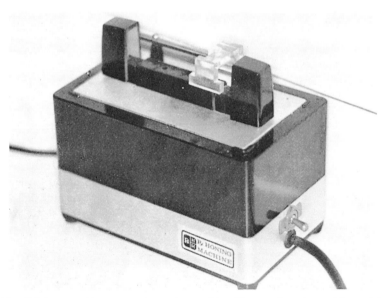

Fig. 18.2 A powered instrument sharpening machine. There are interchangeable revolving stones for different instruments.

available (Fig. 18.2), which have the additional advantages of guides to hold the instrument at a predetermined angle, and diamond attachments for use with tungsten carbide instruments (Table 18.2).

Table 18.2 Sharpening equipment

Sharpening stones are made of abrasive particles compressed into a solid piece which grinds the blunt working tip. There are two general types of stones: mounted and unmounted. Sharpening should always take place in a suitable area equipped with a magnifying viewer, a light source and appropriate sharpening materials which include

- Sharpening stones, mounted or unmounted.
- Mechanical or powered sharpeners.
- Lubricating fluids, such as light mineral oil or water.
- Acrylic test stick.
- Gauze.

Steps in the effective care of instruments

- Clean after use: remove blood and debris under running water.
- Sterilize before storage.
- Test for sharpness and sharpen regularly.

Sharpening techniques

The inexperienced beginner would be well advised only to sharpen instruments with an unmounted stone and for that reason that method is the one described here. There are two basic ways of using unmounted stones: the first and commoner method is to use a stationary stone/moving instrument technique. However, it is equally permissible to use a moving stone/stationary instrument approach, but as this method is more difficult to master, only the former technique will be described.

The sickle scaler

Two stones are used: a flat and a cylindrical Arkansas. Both are lubricated before use with a light mineral oil. The stone is held with the non-working hand (the left in the case of a right-handed individual) and the handle held with a modified pen grasp, so that the top face is at an angle of approximately 110° to the surface of the stone. It should be noted that it will be necessary to adjust the angulation at which the handle of the sickle is held depending upon whether an H6 or H7 sickle is being sharpened. Because the sickle is a curved instrument, the entire cutting edge cannot be sharpened at one time (Fig. 18.4). A rolling action is used to rotate the instrument and thus sharpen from the shank end to the tip. The instrument is moved in an elliptical action across the stone towards the operator, maintaining the 110°

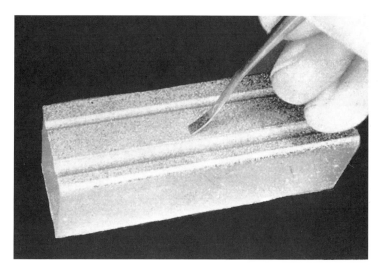

Fig. 18.3 Sharpening a push scaler.

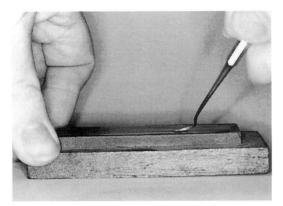

Fig. 18.4 Sharpening a sickle scaler.

inclination. Care must be taken to ensure that the final one-third of the tip is efficiently sharpened. The sharpening movement is continued until the cutting edge appears bright sharp. This procedure is then repeated on the opposite lateral edge with the tip now pointing in the opposite direction. Next a round stone is used to remove any swarf (loose metallic material) from the top face using the cylindrical stone. This will be aided by the use of the magnifying viewer to check the cutting edge. After sharpening, a piece of gauze is used to remove any oil and check by the absence of snagging that all the swarf has been eliminated. Finally the instrument is tested against the acrylic test stick.

The push scaler

For this a flat lubricated Arkansas stone is needed. The flat cutting tip is placed against the surface of the stone, and pushed slowly forward across the stone, maintaining the initial angle. The cutting edge is always pushed against the stone, not with it (Fig. 18.3). Finally the instrument is placed flat against the stone and one or two gentle strokes made to remove any swarf. The cleaning and checking procedures are undertaken in the same way as for the sickle.

The curette

Using a modified pen grip the curette is held against the stone at an angulation of approximately 110° between the top surface and the stone. The instrument is moved towards the operator in an arc whilst it is rotated to drag the cutting edge from the shank to the tip across the stone. The pressure is then released and the

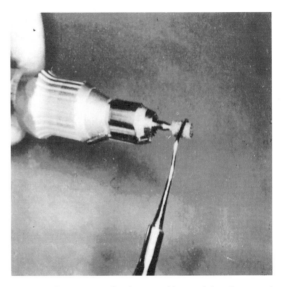

Fig. 18.5 Curettes may be sharpened by applying the curved inner surface to a slowly revolving cylindrical carborundum stone in a handpiece.

instrument slid back before repeating the motion until the edge is sharp. The instrument is then turned over and the other edge sharpened in a similar manner. Finally the toe is rounded by lightly dragging this across the stone. Any swarf present can be removed with a round Arkansas stone rotated against the top edge and oil and loose material cleaned away with gauze (Fig. 18.5).

Tungsten carbide tipped instruments are difficult to sharpen and should be replaced when blunt. All instruments should be resterilized before storage.

Sharpening techniques for
- Sickle scalers: flat and round Arkansas stone.
- Push scalers: flat Arkansas stone.
- Dental curette: flat and round Arkansas stone.

Storage of instruments

Instruments should be stored in dry, air-tight conditions, to discourage corrosion and contamination by air-borne organisms. The ideal method is to use a sealed autoclave bag, taking care that it does not get torn or wet. If this does occur then the instrument must be resterilized before use.

Instruments that become corroded or dull after a period of use can often be repolished on a dental lathe with a soft mop and metal polish, before being cleaned and resterilized.

Scaling techniques

A variety of acquired deposits are found adhering to tooth surfaces including salivary pellicle, dental plaque, calculus and a multiplicity of stains. Scaling is the procedure by which these deposits are removed from the tooth surface. Scaling differs from root planing in that this latter procedure consists of instrumentation, not only to remove surface deposits, but also to smooth the root surface and remove a thin layer of cementum, thus reducing the endotoxin burden. Some authorities do not feel that effective scaling can be carried out subgingivally unless followed by root planing.

Scaling and polishing

During scaling a sharp working edge is placed on the tooth surface adjacent to the calculus and moved along that surface to dislodge the calculus and any adherent soft deposits. The angle at which the working tip is held against the tooth surface is important as scaling is more efficient if it leans back from the direction of movement than if it leans forward. However, in practice most scaling is performed with the tip at 90° or less to the tooth surface. The techniques of scaling are outlined together with the description of each instrument.

Root planing

Root planing is undertaken when, after routine scaling and polishing and in the presence of effective home care, the inflammation in the pockets persists. It is probable that root planing, as opposed to scaling, reduces the level of cementum-bound endotoxin to a biologically acceptable level and thus allows healing of the adjacent periodontal soft tissues. However, recent work has shown that endotoxin may be reduced to the level seen on healthy root surfaces by very light root planing or even polishing the root with a mild abrasive, provided that the root surface in the pocket is instrumented in a thorough, systematic way. It may well be that the only differences between scaling and root planing is the overall reduction in root surface contaminants and this has to be lower in some patients than in others, who have less resistance to the influence of dental plaque and its by-products. There are, of course, differences in the instruments used in scaling, which is often a supragingival procedure, and root planing, which is always carried out in subgingival sites.

When carrying out root planing, some analgesia will usually be required. Often the use of a topical anaesthetic cream will suffice, particularly when at least 2 min is allowed to elapse between application and scaling, so that maximum anaesthesia is achieved. When topical anaesthesia is inadequate, block or infiltration anaesthesia will be required: some patients will even need this reinforced with inhalation relative analgesia. Pain control is described in Chapter 22.

The first step in root planing is to explore the pocket with a light instrument such as a Cross calculus probe or a WHO probe, so that a clear picture can be built up of the outline of the lesion. The next stage is to use an ultrasonic scaler to remove any gross debris and flush out the pocket. This should be followed by a heavy subgingival scaler, such as a periodontal hoe, which is inserted to the base of the pocket. Lateral pressure is then applied to hold the instrument against the root and the scaler advanced out of the pocket with a firm but controlled movement. This is repeated using a series of short overlapping strokes until the whole area of the root involved in the pocket has been instrumented. This procedure is repeated with a suitable file and finally a curette is used to smooth the surface. The pocket is then flushed carefully using the ultrasonic scaler for debridement and finally irrigated with some chlorhexidine solution inserted from a syringe with a blunt-nosed needle (Fig. 18.6).

Hand instrumentation

There follows a general outline of the use of the main types of hygienist scaling instruments. As the use of these instruments is best learned by practical demonstration and practice at the chairside, this description is of necessity limited.

It is important to hold the instrument in an appropriate way as this will determine the amount of control over it and thus the stability

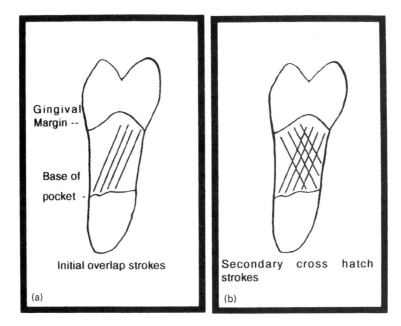

Fig. 18.6 Technique for root planing: (a) initial overlapping strokes, (b) secondary cross hatch strokes. This method ensures that each area is instrumented at least four times by the instrument.

and effectiveness in use. There are two possible ways to hold a scaler. The modified pen grasp is the most commonly used and this variation of the standard pen grip is used for many procedures. The instrument is held as in writing, with the side of the mesial side of the middle finger and the terminal pad utilized on the shank of the instrument. On rare occasions during scaling the palm grip is used to give more power, but at the price of decreased control and visibility. The handle of the instrument is held in the palm of the hand with the fingers grasping the handle and the thumb placed on the shank to control movement.

As well as an appropriate instrument grip it is also important to establish a finger rest to ensure stability and lessen the possibility of slipping when applying pressure. The third or ring finger is the main source of the finger rest and the fourth or small finger is often used in addition.

The sickle scaler

The method of use is usually by rotation of the handle to activate the cutting edge. Sickles have two cutting edges which are formed by the convergence of the top surface and the two lateral surfaces (Fig. 18.7). The cross-section of the working tip is triangular in shape. The sickle is used mainly for supragingival scaling or scaling and root planing just beneath the gingival margin, provided the gingival pocket is fairly loose. This instrument should not be inserted too deeply into a pocket as the sharp tip will lacerate the soft tissue wall.

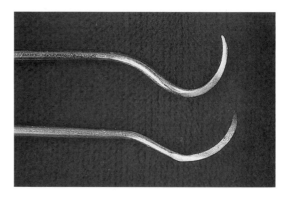

Fig. 18.7 The H6 and H7 sickle scalers.

Method of use

The cutting edge is placed against the tooth at 90° to the surface and then moved upwards with a pull stroke.

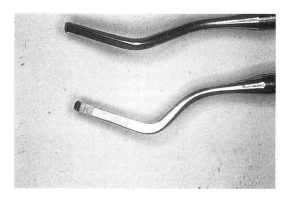

Fig. 18.8 MacFarlane hoes.

The periodontal hoe

This has a straight cutting edge on a short wide blade projecting at right angles from the shaft. The hoe is the principal instrument for removing heavy deposits of subgingival calculus from beneath the gingiva and for root planing. It may also be used to remove heavy deposits of supragingival calculus.

Method of use

The working tip is slid down the root surface over the calculus until its bottom edge is felt. Pressure is applied to hold the hoe against the deposits and the shank against the crown. The instrument is then moved towards the crown to plane away the calculus (Fig. 18.8). When root planing, multiple overlapping strokes are used.

The periodontal file

The file has a series of cutting edges set at right angles to the shank on a round, oval or rectangular base. It is used for subgingival scaling and root planing, but will not cope with heavy deposits which must be removed with a hoe scaler first (Figs 18.9–18.10).

Method of use

The instrument is slid down the root surface to the lower edge of the calculus. Pressure is applied to hold the cutting edges and the shank against the tooth and the instrument moved towards the crown, removing the deposits. The design of a file requires repeated strokes to be made whilst instrumenting an area, especially when it is used for root planing.

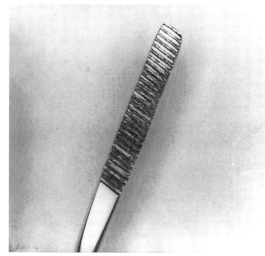

Fig. 18.9 Close-up view of the working surface of a Bunting periodontal file which may be used for root planing.

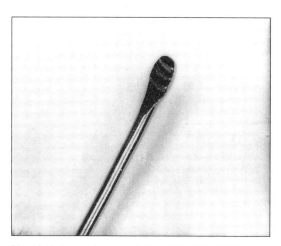

Fig. 18.10 A round type periodontal file (Hirschfeld) used for root planing after the removal of gross calculus deposits.

The push scaler

The push or chisel scaler has a single straight bevelled cutting edge set at right angles to the shank. It is used to remove heavy deposits of supragingival calculus from the interdental surfaces of the anterior teeth. It should only be used when the embrasure spaces are open and sufficient space is present.

Method of use

The cutting edge is placed from the labial aspect against the tooth surface and pressure applied to cleave away adhering calculus deposits.

The dental curette

This has a spoon-shaped working tip with two curved cutting edges. The curette is the principal instrument for fine subgingival scaling, root planing and root surface smoothing. There are two types, the universal with two cutting edges and the site specific which has a cutting edge on one side only (Figs 18.11–18.13).

Method of use

The working tip is inserted to the base of the pocket and tilted to give an angle of more than 90°, then used with a pull stroke towards the occlusal surface. Repeated, overlapping strokes are used.

Instruments for scaling and root planing

- Sickle scaler: used mainly for supragingival scaling or scaling and root planing just beneath the gingival margin.
- Periodontal hoe: used for removing heavy deposits of subgingival calculus from beneath the gingiva and for root planing.
- Periodontal files: used for subgingival scaling and root planing.
- Push scaler: used to remove heavy deposits of supragingival calculus from the interdental surfaces of the anterior teeth.
- Dental curette: the principal instrument for fine subgingival scaling, root planing and root surface smoothing.

Ultrasonic scalers

Since the introduction of the first ultrasonic scaler in 1955, the use of these automated scaling instruments has made the life of the operator so much easier and for many patients made the scaling procedure more acceptable. Ultrasonic scalers operate above 20 kHz (20 000 vibrations a second) and modern machines work at 30 kHz. There are two different types available on the market. The magnetostrictive types use a core or stack of magnetic material which is acted upon by electrical windings in the handpiece which produce an alternating magnetic flux. When the stack is magnetized it contracts and as the stack is connected to the working tip this mechanical change is relayed to the tooth surface. The piezoelectric types utilize the ability of small electrical currents to alter the dimensions of a quartz crystal to produce the vibration. Although it has been said that these scalers cannot perform root planing, they have a valuable role in the removal of gross deposits and flushing out the pocket (Fig. 18.14 and Table 18.3).

Air or sonic scalers

Sonic scalers are operated by the airline usually connected to the air turbine. The air is passed over a reed in the handpiece which then vibrates in a similar manner to a musical instrument. Sonic scalers operate at frequencies below that of the limit of hearing, typically in the 5–10 kHz range. As with the ultrasonic scaler, this type of instrument needs a water spray as heat is produced during use at the working tip and the cooling spray has the additional advantage of washing away dislodged deposits, but also the distinct disadvantage of producing an aerosol (Fig. 18.15).

Technique of use of sonic or ultrasonic scalers

- Preparation of the instrument. The scaler should be adjusted according to the manufacturer's specifications, using the lowest possible setting at which atomization of the water takes place. The instrument tips should be blunt: if sharp, they will gouge or nick the root surface.
- Preparation of the patient. The patient's medical history must be reviewed, since the use of ultrasonic scalers is contraindicated in
    patients who are known to be carriers of hepatitis, since the aerosol spray caused would increase the droplet zone and hence the risk of cross-infection
    patients who have been fitted with a cardiac pacemaker, since it is felt that the ultrasonic vibrations might upset the rate of the pacemaker
    patients with a hearing aid will often be more comfortable if it is turned off.

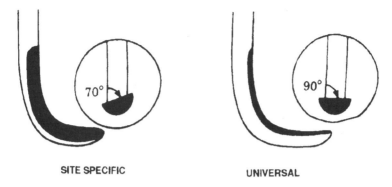

Fig. 18.11 A comparison of a site specific curette, such as a Gracey, with a universal, for example a Langer. The angle of the working tip to the shank is shown in the inset.

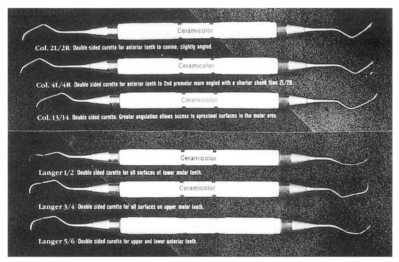

Fig. 18.12 Universal curettes: Columbia and Langer (courtesy of Dentsply Plc).

Table 18.3 Mode of action of ultrasonic scalers

The ultrasonic unit converts high-frequency electrical energy into mechanical energy in the form of very rapid vibrations. A water spray is needed as heat is produced during use in the handpiece stack and at the working tip, and the cooling spray has the additional advantage of washing away dislodged deposits. The removal of calculus and other deposits is achieved in three ways

- **Mechanical abrading action**. The action is a mixture of back-and-forth and circulatory movements and this mechanically abrades and chips away at the deposits on the root surface. A variety of differing shaped tips is available to achieve this result; some are shown in Fig. 18.15.
- **Cavitational effects**. All ultrasonic scalers are provided with a flow of cooling water directed at the tip to remove any heat caused by friction between the tip and the tooth surface. The water contains minute air bubbles which are expanded by the energy in the vibrating tip which causes them to have a negative internal pressure for a fraction of a second and then implode, releasing large shock waves. Such forces have been shown to remove plaque and calculus from the tooth surface. One of the side-effects of the water flow and cavitation is the generation of a large aerosol: precautions should be taken against this, as described later.
- **Acoustic streaming**. Ultrasonic scalers set up vigorous movements of the water around their tips and this is termed acoustic streaming. This assists in the removal of some of the tooth-surface deposits and in the disruption of plaque colonies.

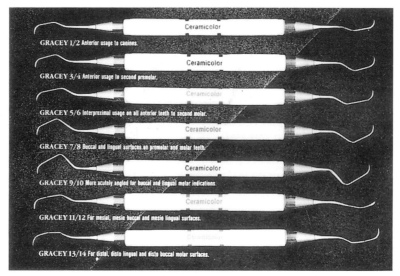

Fig. 18.13 Gracey site specific curettes (courtesy of Dentsply Plc).

This will also prevent the risk of feed-back occurring.

- Many operators believe that an antiseptic mouthwash (such as chlorhexidine) should be given to patients 3 min before using an ultrasonic scaler, to reduce the oral bacterial count and hence the bacterial count of the aerosol spray.
- An all-covering protective towel or bib and high-speed suction is needed to cope with the water spray.
- Preparation of the operator. It is sensible for the operator to take additional precautions when using the ultrasonic scaler, because of its spray. At least a well fitting mask and probably a pair of protective glasses should be considered.
- Instrumentation. A modified pen grasp is recommended with a fulcrum on the nearest comfortable tooth. The working end should be applied as nearly as possible parallel to the tooth surface and, at worst, no more than 15° to the surface. The angulation has to be continually altered to adapt to the tooth morphology and this requires practice, but a greater angulation than 15° will result in scratching of the tooth surface.

The tip should be kept in motion the whole time to avoid overheating any area and the water supply must always be able to reach the tip. A brushing stroke, like that used with a

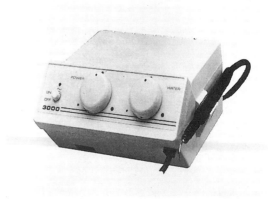

Fig. 18.14 The Dentsply/Cavitron 30K ultrasonic scaler.

paint brush, should be used with the minimum of pressure. Since the spray makes vision awkward, frequent stops are needed to assess the situation and these will also aid water control and prevent overheating (Tables 18.4 and 18.5).

Characteristics of ultrasonic scalers

- Operate at 30 kHz.
- Two types: magnetostrictive and piezo-electric.
- Mode of action: mechanical, cavitation and acoustic streaming.

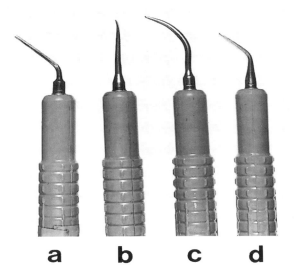

a   **b**   **c**   **d**

Fig. 18.15 A selection of useful inserts for the Dentsply/Cavitron ultrasonic scaler.

Table 18.4 Advantages of ultrasonics

The advantages of ultrasonic scalers include

- Heavy calculus deposits can be removed more quickly and with less effort, allowing more time to be devoted to more detailed manual scaling.
- Debridement is accomplished more effectively because of the spray.
- The patient may experience less pain with scaling of gross deposits than with manual scaling.
- For the above reasons, the ultrasonic scaler is particularly suited to the initial treatment of acute necrotizing gingivitis.

Table 18.5 Disadvantages of ultrasonics

The disadvantages of ultrasonic scalers include

- Visibility is often a problem.
- Water control is difficult without a four-handed approach.
- The noise and spray may be unacceptable to some patients, especially elderly and mentally handicapped patients.

Further reading

Nield-Gehrig J. S., Houseman G. A. (1996) *Fundamentals of Periodontal Instrumentation*. Baltimore: Williams & Wilkins.

Schoen D. H., Dean M. C. (1996) *Contemporary Periodontal Instrumentation*. Philadelphia: Saunders.

19

Rubber dam application

The purpose of rubber dam

All too often, dental procedures are carried out on teeth contaminated by saliva and plaque and, soon after the start of the operative procedure, there may be additional contamination by blood and crevicular fluid. There are many procedures which ideally should be carried out on clean dry teeth, but such conditions are not always possible to achieve, especially for the periodontist or hygienist. When carrying out scaling and root planing it is impossible to avoid damage to the gingiva at all times and limited moisture control may be all that is possible. Nevertheless, while moisture control using such items as aspirators and cotton wool rolls can be adequate for procedures such as prophylaxis, scaling and root planing, for other procedures higher standards are needed.

The ideal method of moisture control is the application of rubber dam, a method obligatory in endodontics where it gives the additional advantages of preventing cross-infection and protecting the patient's airway. In the dental hygienist's practice, rubber dam is of main benefit when placing fissure sealants, but is also of value in the application of certain desensitizing agents and some forms of topical fluoride.

Rubber dam is helpful in other ways apart from preventing moisture contamination. It protects the working field, the operator and the operator's instruments from contamination by the patient's oral flora and is especially indicated for patients with diseases such as

hepatitis B where cross-infection is a great danger. These advantages outweigh any possible disadvantages which might include the inconvenience of fitting the dam, a reduction in the amount of communication possible with the patient and an occasional complaint of claustrophobia. Residues of the chemicals used in the processing of latex may produce an allergic response in a very small number of patients and its use is, of course, contraindicated in patients giving a history of such an allergy.

Advantages of using rubber dam
- The ideal method of moisture control.
- Protection of the soft tissues.
- Prevention of cross infection.
- Control of the tongue.

Disadvantages of use
- Time and inconvenience in fitting.
- Reduction of communication with the patient.
- A feeling of claustrophobia in some cases.

Equipment

The rubber dam itself is a thin sheet of latex which forms a watertight junction around the cervical margin of the tooth, so excluding moisture from the operative field. The necessary equipment for its application includes a rubber

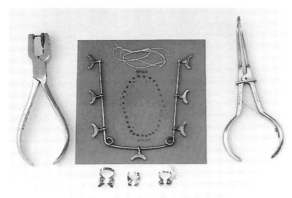

Fig. 19.1 Rubber dam equipment: punch, forceps, sheet of rubber dam, floss silk, Fernauld frame and selection of clamps.

dam punch and frame, rubber dam forceps, an assortment of clamps and a supply of waxed floss silk (Fig. 19.1). A lubricant, most conveniently topical anaesthetic gel, is useful for helping the rubber dam pass through tight interdental contacts.

Rubber dam is generally supplied in 15 cm black or green squares of which medium thickness is the most popular. Recently it has become available in a range of pastel shades and pleasant tastes. At an appropriate position a hole is punched in the dam through which the selected tooth crown passes, so isolating the tooth from the rest of the mouth. Until experience is acquired a rubber dam stamp is useful and serves to pre-mark the dam with the sites of teeth in their arches. Once applied, provided that the punched hole is narrower in diameter than the cervical margin of the tooth, the dam will be retained mechanically. For some procedures the dam at the cervical margin of the tooth is encouraged to enter the gingival crevice, so exposing the maximum clinical crown. If desired the edge of the dam can be inverted into place with a small flat plastic instrument.

While rubber dam punches and forceps are of standard form, rubber dam frames are of two types. The original metal Fernauld frame is a U-shaped piece of thick wire to which the dam is attached by being stretched over short T-bars extending outwards. Modern forms are made of plastic and the dam is attached by stretching it over short 'spikes' protruding from the periphery.

Rubber dam clamps consist of two blades engaging the cervical margin of the tooth and joined by a connector of springy steel. They are of various sizes depending on the tooth to

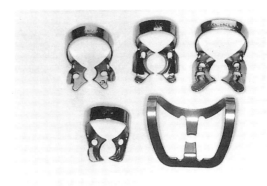

Fig. 19.2 Selection of rubber dam clamps: (top left to right) winged premolar clamp, large and small winged molar clamps;(bottom left to right) small wingless clamp and Ferrier anterior tooth clamp.

which they are to be attached (Fig. 19.2). Rubber dam clamps do not always fit precisely and usually we have to be satisfied with two point contact between the blade and the tooth. Depending on whether the edge of the blade is straight or curved downwards to enter the gingival crevice, the clamp will be suitable for fully erupted or partly erupted teeth.

On the clamp, next to the blades, are found points of attachment, either holes or notches, for the rubber dam forceps and using these the clamp is applied to the tooth and removed afterwards. Most clamps also possess small projections or wings, which serve for temporary attachment of the dam to the clamp during its manipulation outside the mouth. They are found adjacent to the site of application of the forceps. When repeatedly trying in clamps to check their fit, secure them with a piece of floss silk or by attaching their wings to the rubber dam. Clamps have been known to fracture in use and hence should not be placed in the mouth unless secured. In this way the pieces cannot be swallowed or inhaled. Wingless clamps are available and are used, after initial application of the dam, to improve access by securing the dam to more distal teeth. Extra holes are then unnecessary.

> Rubber dam equipment
> - Rubber dam (15 cm squares of latex).
> - Various clamps.
> - A frame to support the dam.
> - Floss silk for securing the clamps.

Application

The method of application of rubber dam varies slightly according to the number and type of teeth to be isolated and methods appropriate to each will be described. Before any attempt to apply rubber dam, however, any interproximal contacts through which the dam must pass are tested for patency with waxed floss silk.

Application to a single molar or premolar tooth

A sheet of rubber dam is selected and a hole punched in the appropriate place using one of the larger guides on the punch. Sometimes, for large molars, two interconnected holes are needed. A suitably sized, winged clamp is chosen and placed in the punched hole retaining the dam on the clamp wings, with the connector to the back. After the frame has been attached to the dam, the clamp is engaged by the forceps (Fig. 19.3) and the entire assembly picked up and placed on the tooth (Fig. 19.4). When the clamp is secure the dam is slipped from the wings to seal the cervical margin (Fig. 19.5). After completion of the procedure the rubber dam is removed after first removing the clamp.

Application to a single anterior tooth

A hole is again punched at the appropriate place in the rubber dam and the sheet of dam

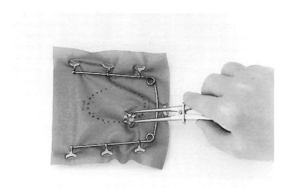

Fig. 19.3 Dam assembly ready for placing on the tooth.

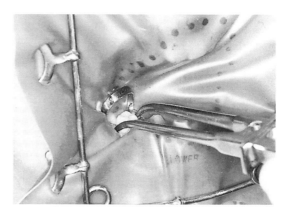

Fig. 19.4 United dam, frame and clamp placed on the tooth.

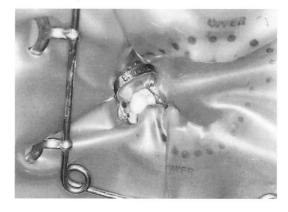

Fig. 19.5 Forceps disengaged and dam removed from wings

attached to the frame. The tissue side of the hole in the dam is lubricated with a small amount of topical anaesthetic gel and the dam placed in position over the tooth, passing the

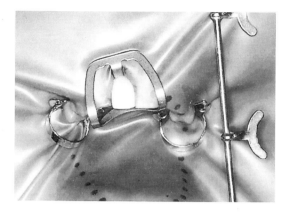

Fig. 19.6 Dam secured on anterior tooth with Ferrier clamp.

edge of the dam through the interdental contacts. To ensure that the sheet of rubber dam is retained on the tooth and that the edge of the dam enters, and is retained in the gingival crevice, a floss silk ligature is applied. A piece of waxed silk approximately 25 cm long is passed twice round the tooth. Holding the free ends firmly in one hand and using a small flat plastic instrument, the ligature is pushed down to the cervical margin of the tooth, carrying the dam with it. Once the ligature is sufficiently far cervically it will be retained at the narrowest point of the tooth and is secured by a double hitch.

Alternatively a clamp can be used. After placing the dam on the tooth by hand it is drawn up with the fingers to expose the cervical margin, at which point a clamp is applied. A Ferrier type clamp is the most useful.

Whichever method is used, for further security and improved access the dam can be held down by clamps in the premolar region.

Small, winged or wingless clamps are applied to a premolar tooth, on each side, over the dam. It is unnecessary to punch a hole beforehand (Fig. 19.6).

Application to several posterior teeth

A number of holes are punched in the dam according to the site and number of the teeth to be isolated. For best access include, if possible, the tooth distal to the operative site. As before, a clamp is engaged into the most distal hole, by its wings, and the frame attached to the dam periphery. After lubricating the internal surface of the punched holes, the clamp, frame and related dam are applied to the tooth, the dam freed from the clamp wings and pushed down over the crowns of the teeth to be isolated, each in its appropriate hole. Floss silk is used to pass the lubricated dam through the contacts. If, after application, the dam does not pass immediately into the gingival crevice it can be inverted into place with a flat plastic instrument.

To improve access a clamp can be applied over a tooth on the contralateral side (Fig. 19.7). Where lip activity is marked and it is feared that it might displace the dam, a further clamp can be applied over the dam, on the same side, but anterior to the site of operation.

Application to several anterior teeth

The ligature method is used as for application to a single anterior tooth. The correct number of holes are punched and after the teeth have been pushed through the dam, small wingless clamps are applied over the premolar teeth in order to secure the dam firmly before ligatures

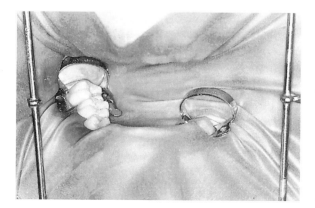

Fig. 19.7 Access to isolated mandibular teeth improved by placement of a clamp over a contralateral premolar.

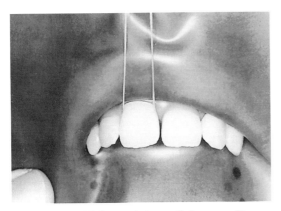

Fig. 19.8 Floss silk ligature being applied to a maxillary central incisor.

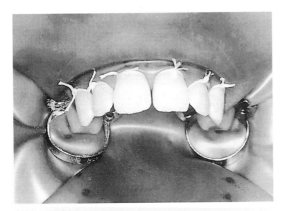

Fig. 19.9 Floss silk ligatures and premolar clamps securing dam.

Placement of rubber dam
- Check contact points with dental floss to ensure patency.
- Punch a hole of the correct size in the dam.
- Attach suitably sized clamp in the dam.
- Attach the frame to the dam.
- Slip the clamp with dam over the tooth.
- Slip the dam off the wings of the clamp to seal the cervical margin.
- Modify technique for single or multiple, posterior or anterior teeth.

Final points

If ever a bridge has to be involved in the rubber dam, application is more difficult. Holes are punched as normal but those holes related to the bridge abutments are joined by a scissors cut. The rubber dam will now fit over the bridge and protect the airway but unfortunately some moisture contamination can occur from the gingival crevice. Because the attachment is relatively less secure, application of clamps on either side of the bridge is advisable.

Although the application of rubber dam is a painless procedure in the hands of a skilled operator, some discomfort can arise if it is to be in place for longer than a few minutes. To prevent maceration of the skin after the dam has been applied, use a saliva ejector and place dental napkins between the patient's lips and the edges of the dam.

Some interference with breathing can occur and it is best to cut away the dam around the patient's nostrils. Patients who are mouth breathers may be inconvenienced if there is a good seal between the lips and the dam. To aid breathing in such cases, accessory holes can be cut in the upper part of the dam, but ensure that none is as large as the smallest instrument to be used.

are applied. When the dam is fully in place, ligatures are applied to all isolated teeth (Figs 19.8 and 19.9). By inserting wedges interdentally, additional security is given for ensuring that the dam remains in the gingival crevice.

Removal of rubber dam

To remove the dam all retaining clamps ligatures and wedges are removed. If a single tooth has been isolated the dam can then be drawn away from the crown. When several teeth have been isolated the dam may still resist removal. The dam is then pulled buccally or labially away from the cervical margins of the teeth and the connections between the punched holes cut with scissors, taking care to avoid damage to the lips or cheeks.

Further reading

Kidd E. A. M., Smith B. G. N., Pickard H. M. (1996) *Pickard's Manual of Operative Dentistry*. 7th edition. Oxford: Oxford Medical Publications.

20

Prevention of dental diseases

Introduction

An important part of the job of the dental hygienist is the delivery of oral health education to patients. This might be on a one-to-one basis in the dental clinic, or it may involve speaking to people in a group. Mostly dental hygienists provide oral health information to patients in the dental clinic. Therefore, the practice of health education in dental practice should reflect the developing challenge of the preventive approach which reflects the general health context. Providing information should have the aim of improving health literacy. This means moving beyond the awareness of an issue such as toothbrushing to a deeper understanding of the importance of the timing of toothbrushing together with such factors as the design and shape of the toothbrush.

In addition, it is important to recognize that there are opportunities for more general health promotion in dental practice. A good example of this would be to provide tobacco risk information and for those dental patients who are interested, a tobacco control programme would help to emphasize the oral health benefits in addition to the general health gains of stopping smoking. Research has shown a link between poor periodontal health and coronary artery disease and this could be another area where the dental hygienist could link the benefits of good oral health with its potential impact on general health.

Further opportunities for health promotion could include the selling of toothbrushes and dental floss to underpin the importance of the information given to patients. Another opportunity would be to provide information and facilities for use by self-help and pressure groups. For example, slimming groups may have a vested interest in diet control with which caries reduction can be associated. There may be a pressure group wishing to move confectionery displays away from the cashier in supermarkets. Oral health promotion is going to be an increasingly important part of the dental hygienist's work and as health care systems move towards prevention, the financing of health care will change to reflect this.

The reader is encouraged to explore oral health education in greater detail by referring to Chapter 23 and by reading one of the recommended texts at the end of this chapter.

Prevention of dental disease

The prevention of disease may be described as being either passive or active: it may involve no effort on the part of the patient or it may require their active co-operation. The more passive the preventive measures are, the more successful they tend to be. Consequently, diseases for which there are effective vaccines have been largely eradicated (for example whooping cough and smallpox), whereas diseases such as those caused by over eating or over drinking, which can only be avoided with the active effort of the individual, are more of a problem than ever.

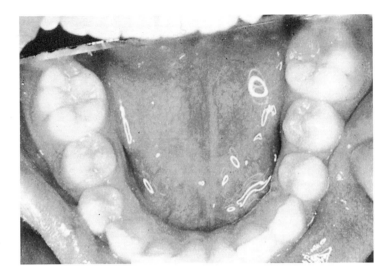

Fig. 20.1 This young patient has never had any carious cavities and therefore has never experienced the dental drill. Regular attendance (three times annually) for topical fluoride since the age of 3 years has probably helped!

One of the most effective passive dental preventive measures is water fluoridation. Most other dental measures involve a good deal of active patient co-operation. This is the main reason for their limited success and underlines why improving health literacy is so important.

Prevention of disease can be classified in three phases: primary, secondary and tertiary prevention.

- **Primary prevention**: procedures carried out to ensure that disease does not occur (Fig. 20.1).
- **Secondary prevention**: the early detection of disease, halting its progress by simple repair or remedial measures. Full recovery to normal may be possible and recurrence prevented.
- **Tertiary prevention**: the treatment of established disease in order to minimize or eliminate the gross destruction. At this stage prevention procedures will help to resist further damage from the disease.

The approach is usually the same, whatever the disease, but the major portion of our present prevention of dental disease is in phase 2. Ideally, we should try to succeed in phase 1 but patients, especially the young, are difficult to convince of the importance of prevention until some problem has occurred.

Periodontal screening and monitoring

The dental hygienist is the main link in the management of patients suffering from inflammatory periodontal diseases. One of the more important procedures she or he can undertake is to screen patients attending the practice for signs of inflammatory periodontal diseases. The community periodontal index of treatment needs (CPITN) has been developed as a screening tool, most notably by the British Society of Periodontology (BSP). As the CPITN is a poor treatment-needs indicator, and is rarely used by community services, it has recently been suggested that the term 'basic periodontal examination (BPE)' should be used in its place. This screening index is explained in Chapter 12.

The BPE needs to be complemented by appropriate radiographs. For the patient without any signs of overt disease, bitewing radiographs or an orthopantomograph will give information on the posterior bony contour, and these should be supplemented by periapical views of the anterior teeth, taken by the long cone parallel technique.

The BPE screening system is not intended to be used for monitoring purposes during treatment and readers can refer to the BSP policy document for more details of recording and monitoring methods. The recommended investigations should include the following assessments.

- Plaque deposits, using a plaque index.
- Gingival health using a bleeding or gingival index.
- Probing depths.
- Mobility using a mobility index.
- Furcation involvement using a furcation index.

Gingival, plaque and mobility indices and periodontal probing techniques are described in Chapter 12.

Oral health promotion will play an increasingly important role in dentistry.
- Prevention of dental disease can be primary, secondary or tertiary.
- Basic periodontal screening may be undertaken using the BPE.
- The BPE should be supported by other indices of measurement such as plaque index, gingival or bleeding index and pocket depths where necessary.

Control of dental plaque

The prevention of dental disease is not, as the name might suggest, a single subject. The two major dental diseases, caries and periodontal disease, have quite different causes and the prevention of each is markedly different from that of the other although there is some overlap. This is particularly true of the part played by plaque control in their prevention.

There is evidence that plaque control alone has little effect on the caries rate and that overall preventive management, including plaque control, dietary modification, fluorides and fissure sealants, is needed to produce a dentition such as that illustrated in Figure 20.1. The reasons why plaque control alone has little effect are as follows.

- Several areas of the dentition cannot be readily kept plaque-free, such as the fissures, pits and contact areas.
- Plaque immediately starts to reform after removal and this consists of the microorganisms which are most involved in caries, such as *Streptococcus mutans*.

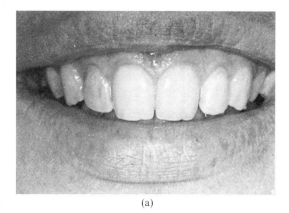

(a)

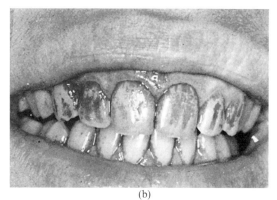

(b)

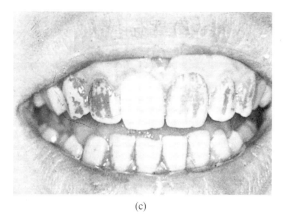

(c)

Fig. 20.2 Photographs of the anterior teeth, showing plaque (a) before disclosing (b) after disclosing and (c) after the upper right central incisor had been brushed free of plaque and the disclosing agent reapplied.

However, plaque control is the single most important aspect of the prevention of inflammatory periodontal disease, and thorough removal of plaque from all surfaces of all teeth even once a day will prevent the accumulation of mature plaque and therefore prevent the progression of periodontal disease. Consequently, in relation to periodontal disease, the thoroughness of plaque removal is much more important than the frequency of toothbrushing.

Disclosing agents

Most patients cannot see the bacterial film on their teeth and frequently the dentist is also unaware that apparently clean looking teeth have significant deposits. It is essential to make these deposits visible if the patient is to be adequately motivated towards their removal (Fig. 20.2). The subject of motivation is dealt with more thoroughly in Chapter 23 but the first stage in motivation must be an awareness that a problem still exists. This is one of the indications for using disclosing agents. Another is for patients and hygienists to assess the quality of plaque removal after toothbrushing or scaling and polishing respectively. The desirable properties of a disclosing agent are shown in Table 20.1.

Table 20.1 Disclosing agents

Effective disclosing agents need to have

- The property of staining plaque selectively to highlight retentive areas.
- The lack of staining of tooth coloured restorative materials.
- The absence of prolonged staining of oral structures such as lips and cheeks.
- An acceptable taste.
- A lack of harmful effects if swallowed including no allergic reactions.

Types of disclosing agent

Iodine

Formerly this was used to disclose plaque. Its staining effect is quite dramatic, but it has two important disadvantages, it has an unpleasant taste and it can cause allergic reactions.

Erythrocin

Although any food dye may be used to disclose plaque, erythrocin is the active ingredient of red food dyes and is the most popular agent used. It is present in many different brands and solutions.

Two-tone agents

Disclosing agents which disclose 'new' and 'old' plaque by different colours or shades are also popular.

Fluorescent agents

Agents that are only visible with the aid of a special light are on occasions particularly helpful. For example, when conducting epidemiological surveys it may not be possible to polish off the plaque after it has been stained. The Plaklite® is a system where a light is shone through a special filter. After rinsing with a fluorescein based solution the special light will cause any plaque present to glow greenish yellow.

Toothbrushing

In the past, an inordinate amount of time has often been devoted to discussing toothbrush design and toothbrushing techniques, at the expense of patient motivation. Too often formalized brushing instruction was not related to the patient's own dentition with its own particular problems or neglected areas. However, it is clearly important that the dental hygienist should be able to discuss the design of toothbrushes, the methods of toothbrushing, the frequency of brushing and the role of dentifrices. Each of these subjects is considered separately in the following pages.

Toothbrush design

There is a multitude of different shapes, textures and sizes of toothbrushes available to the public. Some brushes seem to be quite inappropriate for tooth cleaning, but this is one area in which progress does seem to be being made (Fig. 20.3). Several firms produce perfectly satisfactory brushes and fewer of the larger size, hard, natural bristle brushes are to be found on chemists' shelves.

It would be wrong to be too pedantic about toothbrush design in view of the shortage of experimental evidence to support any details of design. Nevertheless, some statements would seem justifiable on purely clinical grounds.

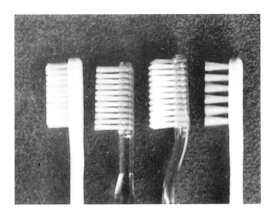

Fig. 20.3 Oral hygiene aids: some suitable toothbrushes for the average adult.

Size

The dentition is considerably more complex than the average person realizes and it has several moderately inaccessible areas. Clearly a brush must not have too large a head to fit into awkward corners, but too small a head would make toothbrushing too time-consuming. Most dentists tend to agree that a brush with a head of approximately 2 cm length should be recommended for the use of the average adult, with an appropriately smaller head for children.

Material

The fashionable preference for natural bristle toothbrushes is now virtually a thing of the past. Synthetic bristles are superior to natural bristles for the following reasons.

- The quality and size control of synthetic bristles is better.
- Plastic bristles are potentially cleaner than natural bristles, since they do not readily absorb fluids or micro-organisms.
- The texture of synthetic bristles is not affected by wetting, whereas natural bristles are softer when wet. There is a general acceptance that multi-tufted synthetic bristles are the most effective. Such bristles have numerous small tufts of bristles, rather than fewer, larger tufts. The individual bristles usually have diameters in the range of 0.18–0.28 mm.

Texture

Medium-textured brushes are commonly recommended. A brush which is too firm may

possibly cause gingival recession and dentinal abrasion. Furthermore, if the bristles are too firm there may not be enough give for them to reach into the embrasures between teeth and other similar areas. Nylon 6/10 is frequently used with a 10–12 mm filament length.

Design

In general, the simpler the brush the more suitable it is. Unnecessary complications in the design seem to make plaque control more difficult rather than easier. It used to be suggested that a well designed brush should have a straight handle and a straight trim on the bristles. This opinion is questionable in view of the recently designed brushes with mildly angled handles or slightly curved trims on the bristles. These brushes appear to be equally satisfactory in plaque removal.

Special brushes

There are areas in many mouths which simply cannot be cleaned with a conventional toothbrush and on occasions it may be necessary to suggest the use of specially designed brushes such as a single-tufted brush (Fig. 20.4) or an interproximal brush (Fig. 20.5). The use of such additional oral hygiene aids is quite time-consuming and would only be used by well motivated patients, but where much time and expense has been spent on restorative work, it would be wrong not to attempt to persuade patients to use any necessary items.

Single-tufted brushes

Single-tufted brushes are ideal for instanding teeth, the distal surface of the most posterior tooth and various types of fixed restorations. The interproximal brush is designed for teeth with slight spacing and for areas such as the mesial surface of tilted lower molars and for some types of bridges.

Mechanical brushes

Experience of these brushes leads to the conclusion that only continuously powered, that is rechargeable, brushes are really useful. Brushes with conventional replaceable batteries suffer from the disadvantage of a rapid lessening of torque from the first day of use. All the

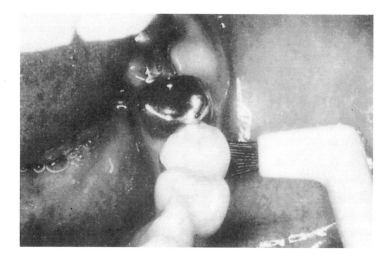

Fig. 20.4 A single tufted brush in use.

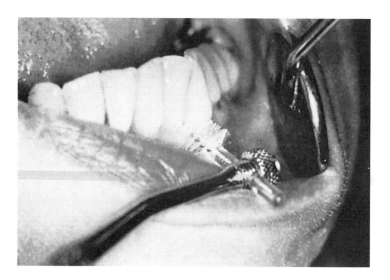

Fig. 20.5 'Bottlebrush' type of interdental cleaner.

powered brushes which are acceptable have quite small heads with multi-tufted bristles.

The potential for damage to the tooth substance or gingiva by powered brushes is limited by the fact that they cannot exert the same pressure as that applied by manual brushes. The automatic brush would stall before excessive pressure could be exerted. However, patients with automatic brushes must be carefully taught how to use them effectively as there is no easy way, even with these brushes. The advantage of the powered brush is that it is easier for the less manually dextrous to achieve an adequate result and once reasonable skill is acquired there is a saving in time over manual brushing. The potential disadvantage of these appliances is that the patient can be lulled into believing that all that has to be done is to purchase one and everything will be done automatically. There appears to be little difference in effect between automatic brushes which use arc oscillations, reciprocal, horizontal movement or a combination of both. A problem with automatic brushes is that of repair and servicing. However, a recent research report has found that automatic brushes can be more effective than manual brushing. It has been recognized for a long time that those patients with mental or physical disabilities may well benefit from using mechanical brushes.

Toothbrushing techniques

The objective in toothbrushing is to remove plaque from every accessible surface of the teeth, without causing damage to dental or soft tissues. The terms 'correct' or 'incorrect' brushing technique should not be used. There is no right or wrong way to brush the teeth: the result is more important than the technique. Too often time is devoted to teaching a formal technique, which may or may not suit the patient, instead of stressing the need for effective brushing.

A purely mechanical demonstration of toothbrushing is doomed to failure with most patients, especially if restricted to dental models. It is necessary to explain to the patient why they are being asked to carry out these procedures and to relate the advice to the patient's own dentition. It is also important to stress that a methodical approach should be adopted, so that all surfaces of all teeth are brushed, and to point out how time-consuming this will be if done efficiently.

If each dental arch is divided into five segments for brushing purposes (right and left molars, right and left premolars and anterior teeth) there will be a total of 10 segments. Each segment has three brushable surfaces: buccal, lingual and occlusal. This gives a total of 30 surface areas to be brushed, and if each surface receives only 2 seconds brushing it will take 1 minute to brush the dentition. Most patients will accept that 2 seconds is a very short time to devote to any area, and this type of discussion might persuade them of the need to devote more time to toothbrushing (few people spend a full minute on toothbrushing!).

From time to time in the past, various dental authorities have developed a toothbrushing technique and recommended it as 'the correct method' of brushing the teeth. This has led to the confusing situation where a patient might well receive contradictory advice from different dentists or hygienists. This is a most unsatisfactory situation, especially when there is no such thing as the one correct technique for all dentitions and abilities. Nevertheless, the dental

hygienist must be aware of these different techniques and their possible advantages or disadvantages.

Horizontal brushing

This is the technique which probably has least to recommend it. The head of the brush is placed on the buccal surface of the teeth with the handle in a horizontal position. The head is brushed back and forward in a mesiodistal direction and the procedure is repeated on the lingual surface. Not only is this technique unlikely to clean adequately in the embrasures between teeth but, if used with excessive force and a hard toothbrush or abrasive toothpaste, it can result in gingival recession and cervical abrasion. Wherever signs of such damage are seen, the toothbrushing habits should be modified appropriately.

Vertical brushing

Because of the problems noted above, it became fashionable to recommend a vertical brushing stroke. The head of the toothbrush is placed on the buccal surface of the teeth with the handle in a horizontal position. The head is brushed up and down over the surfaces of both upper and lower teeth. The procedure is repeated on the inner aspect of the teeth but, obviously, only one arch can be brushed at a time and the handle of the brush frequently has to be held in a more vertical position.

Roll technique

This is a further modification of the vertical brushing stroke (Fig. 20.6). The head of the brush is placed against the buccal surface of the teeth at an angle of 45° to the long axis of the teeth, with the bristles pointing towards the mucogingival line. The handle of the brush is rotated so that the bristles sweep across the tooth surface from gingival margins to occlusal surface. This is repeated three or four times in all areas, buccal and lingual, upper and lower. The principle of the technique is that debris would be swept away from the gingival margin area. Some authorities recommended a roll technique which was the reverse of that already described: the bristles are swept over the tooth surface from occlusal surface to gingival margin. This was meant to represent the

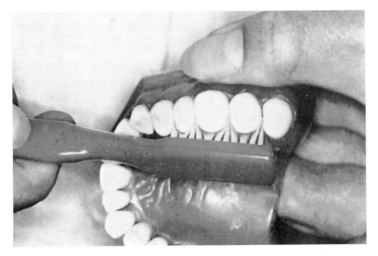

Fig. 20.6 In the roll technique the toothbrush is applied to the teeth , so that the sides of the bristles not the ends contact the teeth. In this way the bristles adapt themselves to the irregularities, embrasures and curvatures, as this figure shows.

physiological action of eating more fibrous foodstuffs. This has been found to be a very ineffective technique.

Charter's technique

This technique was developed in an effort to clean the interproximal surface of adjacent teeth more effectively. The head of the tooth-brush is placed with the handle horizontal and the bristles against the buccal surface of the teeth with the bristles at an angle of 45° pointing towards the occlusal surface of the teeth. They are then vibrated out and in so that they reach into the interdental area, and finally, they are swept over the tooth towards the occlusal surface. This is repeated in all areas of the dentition, but it is obviously much easier to perform on the buccal than on the lingual aspects.

Bass technique

The Bass technique is similar in many ways to the Charter's technique, but in the Bass technique the bristles of the brush, whilst being angled at 45° to the tooth surface, are pointed in a gingival direction. When the head is vibrated in and out, the bristles enter the gingival crevice or the superficial aspect of periodontal pockets as well as the interdental spaces. The ability to remove plaque from these areas has made the Bass technique the one which is probably currently most popular. As in the Charter's technique, the bristles can then be swept over the tooth surface in an occlusal direction (the modified Bass technique). This action is repeated on all buccal and lingual tooth surfaces and the occlusal surface is finally brushed with a horizontal mesiodistal action.

Scrub-brush technique

In this technique no formalized brushing strokes are used; the various tooth surfaces are cleaned with a short scrubbing action. This is the brushing technique used by the majority of people, but it has the possible disadvantage that it may be carried out in a somewhat random way and that various tooth surfaces may be repeatedly missed. This might explain the finding that plaque is more often found in areas which are awkward to brush; for example the lingual aspect of the lower molars. However, care should be taken in deciding to alter a patient's brushing technique. In the words of the character actor Will Rogers: '*If you send somebody to teach somebody, be sure the system you are teaching is better than the system they are practising*'. Usually what patients require is to have their current brushing habits modified so that any deficiencies are corrected. *The Scientific Basis of Dental Health Education* (4th edition 1996, produced by the Health Education Authority) recommends that '*a sensible scrub technique should be advised*'.

No toothbrushing technique should be taught indiscriminately to all patients. The patient's ability to achieve successful plaque removal with the brushing pattern in current use should be evaluated and, in this respect, differences in tooth alignment, arch form and size, manual dexterity and attitude should be assessed. This emphasizes the need for personal 'one-to-one' training and the inadequacy of group teaching in relation to a very personal practical skill such as toothbrushing.

Brushing frequency

As there is no single correct brushing technique, so there is no correct number of times a day for brushing. Obviously patients have to be given straightforward, uncomplicated advice, but the dental hygienist should be aware of the more confusing background theory to the frequency with which the teeth should be cleaned.

It has already been noted that toothbrushing alone has little effect on the caries rate. The total removal of all plaque from every surface of the teeth before each exposure to sugar is simply an unattainable goal. It has become customary to recommend that people brush their teeth at least twice per day: before going to bed and again in the morning. Of these two, brushing before going to bed is considered the more important because of the reduced flow of saliva during sleep. The more motivated patient might also be encouraged to brush the teeth after lunch.

In relation to periodontal disease, the aim must be to prevent the development of mature plaque. In other words, if all plaque is removed from the tooth surface every second day, chronic periodontal disease will not develop in a previously healthy subject. This does imply a total removal of plaque, using both toothbrush and interdental cleaning agents, and those with already established periodontal disease will require more frequent plaque removal. Nevertheless, in relation to chronic periodontal disease the quality of plaque removal is much more important than the frequency. For this reason, those patients who are sufficiently motivated should be encouraged to use floss, tape or interdental brushes once per day. It is easier to establish a daily habit than a once-every-other day habit and, since interdental cleaning is primarily aimed to prevent peri-odontal disease, there is no need to suggest that these time-consuming procedures should be carried out more frequently than once per day.

> - There is no single toothbrushing techni-que that is ideal for every patient.
> - Brushing before going to bed is the most important due to reduced salivary flow when asleep. In the motivated patient brushing three times a day should be encouraged.
> - Interdental cleaning once a day is best to encourage a daily routine.

Dentifrices

A much publicised report by the Consumers' Association in Which (1974) summarized the research carried out into toothpastes and concluded that, other than those containing fluoride, they were of largely cosmetic value. However, the value of fluoridated toothpastes in preventing caries has become more evident. To a large extent, the drop in the caries rate which has been observed in recent years has been attributed to the almost universal use of fluoridated toothpastes. Approximately 95% of all toothpastes sold in the UK contain fluoride. Whether the reduction in caries is due to the topical effect of fluoride or to the repeated ingestion of small quantities of fluoridated toothpaste is a matter of some discussion and research.

Ingredients of dentifrices

Dentifrices contain preservatives and flavour-ings and foaming agents. They also contain a varying amount of abrasive powder. However, it is the action of the brush which is more important in plaque removal than the abrasive powder. The abrasive may aid the removal of stains from the teeth, but the various smokers' dentifrices on the market, are considered by many dentists to be too abrasive and capable of causing gingival recession and cervical wear. Besides flavouring and colouring agents, denti-frices contain a humectant, which is the component which binds all the other ingredients together and keeps it moist.

Fluoridated dentifrices

Different chemical forms of fluoride are present in various toothpastes and the relative merits of these compounds is currently a subject of much research.

Stannous fluoride
This was the initial form of fluoride used in toothpastes in the UK.

Sodium fluoride
Many dentifrices contain sodium fluoride, and other pastes, such as Colgate®, contain sodium fluoride together with sodium monofluorophosphate.

Sodium monofluorophosphate
This compound is the active ingredient of most UK pastes.

Amine fluoride
Elmex, a dentifrice which is available in many European countries but not in the UK, contains both sodium fluoride and amine fluoride.

Other 'active' agents in dentifrices

In the past, a large number of agents have been added to different dentifrices in the hope of reducing caries or inhibiting plaque, mainly without any evidence to support their use and without any proven benefit. Chlorophyll was such an agent, added in the 1950s in the hope of oxidizing bacteria. Emulsifying agents (such as sodium ricinoleate of Gibbs SR®) were early attempts at chemical control of plaque. More recently, dentifrices containing chlorhexidine have been produced (Corsodyl® and Elgydium®), and the plaque-inhibiting effect of chlorhexidine is discussed later.

Desensitizing dentifrices

It has been estimated that 30% of the population have suffered from cervical dentine sensitivity at some time. There is therefore a potentially very large market for dentifrice's which contain desensitizing agents. Currently on the market in the UK are the following.

- **Sensodyne®**, with the active ingredient strontium chloride.
- **Sensodyne F®** with potassium chloride and sodium monofluorophosphate.
- **Sensodyne Gel®** with potassium fluoride and sodium fluoride.
- **Colgate Sensitive Care®** with potassium citrate and sodium monofluorophosphate.
- **Macleans Sensitive®** with strontium acetate and sodium monofluorophosphate.

The filler component in desensitizing dentifrices (usually diatomaceous earth) is also important as it has been shown that this helps to plug up the patent dentinal tubules on the root surface. This topic is dealt with more fully in Chapter 15.

- The caries reduction seen in developed countries is due to the almost universal use of fluoridated dentifrices.
- The use of desensitizing dentifrices will increase as populations age and retain their teeth longer.
- 95% of all toothpastes contain fluoride.
- The other ingredients of toothpastes include foaming agents, preservatives, flavourings, abrasives and a humectant.

Interdental cleaning

The toothbrush can clean facial, lingual and occlusal surfaces of the teeth reasonably well. What is in doubt is the ability of a conventional toothbrush to clean adequately between the teeth, no matter which brushing stroke is employed. The possible use of specially designed brushes has already been discussed and this section deals with the use of dental floss or tape and interdental woodsticks.

It must be remembered that in general the population is 'toothbrush aware' and looks upon the procedure as a natural part of daily routine. Other oral hygiene procedures are not regarded in the same way. An illustration of this is that patients will often apologize for not having brushed their teeth since their last meal. No patient ever arrives apologizing for not having used floss, tape or woodsticks. Therefore, every effort should be made in the use of interdental cleaning aids restricted to those who are more highly motivated. The difficulty of establishing a regular daily habit of interdental cleaning should never be underestimated.

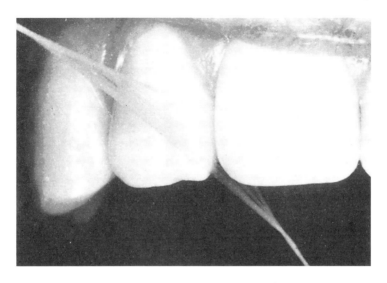

Fig. 20.7 Unwaxed dental floss spreading out against the tooth surface.

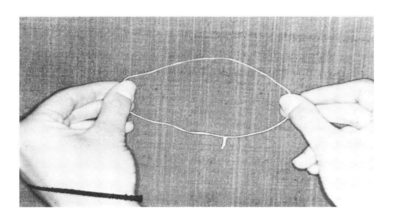

Fig. 20.8 Dental floss formed into a loop for sense of handling.

Dental floss or tape

Dental floss or tape is undoubtedly the most efficient method of cleaning interdentally if used regularly and efficiently. Waxed and unwaxed floss are available and which should be used is largely a matter of choice. The filaments of the unwaxed variety spread out on the tooth surface, as in Figure 20.7. However, this can be a disadvantage in that the filaments may shred when they come in contact with the margins of fillings and become stuck between the teeth. People with numerous large fillings often prefer waxed floss since it is less likely to shred. A wider variety known as dental tape is also manufactured and this is flat when compared to regular floss which is round in cross section. There are other types of floss including nylon and polytetrafluoroethylene (PTFE) floss and also medicated and flavoured varieties are available. There is also one well suited for cleaning the pontics of bridges, known as Super Floss®.

Technique of flossing

Flossing is a difficult procedure to master and requires careful teaching. Two methods have been recommended. One is illustrated in Figure 20.8. A 20 cm length of floss is cut off and the ends tied together to form a loop. This is then held between left thumb and right index finger

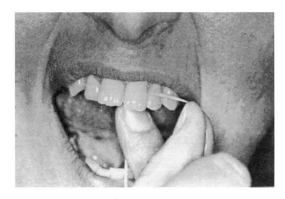

Fig. 20.9 Dental floss being used to clean the upper anterior teeth.

to clean the upper left quadrant (Fig 20.9). The fingers are reversed for the right quadrant. The loop is held between both index fingers for the lower teeth (Fig. 20.10). With the other technique a longer piece of floss is cut off (approximately 30 cm) and the two ends are wrapped around the long fingers of each hand, leaving a working length of approximately 10 cm. This is then used in a similar manner to that already described, using the index fingers and thumbs to control the floss.

Whichever of the above methods is used, the floss is held taut between the fingers and is worked carefully through the contact area of the teeth with a labiolingual sawing action. In this way the floss can be worked through the contact area without snapping down against the soft tissues. Once through the contact area the floss is held firmly round half the circumference of the tooth (Fig. 20.11). In this position the floss can be firmly but carefully rubbed up and down against the tooth. A big advantage of floss is that it can clean plaque from the gingival crevice and at least the more superficial areas of periodontal pockets. The action is then repeated on the surface of the neighbouring tooth. All interproximal surfaces should be systematically cleaned, changing the grip on the floss as necessary.

Where it is not possible to pass the floss through the contact area (i.e. where there are soldered bridge contacts or fixed splints) a floss threader can be used to pass the end of the floss through the embrasure. Flossing devices, such as the one illustrated in Figure 20.12, can be bought, but many people find them more awkward to use than floss on its own.

Interdental woodsticks

Whereas interdental woodsticks cannot remove plaque as thoroughly as dental floss or remove subgingival plaque, their use is considerably less time-consuming and may call for less motivation. The hygienist must assess each patient separately to decide whether it might be better to hope for daily use of woodsticks rather than spasmodic use of floss.

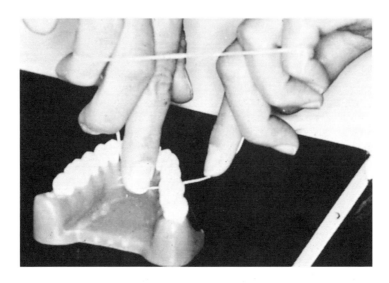

Fig. 20.10 Position of index fingers on floss for cleaning lower teeth.

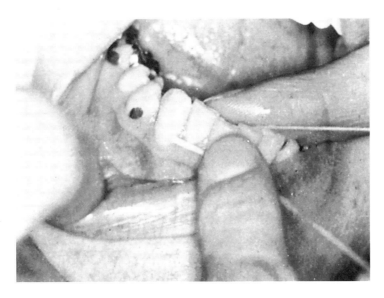

Fig. 20.11 Floss wrapped around tooth to remove as large an area of plaque as possible.

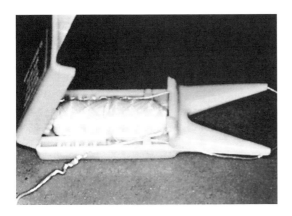

Fig. 20.12 A flossing device.

Interdental woodsticks can only be recommended where there is sufficient interdental space not filled by gingival tissue (Fig. 20.13), but most woodsticks are quite slender and there are few adults who have not experienced a degree of periodontal disease which would allow for the use of sticks. Obviously they cannot be used where there is gross crowding and malalignment of teeth.

Woodsticks should not be used as tooth picks. They are triangular in section, to match the embrasure of the tooth. The stick should be inserted into the embrasure and rubbed in and out several times to remove the plaque from the two proximal surfaces of the embrasure. As always, a methodical approach should be recommended so that no interdental space is omitted. There may be some difficulty reaching the more distal spaces. Most patients can use woodsticks throughout the oral cavity, but some may require to use other aids in the molar region, such as the rubber tips sometimes fitted on the handles of toothbrushes but these are very inefficient and not recommended.

Interdental and interspace brushes

Interdental brushes are very useful and are indicated where there are wide interproximal spaces such as those seen after periodontal surgery or where recession has occurred. They are made in a wide variety of sizes and shapes and some are supplied with handles. They may also be useful for cleaning around precision attachments and dental implants. Generally they have the same indications as interdental wood points but the bristles make their use more efficient enabling concavities on teeth such as the canine fossa on some upper premolars to be accessed.

Water irrigation units

The use of these appliances, which are expensive, has very little justification in oral hygiene. Pulsating water will not remove plaque: it is much too tenacious a film for that. It has been

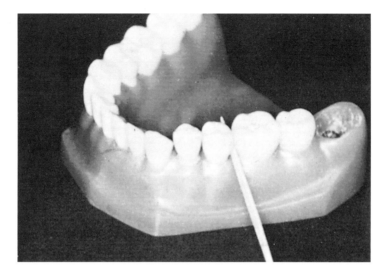

Fig. 20.13 Method of applying a woodstick. Note the angulation.

argued that the water irrigation might alter the bacterial flora of the plaque and make it less harmful, but any benefit gained does not appear to warrant the cost and effort involved.

However, with the development of chemical plaque control agents, such as chlorhexidine, irrigation units have become more important as a delivery system for the chemical agent and they have been shown to be very effective in getting chlorhexidine into periodontal pockets.

For the control of dental plaque
- Interdental cleaning is very important.
- Floss or tape should be used daily to establish a routine.
- Wood sticks can be used if the interdental spaces are large but they are less effective than floss.
- Interdental brushes are very good where interdental spaces are large.
- Water irrigation units can be helpful but are expensive and require an antimicrobial to be added to be effective in plaque removal.

Chemical control of plaque

Considerable interest over the past three decades has been directed to this area, with various antiseptics being investigated. Antiplaque

agents have been delivered by a variety of methods such as mouthwashes and toothpastes. Antiseptics, enzyme preparations and surface energy reducing agents have all been tried. The degree of success with regard to supragingival plaque control has been variable. Combating the subgingival microflora has proved more difficult and the methods tried have included placing antiseptics such as chlorhexidine or antibiotics such as tetracycline into periodontal pockets by means of local sustained-delivery devices such as acrylic or cellulose gels. The incorporated active agent is released over a period of days after contact with moisture. Recently the Periochip® has been marketed which is an effective slow release chlorhexidine device which works over 10 days and is effective in disrupting pocket bacterial metabolism for up to 3 months. This is covered in more detail in Chapter 11.

The antiseptics that have been shown to possess antiplaque properties include cetylpyridinium chloride, sanguinarine, hexitidine, benzalkonium chloride, and various zinc salts. Various mouthwashes are available which contain these agents but the chemical that has been most successful is chlorhexidine in its gluconate or acetate form.

Chlorhexidine

The use of chlorhexidine has been shown in numerous studies to be effective at plaque prevention. It is considered to be particularly effective because it is adsorbed on to the surfaces of teeth, pellicle and the oral mucosa and is released slowly over a long period of time, thereby having a prolonged disruptive effect on the micro-organisms that make up plaque. Unfortunately, there are some disadvantages to chlorhexidine.

- It has an unpleasant taste.
- It can affect the sense of taste for some time after use.
- In some cases it causes extrinsic staining of the teeth, which can be removed only with scaling and polishing (Fig. 20.14a).

For these reasons chlorhexidine is usually reserved for those cases where efficient physical plaque control is not possible: for example, in conditions such as chronic desquamative gingivitis, acute herpetic stomatitis, pregnancy hyperplasia and after oral or periodontal surgery.

Chlorhexidine is marketed as Corsodyl®, which is available as a 0.2% solution for mouthrinsing or a 1.0% gel for brushing. It is also marketed in lesser concentrations as Eludril® solution for rinsing and for toothbrushing. More recently, research has been carried out into the effects of irrigating periodontal pockets with 0.2% chlorhexidine solution. Since solutions used as rinses do not penetrate into periodontal pockets, the plaque inhibition effect can only be obtained by irrigation. This is of particular value in the initial management of lateral periodontal abscesses, but may eventually play a more significant role in the management of chronic periodontitis (Fig. 20.14b).

- Chemical control of plaque cannot replace brushing but it is useful in the short term.
- Chlorhexidine appears to be beneficial in the slow release device Periochip®.
- Various agents have an antiplaque effect and include cetyl pyridinium chloride, hexitidine, sanguinarine, benzalkonium chloride, and zinc salts.

The dental benefits of fluoride

The use of fluorides has been the biggest single development in the prevention of caries. They may be used in either of two ways:

- **Systemic fluoride**. This involves the ingestion of fluoride which is carried to the developing teeth by the blood stream.
- **Topical fluoride**. The fluoride is applied to the surface of the erupted teeth.

It is obvious that systemic fluoride is the more beneficial and the development of topical fluorides has largely been brought about by the difficulties in achieving its use. However, where systemic fluoride is available, there will be additional benefits from topical applications, especially for those with high caries susceptibility.

It is suggested that fluoride reduces the incidence of caries in several possible ways.

The calcium hydroxyapatite of the tooth is replaced by calcium fluorapatite. In Chapter 10 the Stephan curve is discussed and the critical pH at which calcium hydroxyapatite begins to dissolve in acid was stated as being approximately pH 5.5. The critical pH of calcium fluorapatite is estimated as being nearer to pH 4.5, and obviously, the time during which the Stephan curve is at this level is less than below pH 5.5. In fact the pH may not reach 4.5. Teeth containing calcium fluorapatite are therefore much less prone to acid attack than untreated teeth.

Fluoride is also capable of blocking the enzyme systems of plaque bacteria and may inhibit their ability to convert sugars into acids. In addition, there is a suggestion that the teeth which develop in children living in areas with fluoride in the water have fewer and more shallow pits and fissures. This would obviously make such teeth less caries-prone. In Chapter 10 it was noted that the early caries lesion can be remineralized by the action of topical fluoride. More established lesions can be arrested with a high level of fluoride.

History of fluoride use

The value of naturally occurring fluoride in drinking water has been appreciated since the turn of the century. In 1892, Sir James Crichton-Browne suggested to the Eastern Counties branch of the British Dental Association '*that the reintroduction into our diet... of a supply of fluorine in some suitable natural form... might... do something to fortify the teeth of the*

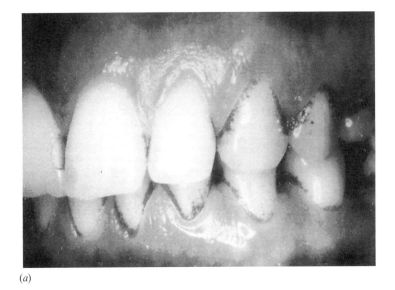

(a)

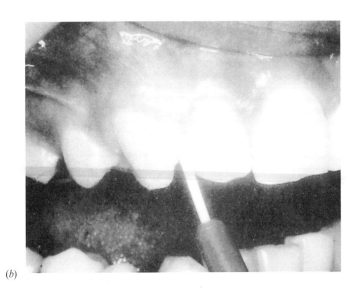

(b)

Fig. 20.14 (a) Chlorhexidine staining, (b) a pocket being irrigated with chlorhexidine.

next generation' (Crichton-Browne, 1892).

Initially the relationship between mottling of the teeth and fluoride in drinking water was observed in various American cities during the early years of the 20th century. This was followed by the discovery that in areas where mottling of the teeth occurred due to fluoride there was a reduced caries rate. Between 1930 and 1940 a great deal of research was carried out into the effects of fluoride in drinking water by Dr H. Trendley Dean. He showed that the severity of mottling of the teeth was affected by the concentration of fluoride in water in the following way:

0.5 p.p.m. = questionable mottling
1 p.p.m. = very mild mottling
2 p.p.m. = mild mottling
3 p.p.m. = moderate mottling
4 p.p.m. = moderately severe mottling

He also showed that a near maximal reduction in the caries rate occurred when water contained 1 part per million (p.p.m.) fluoride and at this level caused only *'very mild mottling*

of no practical aesthetic significance'. He de-
duced that the optimum level of fluoride in
water was 1 p.p.m. (Dean, 1934).

The logical progression from these findings
was to see if the same reduction in caries rate
could be achieved by adding 1 p.p.m. fluoride to
water lacking that ion. In 1945 sodium fluoride
was added to the water of Grand Rapids,
Michigan, and the effect on the caries rate was
compared with that of Muskegan, in which the
water was fluoride-deficient, and with Aurora,
Illinois, which had natural fluoride present in its
water at the level of 1.4 p.p.m. A 50% reduction
in caries incidence was demonstrated, such that
the caries levels in Grand Rapids, which had
previously been similar to those of Muskegan,
eventually approximated those of Aurora. The
evidence was so striking that the authorities in
Muskegan fluoridated their water supply in
1951.

In the UK the beneficial effects of naturally
occurring fluoride have been shown by a
comparison of the caries level amongst children
in North Shields (less than 0.25 p.p.m. fluoride)
and South Shields (up to 2 p.p.m. fluoride). The
mean DMF (see Chapter 10) figures in South
Shields were almost half of those in North
Shields. Initial trials in artificial water fluoridation were begun in 1955 in Kilmarnock (control
town Ayr), Watford (control Sutton) and the
remaining part of Anglesey (control part of
Anglesey). After 5 years a 50% reduction in
caries was demonstrated in all three test areas.
At that stage, because of local opposition, the
fluoridation of the water supply of Kilmarnock
was discontinued and the caries rate gradually
rose to its previous levels.

Since then other areas in the UK have
become artificially fluoridated, including Birmingham (1964) and Newcastle-upon-Tyne
(1968). Unfortunately, a recent decision to
fluoridate the water supply of the Strathclyde
area was opposed in the High Court of Scot-
land and, although the judge ruled that fluoride
was both safe and effective, he found in favour
of the opponent on legal technical grounds.

The beneficial effects of fluoridated water are
only enjoyed by about 10% of the population
of the UK and this is due to a number of
reasons. These include the costs of establishing
fluoridation plants by the water authorities
which are more circumspect now that they are
private concerns. The arguments put forward
by those who are not in favour of water

fluoridation are often very persuasive in their
approach. The silent majority of the population
of the UK cannot be mobilized on a matter
which they see is not a life and death issue.

- The value of drinking water containing
  fluoride has been recognized since the
  beginning of the twentieth century.
- Mild enamel mottling can occur at
  2 p.p.m. and becomes more severe as the
  concentration increases.
- Only 10% of the population of the UK
  drinks optimally fluoridated water

Systemic fluorides

Despite the enormous quantity of research
carried out to establish the safety and cost-
effectiveness of water fluoridation, a vociferous
opposition to the artificial fluoridation of water
supplies has built up. In response the dental
profession has formed the Fluoridation Society.
It is important that the dental hygienist should
be aware of the anti-fluoridation arguments
being put forward at any time and how these
can be countered. Much information and
assistance in this respect can be obtained from
The Fluoridation Society, 64 Wimpole Street,
London WIM 8AL.

The opposition to water fluoridation has
forced the dental profession to make do with
less effective, more costly and less widely
available methods of using fluoride.

Fluoride tablets and drops

Fluoride tablets and drops are widely used in
communities where the level of fluoridation in
the water supply is below the optimum of
1 p.p.m. If conscientiously taken at the correct
dosage throughout the period of tooth formation, the protection against caries approaches
that of water fluoridation. However, it would
be wrong to underestimate the level of co-
operation required of parents to keep up this
daily regimen and few appear to have the
necessary motivation. It is often the children
who require the benefits of fluorides most who
are deprived of it, whereas they would receive
the benefits if the water supply were fluoridated.

The dosage of daily fluoride supplement

varies with the age of the child and has been a
subject of some controversy in recent years. The
current recommended dosages are shown in
Table 20.2.

Table 20.2 Fluoride dosages

*British Dental Association, British Society of Pae-
diatric Dentistry and the British Association for the
Study of Community Dentistry recommended
fluoride dosages*

Birth to 3 years: 0.25 mg fluoride.
3 to 6 years: 0.50 mg fluoride.
6 years and over: 1.00 mg fluoride.

(Published in British Dental Journal 182; 6–7
January 1997)

When giving advice on the method of taking
fluoride tablets, a child should be advised not to
swallow the tablet whole. It is better to allow
the tablet to lie in the floor of the mouth and
dissolve slowly in saliva. In this way, as well as
the systemic effect of the fluoride, the erupted
teeth will receive a topical benefit.

Some debate has also centred on whether or
not fluoride supplements should be given to
pregnant women to provide protection for the
teeth which develop before birth. There should
be no confusion between the entirely laudable
principle of not giving any avoidable drugs
during pregnancy and supplementing the diet
with an ion such as fluoride. For example, few
would question the wisdom of taking calcium
tablets during pregnancy. Although it is likely
that only one third of the available fluoride will
cross the placenta, fluoride tablets, at the level
of 1 mg per day, should be taken during the
second and third trimesters of pregnancy if the
maximum reduction in caries of the deciduous
dentition is to be achieved.

Fluoridated milk and salt

In order to avoid the need for parental co-
operation, the possibility of adding fluoride to
milk supplies has been studied. The Borrow
Milk Foundation is an organization set up to
promote this method of fluoridation. Unfortunately, there are several important disadvantages to relying on the fluoridation of milk.

- If all milk supplies are fluoridated, the
same objections will be put forward as in
relation to water fluoridation. If, on the
other hand, milk is supplied in both
fluoridated and non-fluoridated varieties,
complications arise in relation to ordering,
delivery and possible additional expense.
- Not all children drink the same quantity
of milk: some drink virtually none whilst
other drink a great deal.
- Even if fluoridated milk were used in those
schools which supply milk to pupils on a
daily basis, children under 5 years of age
will be denied the benefits and no fluoride
will be obtained at weekends or during
school holidays.

Similar disadvantages exist in relation to the
fluoridation of table salt.

- It is vital to know the concentration of
fluoride in the local drinking water before
recommending fluoride supplements.
- If the concentration is above 0.7 p.p.m. no
fluoride supplement is required.
- Only a third of the available fluoride from a
daily 1 mg tablet will cross the placental
barrier.
- Fluoridated milk and salt are options
to water fluoridation but they have
marked disadvantages to water fluoridation.

Topical fluorides

Undeniably, the greatest effects from fluoride
will be obtained if it is taken systemically, and
most of the topical fluoride techniques have
been developed as a result of the difficulties
involved in systemic fluoridation. However,
even where systemic fluorides have been used
on a regular basis, topical fluorides can provide
an additional protection to the erupted teeth.
Topical fluorides can also reverse the early
caries lesion and arrest more established caries
lesions (see Chapter 10).

Sodium fluoride solutions

The first clinical study using sodium fluoride
was by Bibby (1942). The technique which he

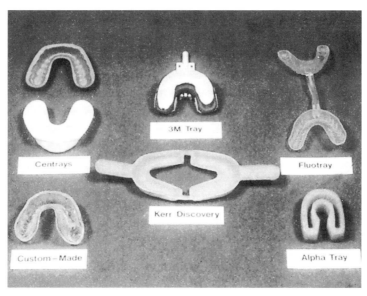

Fig. 20.15 A selection of fluoride applicators available in the UK. These are not very popular now as they encourage fluoride to be ingested.

recommended was first to carry out a thorough prophylaxis and then isolate and dry a quadrant at a time and apply the solution for 4 minutes. Initially, Bibby used a 0.1% solution but later clinicians raised the strength of the solution to 0 2%. The principal objection to this technique, which has largely been superseded by other methods of applying topical fluoride, was that it was time-consuming to carry out.

Stannous fluoride solutions

The use of stannous fluoride was proposed by Muhler and his co-workers in the 1950s. Their findings suggested that it had an enhanced effect in caries reduction over sodium fluoride (Muhler and Day, 1950). However, stannous fluoride is chemically unstable and it has to be mixed freshly for each session. It has a tendency to stain the teeth and some patients find its metallic taste objectionable. Stannous fluoride has been used in 10% and 8% solutions and the technique of applying it was similar to that of sodium fluoride.

Acidulated phosphate fluoride (APF)

APF gel was commonly applied to the whole dentition in specially designed applicator trays (Fig. 20.15) for a period of 4 minutes. It is also available in solution. It contains 1.23% fluoride ion acidulated with phosphoric acid to a level of pH 3. It has long been recognized that lowering the pH will increase the uptake of fluoride by enamel. Consequently, the two main advantages of APF gels are that they are relatively quick to apply and that a greater uptake of fluoride by enamel might be expected. The principal disadvantages of APF systems is that they are somewhat expensive to use and they can be easily adsorbed through the floor of mouth mucosa and quickly give rise to a toxic dose of fluoride. Because of this problem the method of tray application for APF is no longer favoured. It is better to apply them to a few teeth at a time with the teeth being isolated with cotton rolls and an effective saliva injector in place.

There seems to be no particular basis for applying APF gels for 4 minutes. This time appears to have persisted since the initial recommendations of Bibby (1942) in relation to sodium fluoride. However, the greatest uptake of fluoride occurs at the beginning of the application and it gradually tails off with time, and so the hygienist should not be discouraged from applying gels for a shorter period of time if a child is restless or unable to cope with the full application time.

The optimum frequency with which APF gels should be applied has yet to be established. It has become customary to apply the gels twice per annum and the evidence available would suggest that less frequent application than this is of questionable value. The benefits of APF gels are considerably increased if more frequent applications are used, but recent research into the quantities of fluoride ingested during such applications have cast doubts on the wisdom of very frequent applications. For this reason some now frown on the use of APF solutions.

Fluoride varnishes

Whereas a reduction in the rate of caries has been reported with up to three applications of fluoride varnish per year, the evidence would suggest that their use in this way is less cost-effective. Their use as a topical agent is favoured by some particularly when applied to fissures of newly erupted teeth and in the management of dentine sensitivity. In the UK the most widely used commercially produced fluoride varnish is Duraphat® which contains 2.26% of available fluoride. The fluoride varnish can be easily applied to the fissures of teeth using the brush applicator that is supplied for applying acid etchant when undertaking a bonded composite restoration.

Fluoride mouthrinses

Clinical trials of mouthrinsing with sodium fluoride solution have produced between 25% and 50% reduction in caries. Two principal regimens have been used: once-daily rinsing with a 0.05% sodium fluoride solution, and once-weekly rinsing with a 0.20% sodium fluoride solution. In both cases 10 ml of solution is rinsed round the oral cavity for 2 minutes. The daily rinsing is undoubtedly preferable, but either good parental co-operation is needed or, if a school-based programme is used, the daily regimen results in high costs with regard to time, materials and supervision. Some concern has been expressed about the ability of younger children to rinse for 2 minutes without swallowing or spitting out large amounts of the solution.

Fluoride dentifrices

These have already been discussed earlier in this chapter. Much of the credit for the reported reduction in caries in the UK has been

attributed to the almost universal use of fluoridated dentifrices. In 1970 it was estimated that 5% of all dentifrices sold were fluoridated, whereas in 1980 it was estimated that 95% of those sold were fluoridated. In clinical trials with fluoridated dentifrices, caries reductions of between 20% and 30% have been recorded.

The concern which has been expressed in relation to the possible ingestion of fluoride dentifrices has already been discussed with regard to the taking of fluoride tablets or drops.

- Use of fluoride dentifrices produces a reduction in caries incidence of between 20% and 30%.
- Sodium fluoride solutions can be used for caries prevention at concentrations of 0.2% for a weekly rinse or 0.05% for a daily rinse.
- Stannous fluoride is less popular than sodium fluoride in caries prevention due to its poor shelf life.
- APF solutions and gels are readily adsorbed from the floor of mouth mucosa so care is necessary when using them.
- Fluoride varnishes such as Duraphat® are popular to use as a topical agent to apply to fissures of newly erupted teeth.

Fissure sealants

The effectiveness of fluoride in reducing caries is not uniform throughout all surfaces of the teeth: it is most effective in reducing caries of smooth surfaces and least effective in preventing pit and fissure caries (Fig. 20.16). Furthermore, when one looks microscopically at the morphology of pits and fissures, it is evident that even the finest toothbrush bristle could not eliminate plaque from their depths.

A previous preventive procedure for these vulnerable areas was prophylactic odontotomy, cutting out the fissures and pits with burs and filling the defects with amalgam. In the early 1970s fissure sealants were developed and their value tested clinically, initially by Buonocore. Fissure sealants are designed to fill fissures and pits with a plastic material, without cutting into the enamel surface. The plastics used are

Table 20.3 Fissure sealing

Technique for fissure sealing a tooth

- Polish the teeth with an oil-free paste and bristle brush.
- Thoroughly wash the tooth surface free of paste, preferably using a wash bottle rather than the three-in-one syringe to avoid contamination with oil.
- Thoroughly isolate and dry the tooth surface. Cotton wool rolls and high-speed suction are required throughout or ideally isolate with rubber dam.
- Etch the tooth surface. This is usually done with between 30% and 50% orthophosphoric acid applied to the tooth surface for 20 seconds. It was usual practice in the past to etch for 60 seconds, but the reduced time of etch has been shown to be more effective.
- Wash and dry the tooth surface. It is important to avoid contamination with saliva at this point. The surface should be washed clear of acid with water from a wash bottle and the tooth surface dried with air from a three-in-one syringe. Oil contamination in the air flow of these syringes is common and this can be responsible for poor retention. The air supply can, however, be fitted with an oil-and-water filter.
- Apply the sealant using a plastic filling instrument, flowing the solution in one direction across the surface to avoid trapping air bubbles. A straight probe is then ran along the fissure to remove any air bubbles.
- Polymerize the sealant.
- Ensure that the sealant is not interfering with the normal occlusion of the teeth: if it is, adjust it as necessary.

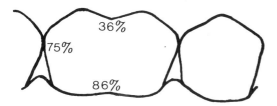

Fig. 20.16 The effectiveness of systemic fluoride in preventing caries of the occlusal surface (36%) interproximal surface (75%) and buccal or lingual surfaces (86%)

bisphenol-glycidylmethacrylate resins (Table 20.3).

Types of sealants

Depending on the way in which they are polymerized, sealants can be divided into three groups.

- **Self-polymerizing**. Two solutions are mixed together and they polymerize by a chemical reaction. Some operators feel that they polymerize too quickly for careful application.
- **Ultraviolet light polymerized**. Once the solution has been applied it is exposed to an ultraviolet light to polymerize it. In the early 1980s some disquiet existed regard-

ing the safety of using an ultraviolet light system, although no real evidence of risk existed. For this reason ultraviolet lights have now largely been superseded.

- **White light polymerized**. Lights which use the blue spectrum from a quartz halogen bulb have now largely replaced ultraviolet lights. This method is often called command set.

Sealants can also be divided into two groups depending on whether they are filled or unfilled. In order to make them more resistant to abrasion, some sealants are filled with lithium alumina silicate. This appears to prolong the life of the sealant and also makes them easier to see.

Effectiveness of sealants

Initially there was a dramatic variation in the rate of success between operators, ranging from 99.5% to 4% retention after 1 year. Many of the poor results were due to problems such as oil and saliva contamination or inefficient light sources for polymerization. Many recent trials have shown that good retention of the sealants is found where careful application techniques are used.

Some concern was previously expressed that

caries might inadvertently be sealed into the fissure and then progress unseen. Fortunately research suggests that if early caries is sealed its progression is halted, and the clinician might be encouraged to adopt the maxim 'when in doubt, seal'. There is also evidence that acid etch applied to enamel does not make it more susceptible to caries and therefore, if the sealant is lost, no damage will have been done to the tooth.

Most authorities would agree that it is important to seal teeth immediately after eruption if the maximum benefit is to be gained, despite the additional difficulty in applying sealants to teeth not fully erupted.

Doubts have been expressed about the cost-effectiveness of sealants and it is difficult to decide what price is justified in preventing disease. Sealants are not a cheap measure. However, recent research suggests that the cost of sealing teeth is less than the cost of repairing the damage caused by caries.

> - Fissure sealants require a dry enamel surface before application.
> - They can be self-polymerizing or light polymerized.
> - The filled ones are more resistant to abrasion.
> - Sealants are not a cheap measure and tend to be used particularly for high-risk groups.

Diet

Diet can influence the health of dental tissues in four ways.
- The role of sugar in the aetiology of caries.
- The effect of the diet on plaque formation.
- The cleansing action, if any, of fibrous foodstuffs.
- The nutritional requirements for healthy teeth and periodontium.

Sugar and caries

The aetiological role of sugar in caries has been fully described in Chapter 10. Based on these facts, the dietary advice to patients should be centred on reducing the frequency with which sugar is eaten and particularly avoiding sugar-containing snacks.

The danger of snacking

It is important that the dental hygienist should understand the need to give advice which is in agreement with that being given by other health educators. Reducing or avoiding snacks, especially those containing sugar, fits in well with the advice given by health educators in relation to the dangers of being overweight. It is foolish to suggest that patients avoid refined carbohydrates, when sugar is really what is meant. Many unrefined sugars are very cariogenic, for example those in honey, and the term 'carbohydrate' is both inaccurate and unnecessarily complicated. Furthermore, many nutritionists would prefer people to eat relatively harmless carbohydrates (not sugars) rather than the potentially harmful alternative of fat.

If people are unable to avoid snacks altogether, it may be necessary to suggest less harmful substitutes than sweets, biscuits, cakes and sweetened drinks. However, care is needed to ensure that this advice is in agreement with that being given by dieticians and health visitors. Not only are foodstuffs which contain fat not cariogenic, but they will actively reduce the development of caries. The temptation is, consequently, to recommend that peanuts and cheese be substituted for sweet snacks: this would be totally contrary to the advice of dieticians and nutritionists. It is important to realize the harm done when two separate health specialists give contradictory advice to, for example, a pregnant woman. There is a risk of the medical opinion being believed in preference to the dental advice, with the consequential loss of confidence and, possibly, total rejection of all the advice given in relation to dental health.

Hidden sugars

The term 'hidden sugar' is used to describe the sugar present in food which would usually be considered to be savoury rather than sweet. Many products, such as bottled sauces and tinned vegetables, contain a good deal of sugar and it is a depressing lesson to read the contents listed on the labels of a large number of packets, tins and jars. It is wrong merely to stress the need to avoid sweets, when most people are unaware of the problem of hidden sugars.

Sugar substitutes

The use of sugar substitutes is increasing, partly because they are virtually non-cariogenic and partly because their low calorific value makes them virtually non-fattening. There are many such substitutes, but xylitol which is entirely non-cariogenic, sorbitol, mannitol and saccharin which are all much less cariogenic than sucrose are among the most commonly used. Fortunately, many medicines are now sweetened with these agents rather than the sugars used previously. Many people object to the different flavour or the after-taste of artificial sweeteners, but there seems little doubt that they could be more widely used than at present.

Added sugar

It is often difficult for people who have become used to the flavour of sweetened tea, coffee, cornflakes, grapefruit, etc. to break the habit of adding unnecessary sugar in this way, despite the fact that many would prefer not to take all this sugar often for weight reasons. The dental hygienist should try to convince pregnant women or mothers of young children that sugar is not equal to kindness; it is not necessary for healthy child development; food is not less enjoyable without added sugar; it is not depriving children not to add sugar to their food, but quite the reverse. Far from feeling deprived, most adults who have grown up without the habit of adding sugar to tea and coffee are grateful for the fact.

Diet and plaque formation

The effect of sucrose on the development of plaque is described in Chapter 9.

The cleansing action of foods

For many years it has been fashionable to recommend that patients conclude a meal with an apple in order to clean the teeth, despite the ample evidence that fibrous foods do not remove plaque from the teeth to any significant degree. Whereas apples are undeniably less harmful than sweet, sticky snacks it is quite wrong to suggest that they are good for the teeth. Not only do they not remove plaque, they also contain sugar and may produce a pH drop in plaque.

Advising people that apples clean the teeth can in fact be harmful. If a child decides not to clean the teeth before going to bed because he or she had just eaten an apple, this misleading advice is potentially damaging. In addition apples are acidic with high levels of fructose. With this in mind, it is hard to see any justification in the preoccupation dental health educators seem to have with raw carrots!

An apple might reasonably be suggested as a less harmful snack than sweets or biscuits, but it should not be recommended as having a cleansing effect, nor should it be claimed to be good for the teeth.

Nutrition and the dental tissues

Dental hygienists are not dieticians, nor are they trained as such. It is not the dental hygienist's role to advise people about a balanced diet, since this is a complex subject well removed from the prevention of dental disease. It is wrong to suggest that a balanced diet will lead to healthy teeth: few children dying of starvation in underdeveloped countries have caries, but the well fed children of civilized societies do! It is, of course, necessary for the hygienist to understand what comprises the diet and how it might affect the teeth or supporting tissues. This is covered in Chapter 3.

Further reading

Bibby B. G. (1942) A new approach to caries prophylaxia. *Tufts Dent. Outlook*, **15**, 4.

British Society of Periodontology (1986) *Periodontology in General Dental Practice in the United Kingdom. A First Policy Statement.* The Secretary, British Society of Periodontology, Newcastle Dental School, Newcastle-upon-Tyne NE2 4BW, UK.

British Dental Association (1997) Policy Statement on Fluoride Supplement Dosage. *British Dental Journal*, **182**, 6–7.

Crichton-Browne I. (1892) Address to the Annual General Meeting of the Eastern Counties Branch of the British Dental Association. *British Dental Journal*, **13**, 4–16.

Dean H. T. (1934) Classification of mottled enamel diagnosis. *J. Am. Dent. Assoc.*, **21**, 1421–1426.

Grace A. M., Smales F. C. (1989) *Periodontal Control: An Effective System for Diagnosis, Selection, Control and Treatment Planning in General Practice.* London: Quintessence.

Lock H., Kleinmann D. U. (1986) *Dental Plaque Control Measures and Oral Hygiene Practices.* Oxford: IRL Press.

Muhler J. C., Day H. C. (1950) Effects of stannous fluoride, sodium fluoride on incidence of dental lesions in rats fed carious producing diets. *J. Am. Dent. Assoc.*, **41**, 528.

Murray J. J. (ed.) (1989) *The Prevention of Dental Disease.* 2nd edition.
Oxford University Press.

Murray J. J., Rugg-Gunn A. J. (1982) *Fluorides in Caries Prevention.* 2nd edition. Bristol: Wright.

Schou L., Blinkhorn A. S. (1993) *Oral Health Promotion.* Oxford University Press.

Health Education Authority (1996) *Scientific Basis of Dental Health Education.* 4th edition. Health Education Authority.

21

Dental radiography

Introduction

Radiographs are the images produced by X-rays coming in contact with an appropriate film, in a similar manner to the production of photographs by light rays. Dental radiographs are taken by passing X-rays through the teeth and jaws and recording the resultant shadow on an X-ray film.

When a photographic camera is pointed at a scene and the shutter release pressed, light enters through the lens and is recorded on the film as an image. If, by some misfortune, your hand happens to be in front of the lens at the time of shooting, a shadowy image of this appears on the film. If instead of your hand you held a more transparent object in front of the lens, such as a glass rod, the shadow would not be so dark. In a similar way, X-rays emitted from an X-ray machine and directed at an X-ray film will record the shadow of anything in the path of the rays. X-rays are useful because they can penetrate many objects without leaving a shadow, but the denser a substance, the more likelihood there is of it casting a shadow on the film. The more dense an object is, the more complete will be the shadow: the enamel of a tooth will produce a more marked shadow than will dentine and an amalgam restoration will have an even more marked shadow than enamel.

A large number of terms used in radiography have the prefix 'radio-': such as radio-opaque, which describes an object through which X-rays cannot pass and which therefore casts a shadow on the film, and radiolucent, which describes an object through which X-rays can pass and which therefore does not cast a shadow on the film.

Production of X-rays

Primary rays are produced in the X-ray machine when a stream of electrons strikes a target area made of tungsten (Fig. 21.1). The electrons are produced in a similar manner to those inside a television set, with a very high voltage produced through conversion from the normal domestic power supply. The electrons are emitted from a glass tube which is usually suspended in oil for heat absorption. The primary rays are highly penetrating and these produce the required image on the film. However, some rays are reflected from more solid objects which they cannot penetrate and may be scattered in different directions. This scattered radiation is an undesirable feature of an X-ray examination.

Precautions

X-rays are a boon to mankind if used carefully and sensibly. Repeated and excessive exposure of the same regions of the body to the X-rays will eventually bring about changes which are cumulative and may thus do a great deal of damage. The X-rays themselves do not 'add up' in the body but the slight changes that excessive exposure produces in the affected cells remain,

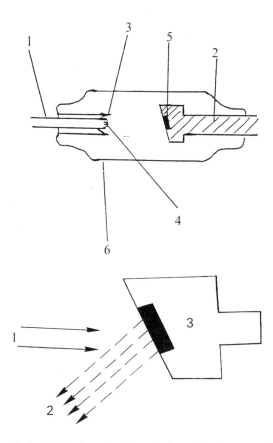

Fig. 21.1 (a) **1** The cathode (negative) provides the source of the electrons. **2** The electrons are attracted by the anode (positive). **3** The focusing device to direct the stream of electrons to the anode. **4** The heated filament of the cathode is the source of the electrons. **5** The target area of the mode is made of tungsten and is where the stream of electrons hit. **6** The tough glass container of the apparatus. (b) The electron beam **1** hits the target area of the anode **3** and this then liberates X-ray photons **2** from the target area.

and eventually the cells may be irreversibly altered. The taking of dental radiographs is relatively safe, since the amount of radiation used in dental radiographs is much less than that used in most medical views. It is the operator who is principally at risk, rather than the patient, since the operator may be repeatedly exposed to small levels of radiation over a long period of time which may give rise to malignancy. Therefore, sensible precautions should be taken to ensure there are no unwanted side-effects.

The precautions that need to be taken when using radiographs are governed by the Ionising Radiation Regulations 1985. The Ionising

Radiation (Protection of Persons Undergoing Medical Examination or Treatment) Regulations 1988 (the POPUMET regulations) extend the provision to patients and there is an approved code of practice published by the Health and Safety Executive. Dental hygienists should be familiar with the advice given in these documents which are listed, together with other relevant material, at the end of this chapter in the appendix.

- X rays are produced as photons when rapidly moving electrons hit the target of the anode.
- X-rays can produce genetic and somatic effects on the body which are cumulative.
- The use of X-rays in the UK is governed by the Ionising Radiation Regulations 1985.

Dental films and their uses

Dental films are supplied as film packets of various sizes. Each packet is in fact a light-sealed envelope of a soft plastic material containing a film, a sheet of black paper protecting against light leakage, and a sheet of lead foil. Any rays striking the lead foil have already passed through the subject and the film and are therefore no longer useful. Thus the lead foil performs the function of absorbing these excess primary rays as well as preventing secondary rays being reflected back by scattering on to the film. Care must be taken that films are not sharply bent or the outer packets torn. A sharp bend induced by a finger nail will often show up on the developed film as a black line or crescent-shaped mark (Fig. 21.2). A torn packet will let in light which will affect the film in a similar manner to X-rays. It may be necessary to bend the film, however, for it to be accommodated by the shape of the mouth, but the bend should be no more than a gentle curve. There are several sizes and types of dental films (Fig. 21.3).

Periapical films

There are several sizes and types of periapical films. The most usual size, called standard, is

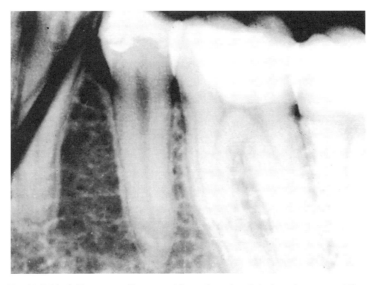

Fig. 21.2 Black line across film caused by a sharp bend during placement of film. Sometimes a similar fault is seen as a crescent shaped mark due to finger nail damage.

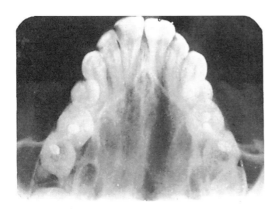

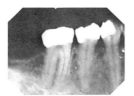 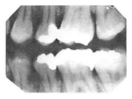

Fig. 21.3 Three types of intraoral film: (a) occlusal, (b) periapical, (c) bitewing.

on a standard film. They are useful for detecting the following.

- The state of the alveolar bone supporting the teeth. Periapical views are particularly important in the assessment of the severity of chronic periodontal disease.
- Changes around the apex of a tooth. This may denote the presence of a chronic abscess and other abnormality.
- The length of a root canal in endodontics and the position of a root canal filling in relation to the apex.
- Fractures of the roots and retained root tips.
- Missing or unerupted teeth.
- Supernumerary teeth.
- Impacted teeth.
- Malformation of the roots which may make an intended extraction more complicated.

Bitewing films

These may be the same as periapical films with the addition of a tab placed centrally on the face (Fig. 21.3c), towards the tube, so that the patient holds this between the teeth (hence bitewing) and the X-ray beam is directed along the axis of the tab.

3.2×4.1 cm. There is a smaller size, 2.2×3.5 cm, often called child-size, but these are frequently used for taking radiographs of adult anterior teeth.

The periapical film shows the entire tooth, and usually up to 3–4 teeth are accommodated

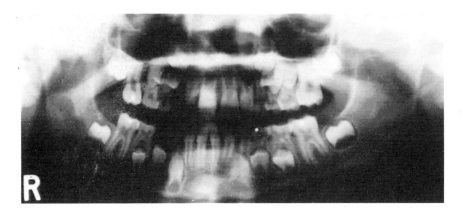

Fig. 21.4 A panoramic radiograph: these are commonly called OPGs or OPTs.

There is a longer film, the number 3 bitewing, which measures 5.4×2.7 cm. This covers all the posterior teeth, but distortion is possible.

Bitewings show only the crowns and cervical portion of the roots of the teeth, but have the advantage of showing both upper and lower teeth at the same time. This means that, if the radiographs are being taken to examine the crowns (e.g. for interproximal caries), one bitewing will show the same area as two periapicals, that is only half the amount of exposure to X-ray is needed. Bitewings, therefore, are mainly used for full-mouth surveys to check for caries or early bone loss in periodontal disease.

Occlusal films

These are somewhat larger, 5.7×7.6 cm (2.5×3 in), and are placed between the teeth in the occlusal plane (Fig. 21.3a). Their purpose is to show all or a large part of the mandibular arch or the maxilla in one film. They may be used to detect abnormalities such as salivary duct calculi in the floor of the mouth, or to localize a tooth or an object in another plane of the jaw. They are often taken to record the position of buried teeth, such as upper canines or lower third molars. It is possible to discover and identify the shape and extent of cysts, fracture lines in the jaws and other abnormalities of the bones such as tumours, both benign and malignant.

Panoramic radiographs

These are the most common extraoral radiographs with which the dental hygienist will come in contact and are frequently referred to as OPGs or OPTs (Fig. 21.4). They are larger films, measuring 30×15 cm, placed in a curved holder and designed to give a panoral picture of the entire dentition on the one film. The film is placed on one side of the head and the X-ray source is set on the other side. The source moves round in an arc, exposing a thin line of the film as it does so. In this way a flattened-out view of the entire dentition and the surrounding structures is produced. These films are extremely useful in making an overall assessment of the patient's dentition, but they have the disadvantage of lacking the clarity of detail found in periapical views.

The radiation dosage involved in taking an orthopantomograph is only 50% of that involved in a full-mouth periapical survey.

Other extraoral films

There are many other extraoral films used in dentistry, especially in oral surgery and orthodontics. However, the dental hygienist probably will not be very involved with any of these views. It is unlikely that the hygienist would be required to take such views and they are unlikely to contain information which the dental hygienist would wish to have. If further information is required about these views, the student is referred to standard texts on dental radiography.

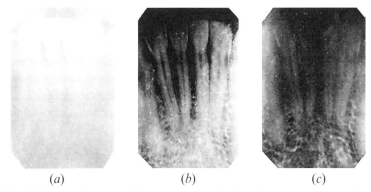

Fig. 21.5 Three radiographs of lower anterior teeth: (a) underexposed, (b) correctly exposed, (c) overexposed.

- Intraoral films include periapicals, bite-wings and occlusals.
- Extraoral films include panoramic films which are the ones of most use to hygienists.
- The radiation dosage from a panoramic film is about 50% of that from a full mouth periapical survey.

Exposing the film

Little is to be gained by detailed written descriptions of the techniques of using dental X-ray machines. Practical skills are best taught by demonstration and practice under supervision. However it is necessary to know the factors which influence the density of the image on the film and to understand the principles behind the two basic techniques for taking periapical radiographs.

The density of the image

This means the darkness of the pictures on the film. This is influenced by the following factors.

- **Kilovoltage**: the greater the kilovoltage, the denser the image.
- **Current**: the greater the current, the denser the image.
- **Time**: the longer the exposure, the denser the image (Fig. 21.5).
- **Film**: the faster the film, the denser the image.
- **Distance**: the nearer the film to the source, the denser the image.

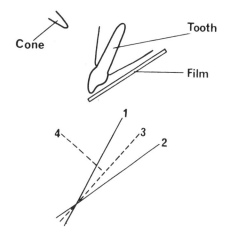

Fig. 21.6 Diagram of the bisecting angle technique showing: **1** the long axis of the tooth, **2** angulation of the film, **3** the bisection of the angle, **4** the direction of the X-ray beam.

Basic techniques for periapical radiographs

Periapical films may be exposed by either the bisecting angle technique (short cone technique), or the paralleling technique (long cone technique).

Bisecting angle technique

This uses a near approximation to obtain an image on the film, which is as little distorted as possible (Fig. 21.6). Because the film, when placed in the mouth does not ordinarily lie parallel to the long axis of the tooth, the most accurate image will be obtained by directing the central ray of the X-ray beam perpendicular to the bisection of the angle between the long axis of the tooth and the film.

Table 21.1 Radiography
Helpful hints when taking dental radiographs
<ul><li>A few patients gag very badly when the film is placed in the mouth, especially on the posterior part of the palate. To overcome this, some operators apply topical anaesthetic to the mucosa of the palate for a few minutes.</li><li>When placing the film in the patient's mouth make sure that the embossed dot on the edge of the film is placed occlusally. Then, when the film is being clipped to a hanger for processing, it can be clipped near the embossed dot with the knowledge that no important part of the radiograph is being damaged.</li><li>Some radiographers prefer the film to be placed with the dot always at the lower edge. In this way, there is never any doubt about whether the film is of upper or lower teeth, which lets the inexperienced orientate the film without the help of anatomical landmarks.</li></ul>

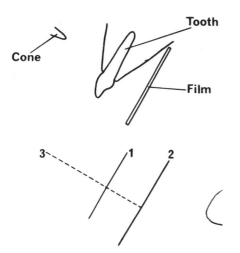

Fig. 21.7 Diagram of the paralleling technique showing: **1** the long axis of the tooth, **2** the angulation of the film, **3** the direction of the X-ray beam.

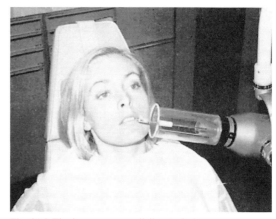

Fig. 21.8 The long cone paralleling technique.

Paralleling technique

If the film is placed parallel to the long axis of the tooth (Figs 21.7 and 21.8) either by interposing a cotton wool roll between them, or by using special film holder, the central ray of the beam can be directed perpendicularly to both film and tooth, producing a more accurate picture. Since the film and tooth are further apart, the source must be placed further away from the film hence the description long cone technique.

Angulation

It is not possible in this text to detail all the angulations and film positions for the numerous different views. Some excellent illustrations and directions for the technique of film placement can be obtained from the X-ray supply companies, especially Kodak® and Rinn®.

Processing the film

It is not the purpose of this text to detail the stages involved in processing a film. These can be learned adequately only by practice. However, the hygienist should have grasped the theory of developing and processing before practising the techniques.

Developing

Once the film has been exposed to the X-rays it contains an invisible, latent image, which is converted into a visible one by the developing solution. The emulsion of the film contains silver salts and the developer acts on those which have been exposed to the X-rays,

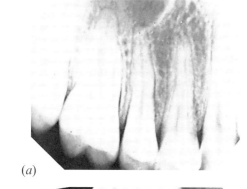

(a)

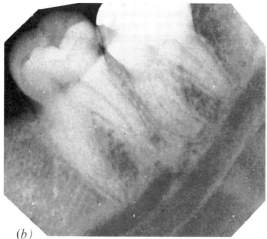

(b)

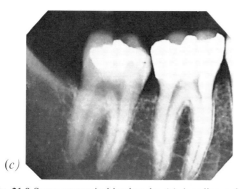

(c)

Fig. 21.9 Some anatomical landmarks. (a) A radiograph of the upper right molars and premolars, in which the maxillary sinus can be seen, overlapping the roots of 65. (b) A radiograph of the lower left molars, with the mandibular canal visible below their roots. (c) A radiograph of the lower right molar teeth in which the lamina dura is clearly visible, especially around the mesial root of the first molar.

precipitating the silver. The density of the image is affected by the following.

- **Temperature**: the warmer the solution, the darker or denser the image.

- **Time**: the longer the film is in the developer, the darker it gets.
- **Strength of the solution**: the more concentrated the developing solution, the darker the image it produces.
- **Age of the solution**: the developer will eventually become 'worked out' if used for too long and the image will be pale and weak.

The various manufacturers of developer give tables of recommended times and temperatures for using their products. The solution should be mixed according to the instructions and the times and temperatures carefully adhered to.

Fixing

The fixing solution serves two purposes: it dissolves off the unused emulsion, thus clearing the film, and it fixes the image permanently on the film, so that it is no longer affected by exposure to light.

The time and temperature of fixing are not as critical as they are for developing. Once the film has cleared it can be viewed briefly in the daylight, without harm, but it should be kept in the fixer for the recommended time before being finally washed and dried. Films can be left in the fixer for longer than the recommended time, but should not be left longer than an hour, or the density of the image may be reduced.

Washing

Thorough washing after processing is essential to remove all chemicals from the film, because if they are left they will cause staining. This can only be done adequately in running water.

- The warmer the developer the darker the image.
- Too long in the developer gives a darker image.
- Too concentrated developer gives a darker image.
- Developer which has been used for too long can become worked out and the image become pale or weak.
- Fixing is the process of fixing the image permanently on the film.
- Time and temperature are not as critical when fixing as they are in developing the film.
- Washing is important to remove all residual chemicals from the film.

Anatomical landmarks

The hygienist's main use of anatomical landmarks is in orientating the film, that is, deciding whether the film is of the upper or lower teeth.

Curve of Spee

From the tip of the canine to the third molar, the occlusal surfaces of the teeth do not form a flat plane but in fact curve upwards towards the back. This is called the curve of Spee and it means that the occlusal plane of the lower teeth is concave mesiodistally, while that of the upper is convex. This is a valuable feature in identification of upper and lower posterior radiographs.

Bone cavities

Maxillary sinus

This is a prominent feature of upper posterior radiographs (Fig. 21.9a). The sinus itself appears darker than the alveolar bone and the wall of the sinus can be seen as a whitish line.

Nasal cavity

A periapical view of the upper anterior teeth often shows the lower part of the nasal cavity, which appears as two dark areas separated by the lighter line of the nasal septum.

Foramina and canals

Mandibular canal

This is sometimes visible on periapical radiographs of the lower molar teeth as a dark band curving downwards and forwards below the roots of the teeth (Fig. 21.9b).

Mental foramen

The mental foramen may appear as a round dark area situated close to the apices of the lower premolars. This may well be mistaken for a dental abscess of one of these teeth.

Incisive foramen

Between the apices of the upper centrals, the incisive foramen may be seen as a round dark area.

Bony ridges and projections

External oblique line

This may show as a wide whitish line curving downwards and forwards and overlapping the roots of the lower molar teeth.

Genial tubercles

On a lower occlusal film the genial tubercles can be seen projecting backwards from the inner aspect of the mandible behind the lower incisors.

Zygomatic arch

The zygomatic arches are visible on an upper occlusal radiograph, curving outwards at the level of the premolars or molars. They can also be seen on some periapical views of the upper molars, overlapping the roots.

Dental structures

The pulp

This is easily recognized as a dark area in the centre of the tooth. The shape of the pulp chamber and root canals can be clearly seen.

Roots

These are another important feature for telling upper molar radiographs from lower ones. Because the upper molars have three roots, their shadows overlap each other on the radiograph, making it difficult to decide how many there are, whereas the lower molars usually have two distinctly visible roots.

Lamina dura

The lamina dura lining the tooth sockets is visible as a white line surrounding the root (Fig. 21.9c) and often the earliest sign of a dental abscess is loss of this line.

Orientation of the film

Dental radiographs are normally mounted on a special card, to match the dental charting of the patient. Accuracy in orientating the films and mounting them correctly is of prime importance. For example, an upper left film mounted

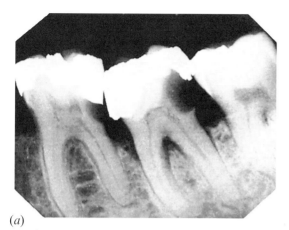

(*a*)

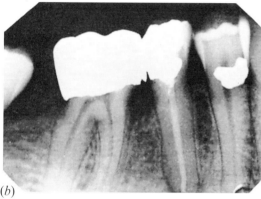

(*b*)

Fig. 21.10 The radiographic appearance of restorations and dental pathology. (a) The lower left molars, with amalgam restorations on three teeth and large distal carious cavities on the first and second molars. There is also bone loss due to periodontal disease, especially around the second molar. (b) The lower right teeth. There are amalgam restorations on the premolars and a gold crown on the molar. The second premolar has a root filling and an area of apical pathology.

in the place of an upper right one could lead the dentist to treat the wrong tooth. There are two stages involved in orientation.

Stage 1: upper or lower?

Using the landmarks previously described, the hygienist soon becomes capable of telling, almost at a glance, an upper radiograph from a lower one.

Stage 2: left or right?

Once it has been decided to which arch the teeth belong, the hygienist should focus attention on the little pimple on the corner of the film. The

convexity of this should point towards the person viewing the film and provided it does, it is easy to tell from the order of the teeth which side the film depicts.

Pathological and other features

It is not the job of the radiographer to interpret the film or to recognize pathology. This is the responsibility of the radiologist, who is, in dentistry, the dentist. However, certain features are so obvious that the hygienist would need to be particularly un-inquisitive not to wonder what they are. Furthermore, there is a need to recognize what is abnormal and to refer it to the dentist.

Pathology

The lesions which are visible on radiographs are those which destroy either tooth substance or bone. Because the calcified tissue has been removed, the X-rays can pass more freely through the lesions which, therefore, appear darker than the surrounding tissues.

- **Caries**: initially a small round dark area which becomes more irregular as the cavity grows bigger (Fig. 21.10a).
- **Chronic periodontal disease**: loss of the interdental septum of bone (Fig. 21.10a).
- **Dental abscess**: a round dark area most usually found surrounding the apex, but which may also occur on the side of the root (Fig. 21.10b).
- **Fractures of root or bone**: the gap between the broken ends shows as a dark line in the root or bone.

Restorations

Most filling materials are radio-opaque and appear completely white on radiographs, for example gold, amalgam, cement and zinc oxide (Fig. 21.10). However, many composites are completely radiolucent and these restorations closely resemble a carious cavity, unless a telltale cement lining can be seen.

Acrylic is naturally radiolucent and would not be seen on a radiograph if it were not for special radio-opaque additives put into the acrylic to make it visible. This is done in case the appliance is inhaled or swallowed, and it

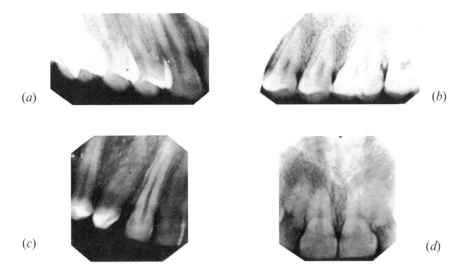

Fig. 21.11 Faults in radiographs: (a) overlapping, (b) cone cutting, (c) elongation, (d) foreshortening.

makes it necessary to remove dentures and orthodontic appliances before taking radiographs. Some acrylic crowns are made with materials lacking the radio-opaque additives and a radiograph of one of these would show a tooth stump apparently covered only by a layer of cement. Glass-ionomers are radiolucent unless they have an additional material added to make them radio-opaque.

Diagnosing faults in radiographs

If a hygienist is to be able to correct faults in her or his technique of taking radiographs, she or he must first recognize the fault and then know what action to take to prevent it happening again. Some of the more common faults are listed below and the remedy suggested (Fig. 21.11).

Overlapping of the teeth

Often, the part of a radiograph of most interest to the dentist is that showing the interproximal area, for example when checking for caries of the contact point or periodontal disease involving the interdental septum. If the teeth overlap each other on the film this area cannot be seen properly and the radiograph may be useless. Overlapping means that the X-ray beam has not passed perpendicular to the line of the teeth

being radiographed, that is, the cone is angled too far back or too far forwards.

Elongation and foreshortening

In general, distortion of the length of the teeth should be avoided when taking a periapical film and this is most easily achieved using the paralleling technique. The bisecting angle technique is generally quicker but does allow distortion of the image to occur. For example, during endodontic treatment, the dentist uses a periapical film to judge how far to ream the root canal and how far to insert the root filling. Elongation or foreshortening of the tooth on the film makes this impossible. Similarly, a radiograph taken to find the depth of an impacted tooth will be very misleading if distortion of the film has taken place. Using the bisecting angle technique, distortion of the length happens when the beam is not perpendicular to the bisection of the angle. Foreshortening means that the beam is angled too far towards the apex and elongation means that it is angled too far towards the crown. This can best be understood by remembering the angulation used for occlusal films, which produce very foreshortened teeth.

Cone-cutting

An X-ray beam, like the beam of light from a

torch, is conical in shape and, just as the torch beam produces a round patch of light when projected on to a wall, so the X-ray beam affects a round area when projected on to a large radiograph. Normally, the small dental radiographs are placed in the centre of the beam, so that the whole film is exposed to the X-rays but, if the cone is not aimed properly, the edge of the beam will cut across the film, resulting in the fault termed cone-cutting. Obviously, the remedy for cone-cutting is to take more care in pointing the cone at the film.

Film too dark

This can result from either overexposing or overdeveloping the film. If only one film of a series is too dark, it must have been over-exposed since they were all developed simultaneously. On the other hand, if all the films are too dark, it is likely that it is the developing which is wrong. A completely dark film generally means that it has been exposed to light during processing or that it was not fixed adequately.

Film too light

This is caused by the opposite of the dark film, that is underexposure or underdevelopment, but the same guide can be used to decide which is at fault. A completely clean film means that either it was not exposed or not developed at all.

Haziness

If the film appears as if it is out of focus either the X-ray cone or the patient has moved slightly during the exposure.

- Overlapping teeth on bitewings can make the film useless for spotting interproximal caries.
- Avoid distortion when taking radiographs if possible.
- Cone cutting is due to the cone of the X-ray set not being aimed properly.
- Too dark a film can be due to over-exposure or over-development.
- Too light a film is due to underexposure or underdevelopment.
- Haziness is often due to patient movement.

Appendix

These regulations are taken form the Ionising Radiation Regulations 1985 and The Ionising Radiation Regulations (Protection of Persons Undergoing Medical Examination or Treatment 1988) often called the POPUMET regulations. They list the precautions to observe when taking radiographs.

1. Primary considerations

a. Only X-ray a patient if clinically necessary. ALARA is the acronym to remember and stands for as low as reasonably achievable. Only take radiographs when absolutely necessary.
b. The radiation protection supervisor (RPS) shall ensure that all staff understand and observe the local rules.
c. Only a trained and competent operator should use the X-ray equipment.

2. Equipment

a. Ensure that the equipment is of adequate tube rating not lower than 50 kV and preferably about 70 kV.
b. The beam diameter should not exceed 60 mm measured at the patient end of the cone.
c. Ensure correct beam filtration: equivalent to at least 1.5 mm of aluminium for X-ray tube voltages up to and including 70 kV and 2.5 mm of aluminium (of which 1.5 mm is permanent) for X-ray tube voltages above 70 kV.
d. Ensure that the equipment is regularly checked and properly maintained.
e. If a fault in the equipment occurs it should be disconnected and the RPS notified.

3. Films and film holders

a. Use the minimum number of films consistent with adequate diagnosis.
b. Use the fastest film available consistent with good film quality. Intensifying screens must be used for extraoral and vertex occlusal views.
c. A film holder should be used if possible. The operator should never hold the film, the patient or the tube housing during exposure.

4. Operating technique

a. Persons whose presence is unnecessary for the examination should be excluded from the X-ray room.

b. The operator must stand outside the controlled area. This will be achieved by being at least 2.0 m from the tube and the patient, and being outside the primary beam.

c. Ensure that the exposure is correctly set and a minimum exposure time is used.

d. Ensure that the exposure is properly terminated – observe the warning signals.

e. Where it is likely that a fetus will be irradiated by the primary beam a protective apron should be used.

f. Personal monitoring of staff should be carried out if their individual workload exceeds 150 intraoral or 50 panoral films per week.

g. Disconnect the X-ray unit from the mains supply after use in order to de-designate the controlled area and to eliminate the possibility of an inadvertent exposure.

h. All films should be correctly processed.

i. Routine checks should be made to detect if any deterioration in the quality of radiographs occurs.

j. In cases of accidental overexposure the recommended procedures must be followed.

5. X-ray room and environment

a. Room size should be large enough to provide safe accommodation for those persons who have to be in the room during exposure. This will be achieved if there is sufficient space to allow the operator to be 2.0 m or further from the tube and patient and well outside the primary beam.

b Additional protective panels: these may be required if the work load exceeds 150 mA/mm per week for panoramic films or 30 mA/mm per week for intraoral films. This is roughly equivalent to 50 panoramic or 300 intraoral films.

c. A dental surgery or any other room should not be used for other work (or as a passageway) whilst radiography is in progress.

d. Radiation warning sign: if the room door opens directly into an area where the instantaneous dose rate is greater than 7.5 μSv/h a radiation warning sign should be displayed.

e. Automatic warning signal: if the controlled area extends to the room entrance an automatic warning signal indicating emission of radiation is required to warn against entry.

f. Persons in all occupied areas outside the X-ray room should be adequately protected.

6. Routine dental radiography

a. Training and competence: a person clinically or physically directing an exposure shall have received adequate training ('clinically directing' means having a clinical responsibility for the decision to effect an exposure. 'Physically directing' means effecting the exposure).

b. Where it is necessary to support a small child or handicapped patient the advice of a Radiation Protection Adviser (RPA) must be sought.

c. Where a film holder cannot be used and the patient is unable to hold the film, a person assisting must observe adequate protective measures in accordance with the advice of a RPA.

d. Exposure values should be checked before using the X-ray machine, particularly if changing between long and short cone techniques.

e. Attenuation of beam: since the beam is not fully absorbed by the patient it should be considered as extending beyond the patient until it has been attenuated by distance or intercepted by shielding such as a brick wall.

7. Panoramic radiography

a. Automatic warning signal: where the controlled area extends to the entrance of the X-ray room an automatic warning signal indicating when the equipment is in the ready state and while radiation is being emitted should be provided at the room entrance.

b. Rotation faults: the irradiation switch should be released immediately if the rotational movement fails to start or stops before the full arc is covered.

8. Cephalometry

a. Cephalometry should not be carried out without prior consultation with a RPA.

b. Ordinary dental X-ray equipment operating at less than 60 kV should never be used for cephalometry. Equipment operating at or above 60 kV may be suitable if used with specially designed auxiliary equipment.

9. Core of knowledge

The following core of knowledge as to radiation protection of patients is what a person physically directing medical exposures is expected to have acquired:

1. The nature of ionizing radiation and its interaction with tissue.
2. The genetic and somatic effects of ionizing radiation and how to assess their risks.
3. The ranges of radiation dose that are given to a patient with a particular procedure. The principal factors which affect the dose and the methods of measuring such doses.
4. The principles of quality assurance and quality control applied to both equipment and techniques.
5. The principles of dose limitation and the various means of dose reduction to the patient including protection of the gonads.
6. The specific requirements of women who are or who may be pregnant and also of children.
7. If applicable, the precautions necessary for handling sealed and unsealed sources.
8. The organizational arrangements for advice on radiation protection and how to deal with a suspected case of overexposure.
9. Statutory responsibilities.
   For those clinically directing medical exposure, the following additional knowledge should be acquired:
10. In respect of the individual diagnostic and therapeutic procedures which the person intends to use, the clinical value of those procedures in relation to other available techniques used for the same or similar purposes.
11. The importance of utilizing existing radiological information i.e.: films and/or reports about a patient.

Further reading

Health and Safety at Work Act (1974) London: HMSO.

Mason R. A. (1988) *A Guide to Dental Radiography*. 3rd edition. Bristol: Wright.

Standing Dental Advisory Committee (1990) *Radiation Protection in Dental Practice*. London: Department of Health.

Smith N. J. D. (1988) *Dental Radiography*. 2nd edition. London: Blackwell Scientific Publications.

The Ionising Radiations Regulations (1985) Approved Code of Practice. London: HMSO.

The Ionising Radiations Regulations (1988) Guidance Notes for the Protection of Persons from Ionising Radiation in Medical and Dental Use. London: HMSO.

22

Local analgesia and pharmacology

Local analgesia

Local anaesthesia is a very safe procedure and the techniques are easily mastered. However, it should only be administered by an operator who is fully conversant with the anatomy of the area and the reader is referred to the appropriate sections on anatomy earlier in this book. The hygienist should also be familiar with commonly used local analgesic drugs and the effect that these have on the body. The local anaesthetics used in clinical dental practice have been available since the 1950s and are known to have few side effects and a low incidence of allergic reactions. In the few patients who report a previous allergic response it may be wise to check with the dentist who could arrange for skin patch tests to be done, either in the dental practice or in conjunction with the local medical practitioner or hospital dermatology department.

Physiology of the peripheral nerve

The process of conduction along the nerve axon is principally dependent on the changes in the electrophysiological status of the axon membrane. When the nerve cell is resting it has a negative potential of about -70 millivolts within the cell with respect to the exterior cell membrane potential. When a nerve impulse or action potential is transmitted along a nerve, the membrane charge increases to $+40$ milli-

volts, an event called depolarization, and a series of changes takes place as described in Table 22.1. The passage of an impulse along a nerve can be likened to the wave which passes down a whip when it is cracked.

Table 22.1 Action potential

Sequence of events in the movement of an action potential along a nerve

- A slow depolarization of the nerve membrane takes place when the nerve membrane becomes less negative as ions are transferred out of the axon.
- When the potential between inner and outer membrane surfaces reaches a certain point the firing level is said to have been reached.
- Depolarization occurs and the interior of the membrane is positively charged with respect to the exterior aspect of the cell membrane.
- The peak of the positive action potential will reach $+40$ millivolts.
- A process of repolarization begins until the resting potential of -70 millivolts is restored again to the inner cell membrane.

Nerve function is dependent on the exchange of sodium and potassium ions across the cell membrane and it is interesting to note that the concentration of potassium ions is higher inside the cell where the concentration of sodium ions is low. This ionic concentration is the opposite of that found normally in the extracellular fluid.

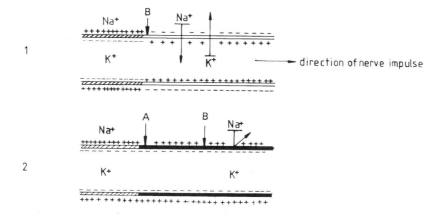

Fig. 22.1 Transmission of a nerve impulse: (1) a stimulus applied at point B causes depolarization of the axon allowing sodium and potassium ions to move in the direction shown, (2) when a local anaesthetic drug is present at point A the movement of sodium and potassium ions is prevented, so that no nerve impulse is generated.

At rest the cell membrane is relatively resistant to ionic exchange but on excitation of the cell permeability increases and there is an influx of sodium ions which accounts for the depolarization phase. When the membrane is maximally depolarized sodium ion passage is arrested and potassium ions pass out of the cell to effect a repolarization of the cell membrane. During the excitation of the membrane the movement of the sodium and potassium ions is passive and along a concentration gradient.

After repolarization there is an imbalance with too many sodium ions intracellularly and too many potassium ions extracellularly. This imbalance is corrected by means of the sodium pump, a mechanism of ionic repatriation which uses energy because it works against the ionic gradient. By this means the nerve cell is returned to its resting state, ready to conduct another action potential when necessary.

The presence of local anaesthetic solution in the vicinity of the nerve will interfere with the ionic exchange that is necessary for nerve conduction. It does this by interfering with the influx of sodium ions so that the critical threshold is not reached and an action potential is not produced (Fig. 22.1). Nerve function returns slowly to normal as the local anaesthetic solution is transported away from the area by blood and tissue fluid and metabolized. For an infiltration this may take up to 2 hours or in the case of a regional block, 3–4 hours.

- Normal nerve function is achieved by the movement of sodium and potassium ions across the axon membrane.
- The nerve impulse itself is called the action potential.
- Local analgesia with lignocaine and prilocaine has been available since the 1950s and is very safe.
- The presence of local anaesthetic in the vicinity of the nerve will prevent the influx of sodium ions into the axon and so stop the critical threshold forming.

Pre-injection topical analgesia

The need for pre-injection topical analgesia is considerably less with the advent of modern disposable needles. However, some patients, particularly those of a nervous disposition, will request it. It is more likely to be required for infiltration injections in the labial sulcus around the upper incisors where the tissues are particularly sensitive or when an injection needs to be given in the palate. The mucosa can be anaesthetized in advance by applying a suitable ointment such as Xylocaine® ointment containing 5% lignocaine, which is applied on a cotton roll and left in the sulcus for about 3 min. Children will particularly appreciate this technique when the topical ointment is bubble gum or pinocolada flavoured! The alternative is to use a topical spray containing 10% lignocaine and this works within 2 min or so but the spray does not taste particularly pleasant. However, use of a careful and slow injection technique will contribute most to painless administration of local anaesthetic solution.

Local analgesic drugs

The drug most commonly used is lignocaine, which is sold under a variety of trade names. A 2% solution is used, together with a small amount of adrenaline (1 in 80 000). The adrenaline increases the duration of anaesthesia by inducing vasoconstriction in the area and thus confining the anaesthetic to the site of injection. It also has the advantage of improving visibility for the operator by decreasing the amount of gingival bleeding that can occur when scaling deep pockets.

The use of adrenaline-containing local anaesthetics may be best avoided in patients with severe ischaemic coronary artery disease, hypertension, or those taking major tranquillizers such as the tricyclic antidepressants, or hypotensive drugs such as beta-blockers, although the use of aspirating syringes will most definitely help to avoid any unfortunate complications.

In patients with coronary artery disease or hypertension, the alternative local anaesthetic is 3% prilocaine together with felypressin as a vasoconstrictor, which is sold in the UK under the brand name of Citanest with Octapressin®. For those patients on medication which may interact with a vasoconstrictor, then prilocaine is available as a 4% solution, although its duration of anaesthesia is very limited. Clinical experience leads to the impression that the duration of analgesia with prilocaine is less than that obtained with lignocaine.

It has recently been suggested that patients should receive no more than 10 mg of lignocaine for dental purposes at any one time (Cannell, 1997). This amounts to about four and half cartridges of lignocaine and is a good guide for dentists and hygienists to follow. The same author recommends that only one 2.2 ml cartridge of lignocaine should be administered for dental purposes in the medically compromised patient. In the case of the dental hygienist when working on a healthy patient only 1–1.5 cartridges would be necessary for quadrant infiltration anaesthesia for scaling purposes (Table 22.2).

Table 22.2 Local analgesics

Contents of a local analgesic cartridge may include the following

- Local analgesic agent: lignocaine (2%), prilocaine (3%), mepivacaine (3%).
- Vasoconstrictor: adrenaline 1 : 80 000, felypressin 0.03 units/ml.
- Reducing agent: sodium metabisulphite.
- Preservative: caprylhydrocuprienotoxin.
- Fungicide: thymol.
- Carrier: isotonic saline.

Equipment

The local anaesthetic is usually provided in a glass or plastic 2 ml cartridge, which has a thin plastic seal at one end and a rubber bung at the other. When the cartridge is placed in a syringe, the double-ended needle pierces the plastic seal. Solution is injected when the plunger at the other end pushes down on the rubber bung. A common mistake of the beginner is to place the cartridge in the wrong way round, the operator should always check that the solution can be ejected through the needle before inserting it into the tissues. In addition it is important to check the expiry date on the cartridge as well as checking that the cartridge itself is not cracked or its contents cloudy.

To reduce the risk of cross-infection, care should be taken not to touch or contaminate the plastic end of the cartridge or the needle itself. The cartridge should be kept in its sealed packaging before use, to reduce contamination by air-borne fomites. After use, the needle should either be resheathed using an Aim Safe (Fig. 22.2) or left unsheathed until disposal. When no longer needed, it should be safely disposed of in a sharps bin.

With modern fine needles there is little risk of fracture, but it would be wise to have a pair of fine haemostats to hand with which to grasp the needle should this eventuality occur when giving local anaesthetics.

Injection techniques

The three main methods of giving local anaesthesia are a nerve block, intra-ligamentary

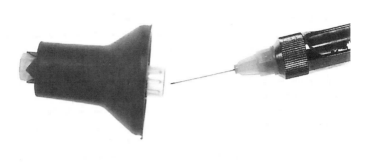

Fig. 22.2 The Aim Safe is a rubber 'mushroom', which is slipped over the needle sheath. It prevents needle stick injury when resheathing the needle.

and local infiltration. As the latter method is the only one that is permitted for UK hygienists, a brief description will be given here. This restriction means that in the upper jaw, both the teeth and gingiva can be anaesthetized, but in the lower jaw, anaesthesia will be confined to the gingiva and the teeth anterior to the mental foramen. Should the hygienist find that anaesthesia of posterior mandibular teeth is required an infiltration can be tried by injecting in the sulcus buccally but if the level of analgesia is insufficient then the supervising dentist should be asked to administer an inferior alveolar block.

A nerve block deposits the anaesthetic solution adjacent to the main nerve, just as it enters or leaves the bone and prevents pain conduction from the whole peripheral distribution of that branch. The principal dental blocks are inferior dental and mental in the mandible, and posterior superior, infraorbital and incisive in the maxilla.

The intra-ligamentary injection uses a fine short needle with a high pressure syringe to deposit a very small amount of local anaesthetic into the periodontal ligament of the tooth to be anaesthetized. As with the nerve block, hygienists are not be allowed to administer this type of anaesthetic. As the intra-ligamentary injection should not be given in the presence of inflammation, perhaps this is fortuitous.

An infiltration local anaesthetic deposits local anaesthetic into the soft tissues of the area to be anaesthetized. The technique may be used for

making scaling and root planing painless, or for the control of excessive bleeding from the gingiva during instrumentation. However, it is not necessary to offer every patient local analgesia, many will be quite happy to have their scaling done without it.

Before giving an injection the medical history should be checked and a brief, sympathetic description given to prepare the patient. Although many operators insist on the patient being placed in an upright position so that the anatomical landmarks are more visible, it is easier for the operator and safer for the patient to be placed horizontal in the chair. The use of protective spectacles for the patient is mandatory. For infiltration injections a short needle is preferred and this, together with the syringe, surface antiseptic such as chlorhexidine or iodine, and a topical anaesthetic, are laid out ready.

The surface anaesthetic, if required, is applied and left for 2 min. The site is then dried and cleaned with the surface antiseptic. The needle is inserted into the mucosa in the base of the sulcus just over the area where anaesthesia is required, as shown in Figure 22.3. It is not necessary to penetrate the tissues deeply and about a cartridge (2 ml) should be sufficient for an area over four teeth (Fig. 22.4). If haemorrhage control is required, then further solution may be deposited into the attached gingiva adjacent to each interdental papilla, after the initial anaesthetic has taken effect. This is required because an injection into attached

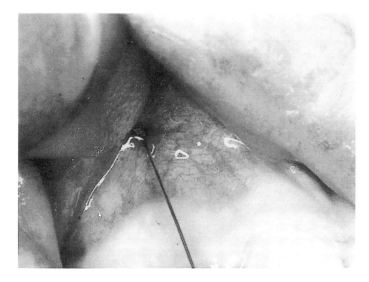

Fig. 22.3 Inserting the needle into the mucosa in the upper labial sulcus, apically to the mucogingival junction.

gingiva can be very painful without prior anaesthesia. If an aspirating syringe has been used the plunger should be withdrawn slightly before injecting the solution. If blood enters the cartridge, then the needle is withdrawn out of the blood vessel and the check repeated.

After the injection the patient is monitored for any untoward effects for about 3 min before work can begin. After completion the patient should be warned about care of the numb area and advised to avoid traumatizing the site or eating excessively hot foods.

- Dental hygienists in the UK can only administer infiltration injections.
- Not every patient needs local analgesia.
- A surface analgesic may be needed for some injections such as for upper incisor teeth.
- If haemorrhage control is needed this is given adjacent to each interdental papilla after an injection into the sulcus.
- Infiltration analgesia takes about 3 min to work for scaling procedures.

Unwanted effects of local analgesia

Although local analgesia does have some

possible adverse effects, it should be remembered that it has been responsible for permitting modern techniques of restoration to be used on countless patients with very few side-effects (Table 22.3).

Contraindications to local analgesia

There are a few contraindications to local analgesia and some have already been mentioned, but those the dental hygienist should bear in mind are shown in Table 22.4. The reader is again reassured about the relative safety of this method which can permit the treatment of many patients who previously found scaling very upsetting.

Drugs used in dentistry

Dentists do not on the whole prescribe many medicaments for home use by the patient and, of the few that are popularly used, even fewer can be administered by the dental hygienist. Nevertheless, although the hygienist may not prescribe many of these drugs, it is important that she or he knows what help might be requested from the dentist.

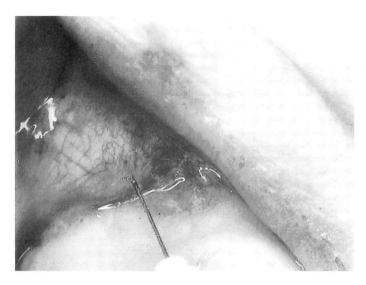

Fig. 22.4 After depositing about 0.5 ml of local anaesthetic solution some mucosal distension and blanching will be seen

---

Table 22.3 Problems with local analgesia

The occasional problems that may be encountered with local analgesia include

- **Fainting.** This is still an occasional problem with a small number of patients but may be reduced by using a confident, sympathetic approach. Placing the patient in a horizontal position also helps to reduce its incidence by preventing blood from pooling in the lower limbs and thus sustaining the cerebral blood flow. The action to take if a vasovagal syncope does occur is given in Chapter 16.
- **Hypersensitivity.** A very small number of patients will claim to be allergic to certain local anaesthetics. The results of patch-testing will reveal that very few are sensitive to one of the constituents of the cartridge but as alternative solutions are available, it is wise to try one of the alternatives if such a claim is made.
- **Facial vasoconstriction.** This may be seen occasionally and is thought to be caused by activation of the sympathetic nerves around the blood vessels in the area. It will resolve eventually, but may be alarming at the time as it may involve the vessels to the orbit, temporarily interfering with vision.
- **Needle-track infection.** Infection in the site of injection is extremely rare provided a careful technique is used. If it occurs then an antibiotic may need to be prescribed.
- **Haematoma** formation where a blood vessel has been traumatized during the injection.
- **Visual disturbance** due to an intravascular injection.
- **The needle** may break in the tissues.

Pain-relieving drugs

Probably the most commonly prescribed drugs are those for the relief of pain (analgesics).

Aspirin (acetylsalicylic acid)

This is the most frequently used pain reliever. In common with the other mild analgesics described in this section, it can be bought in any pharmacy without a prescription. The vast numbers of aspirin tablets consumed throughout the world are an indication of the remarkable safety of this drug. However, it is irritant to the stomach lining and can cause a mild degree of gastric bleeding. For this reason, aspirin is not normally prescribed to those suffering from gastric complaints or from bleeding disorders. It is also recommended that it should not be given to children under the age

---

Table 22.4 Contraindications

Contraindications to local analgesia include

- The presence of infection in the site of the injection will often prevent the achievement of an adequate depth of anaesthesia. There is also a risk of spreading the infection and it is always very painful to inject into an infected area.
- Great care should be taken with patients suffering from bleeding disorders such as haemophilia, Christmas disease or von Willebrand's disease as bleeding may occur internally or externally at the injection site. It would be preferable for the dental surgeon to administer the local anaesthetic after advice from the patient's consultant haematologist.
- Some patients may be hypersensitive to constituents of the anaesthetic and alternatives should be used. Advice from the dentist should be sought in such a case.

---

of 12 years because of the risk of inducing Reye's syndrome. Besides being analgesic, aspirin is also antipyretic, which means that it will tend to lower the temperature of those suffering from fever. A very large variety of proprietary brands of tablets and powders are sold and a common dosage would be two 300 mg tablets every 4–6 hours, although the dosage can be varied a great deal. Some patients take aspirin not for its pain relieving properties but to 'thin' the blood and this is on the recommendation of their medical practitioner. These people have usually had a mild stroke or heart attack and the aspirin will decrease the tendency for their platelets to clot.

Paracetamol

This is an analgesic that is steadily becoming more widely used. It is a less effective pain reliever than aspirin but has less side effects. However, one important disadvantage is that in overdose it can produce irreversible liver damage which can result in death and this property is causing increasing concern in medical circles. Many different proprietary brands can be bought, without prescription, and the usual dosage is two 500 mg tablets, taken every 4–6 hours.

Non-steroidal anti-inflammatory compounds

These have both analgesic and anti-inflammatory properties. Ibuprofen (Nurofen®, Brufen®) has recently been licensed for general sale in the UK. The main side-effects are gastrointestinal and they should not be given to patients with a history of peptic ulceration, asthma or to elderly people. A typical dosage for analgesic use would be 400 mg three times a day, preferably after food.

Codeine compound

These tablets usually contain codeine (10 mg) and aspirin (250 mg), but paracetamol is also sometimes a constituent. Codeine has more potent analgesic properties than aspirin, but is also more toxic. It has a tendency to cause constipation. No prescription is required for these tablets.

Moderate-strength analgesics

Analgesics in this group can only be bought with a prescription from a registered doctor or dentist. Although they are often used in certain branches of dentistry, it is unlikely that dental hygienists would ever have any reason to request a dentist to prescribe them for a patient under treatment. Examples of moderate-strength analgesics include dihydrocodeine tartrate (DF 118).

Strong analgesics

Obviously, there is little requirement in dental practice for strong analgesics and they are included here for the sake of completeness only. They include such drugs as pethidine and morphine.

Anti-microbial drugs

Antibiotics are chemical substances that were originally produced by bacteria which kill or prevent the growth of other species of bacteria.

Obviously, although they can be produced by bacteria, those used therapeutically are now produced by industrial chemical processes.

They are divided into two main groups, according to their mode of action: those which are bactericidal (i.e. they kill bacteria) and those which are bacteriostatic (i.e. they prevent the multiplication and growth of b...   :terio-

of an
fences

ics in
:h as
gingi-
rditis.
treat
:s can
:terial

iscov-
:neral
il and
ver.

h are

sen-
ipter
on in
nore
why
ent's

evel-

ance,
lutely
ole to
icipal
penicillin are

either orally, usually in tablet form for adults, and intramuscularly.

Many different forms of penicillin exist and it is not necessary for the dental hygienist to try to keep informed of all the developments which take place in this respect. Some types of penicillin are more relevant to dental hygienist practice than others but since penicillin can only be prescribed by the dentist, the hygienist need not know all the details.

For the treatment of dental infections, oral penicillin is normally used and 250 mg four times daily for 5 days is the common dosage. One of the commonest penicillins used for dental infections is phenoxymethyl penicillin (V). A popular broad spectrum penicillin called amoxycillin is frequently prescribed in dental practice nowadays because it is effective against a broader range of dental infections than phenoxymethyl penicillin. Amoxycillin in combination with metronidazole may be given to some patients who have severe dental infections. The usual dose of amoxycillin for oral infections is 250 mg three times a day for 5 days

When given to prevent infective endocarditis, penicillin must not be given too far in advance of the treatment since *Streptococcus viridans* is particularly capable of developing resistance. It must also be given in a dosage that will give a high enough level in the blood to kill off any bacteria. Various different regimens have been adopted to satisfy these requirements and the latest development in this field is the use of amoxycillin. This can produce a sufficiently high blood level if given orally in a high dose 1 hour before treatment. The prophylactic dosage of amoxycillin is one 3 g sachet taken orally 1 hour before treatment. Amoxycillin can be administered in this dosage twice in a period of a month for antibiotic cover purposes but no more, due to the danger of resistant organisms developing. In cases where the patient is penicillin sensitive or amoxycillin has already been used twice an alternative regime is necessary. This is provided by the antibiotic clindamycin which again is taken orally in a dose of 600 mg 1 hour before starting scaling.

Tetracycline

This has tended to be the antibiotic of second choice in the treatment of dental infections, as it is a bacteriostatic antibiotic and is not suitable for prophylactic cover. Tetracycline is currently recommended for use in the treatment of juvenile periodontitis usually as a three-week course. More details are given in Chapter 11.

The normal dosage of tetracycline for dental use is 250 mg taken orally four times daily, for 5 days. An unwanted side-effect of tetracycline is that it can cause marked staining of developing teeth, which can be very disfiguring once these teeth erupt. This intrinsic staining is of particular interest to dental hygienists as no amount of polishing can remove it!

Other antibiotics

There is now a very wide and complex range of antibiotics available, but since the dental hygienist does not prescribe such drugs, there seems little point in studying them in depth. When a patient requires antibiotic cover, for example, and is allergic to penicillin, it is the dentist's responsibility to choose a suitable bactericidal alternative. The hygienist can always refer to an appropriate textbook should any further information be required about any particular antibiotic.

Metronidazole

This is not an antibiotic, but its action is similar. It is marketed under the trade name Flagyl® and is the drug of first choice in the treatment of acute necrotizing gingivitis. This has already been discussed in Chapter 12. Metronidazole is administered orally: a 200 mg tablet is taken three times daily for 3 days. It can, in some patients, produce hypersensitivity but to a lesser degree than penicillin and has few unwanted side-effects. It may react adversely with alcohol and should be withheld from a patient who cannot abstain from alcohol. It is also recommended that it should be used with caution in pregnancy, especially during the first trimester.

Chlorhexidine

The use of chlorhexidine as an oral antibacterial agent is increasing dramatically. It has been shown to inhibit the development of dental plaque and the chemical control of plaque is useful where normal mechanical measures are interrupted for some reason. This subject has been discussed in other sections of this book. Chlorhexidine has been marketed as a gel., mouthrinse and oral spray and has been incorporated in toothpaste. In the UK, it is marketed as Corsodyl® (a 1% gel or 0.2% rinse) and Eludril® (a 0.05% rinse, an oral spray and a toothpaste). There are, however, some important disadvantages associated with chlorhexidine. It has an unpleasant taste and may have a prolonged after-effect on the patient's sense of taste. It may also cause heavy extrinsic staining of the teeth which can be difficult to remove. This staining seems to be related to dye elements in our diet and includes such things as coffee and tea drinking. Chlorhexidine definitely has a role in the initial treatment of oral conditions where plaque-induced inflammation is evident but its use instead of mechanical measures should not be recommended.

Agents used to control bleeding

Bleeding from the gingiva increases the difficulty of scaling probably more than any other factor. Controlling this bleeding and keeping it to a minimum is essential if careful fine scaling is to be carried out. Unfortunately, the hygienist can look for little pharmaceutical help with this problem and recognized haemostatic agents are of little value.

The problem of patients with clotting disorders or patients taking anticoagulants has been discussed in the first part of this chapter. The hygienist need only note the patient's medical history and seek appropriate help and guidance and ensure the minimum of trauma during scaling.

The commonest reason for bleeding during scaling is gingival inflammation. One of the earliest signs of chronic gingivitis is bleeding and the more severe the gingivitis, the more of a nuisance will be the bleeding. It has been mentioned that, when treating a new case of acute necrotizing ulcerative gingivitis, the degree of bleeding will prevent all but the gentlest of debridement. The hygienist learns to control gingival bleeding by seeing a patient for multiple visits and carrying out as much treatment at each visit as the vision allows. The tissue resolution that takes place between visits allows a gradually more thorough scaling to be carried out on subsequent visits.

Adrenaline can be used to help control bleeding which is proving to be particularly difficult. It can be applied topically with a cotton wool pledget as a solution of 1:1000. However, the efficacy of adrenaline used topically in this way is questionable. A much more effective use would be as an infiltration injection, using the 1:80 000 adrenaline solution found in many local anaesthetics. In particular, when carrying out deep scaling and root planing of severely periodontally involved teeth, the dental hygienist will find it very beneficial to infiltrate the surrounding tissues with an adrenaline-containing anaesthetic. In such cases, attention must be paid to the medical history, since the taking of certain antidepressant drugs or existing heart disease may contraindicate the giving of adrenaline.

Some patients with haemorrhagic gingiva will benefit from the application of a pressure dressing. A stiff dressing of zinc oxide and eugenol or zinc oxide and Coe Pak® is inserted into the pocket and left in place for 5–7 days. This will usually allow resolution of some of the inflammation and permit fine scaling.

- First choice antibiotic for prophylaxis is amoxycillin 3 g orally 1 hour before scaling. This can be given twice in 1 month to people who are not penicillin sensitive and have not had it for another reason.
- The alternative antibiotic for prophylaxis purposes is clindamycin 600 mg orally 1 hour before treatment.
- Tetracycline is recommended for use in cases of juvenile periodontitis given over a 3 week period.
- Chlorhexidine gluconate has an important role in controlling plaque-induced inflammation, but only for 3 weeks at a time.
- Control of bleeding can be achieved by local means such as pressure or adrenaline can be applied topically or by administering more local anaesthetic solution.

Further reading

Cannell H. (1997) Evidence for safety margins of lignocaine local anaesthetics for perioral use. *British Dental Journal*, **181**, 243–249.

Roberts D. H., Sowray J. H. (1987) *Local Anaesthesia in Dentistry*. 3rd edition. Bristol: Wright.

23

Oral health education

The background to oral health education

The term Dental Health Education (DHE) has been gradually superseded in recent years by Oral Health Education (OHE), reflecting a wider concern than health only of the teeth. For example, the oral health educator could have a role to play in the prevention of oral cancers.

By any standards, the results of several decades of oral health education are disappointing (Table 23.1). The very considerable resources which in the past have been devoted to promoting improved oral hygiene and better dietary habits might not stand up to modern audit procedures in relation to value for money. Of course, there have been improvements in this area, but these are often associated with factors other than OHE. For example, the reduction in caries levels has much to do with the widespread use of fluoridated toothpastes promoted by the manufacturers' advertising and the increasing switch to the consumption of sugar-free drinks owes more to weight-watching than to dental health awareness.

Much attention has been given in recent years to getting the messages of dental and oral health correct. In this respect, the dental hygienist is directed particularly to two pub-

---

Table 23.1 Problems with oral health education

Previous inadequacies in OHE delivery have been attributed to two main faults

- The message which has been contained within the dental health advice has not always been correct and has at times been totally misleading. For example, the suggestion that raw carrots are good for the teeth has been hallowed by long usage, despite the evidence that they do not remove plaque from the teeth in any significant way. There has also been the inordinate attention given to particular brushing techniques rather than concentrating on a methodical, efficient approach to plaque removal. These and other points have been dealt with in previous sections of this book.
- Oral health education has, in the past, frequently been given by untrained personnel: that is, by those untrained in educational techniques. Such people are likely to make so many basic teaching errors that the message will be lost. The untrained may fail to see the need for adequate preparation and may not fully appreciate the value of, for example, correctly used visual aids. Those with an amateurish attitude towards education are often blind to the many pitfalls involved in trying to teach others. An example of this is in the handling of a patient who presents with inadequate plaque control, despite two or three previous oral hygiene phase visits. Such a patient is unlikely to require further brushing or flossing instruction: what is really required is motivation.

lications: 'The Scientific Basis of Dental Health Education' and 'Notes on Oral Health'. These provide an up-to-date review of OHE messages and are designed to standardize the advice given to the public and to ensure that such advice is scientifically sound. Other chapters of this book deal with aspects of the message of OHE, but this chapter is designed to deal with the delivery of that message.

In the past, the need for training in teaching has not always been appreciated by dentists and others in the dental field However, the profession is gradually improving in this respect and more attention is being given to the provision of training courses for potential oral health educators. A person with a good knowledge of a subject does not necessarily make a good teacher. A number of other qualities are required, some of which are inborn, but most of which must be learned with training and experience. No longer are dental hygienists the only members of the dental team to receive training in teaching. This forms part of the undergraduate curriculum for dentists and post-qualification OHE courses are available to dental nurses.

Domains of learning

In OHE, it is only too easy to concentrate on theoretical and practical training at the expense of the motivation aspects (Table 23.2). There is no point in repeatedly telling people why and how they should clean their teeth if they are never persuaded to actually do so!

Table 23.2 Domains of learning

In education it is accepted that there are three domains of learning

- **Cognitive domain**: this relates to the acquisition of knowledge.
- **Skills domain**: this is the learning of practical skills.
- **Affective domain**: this involves the creation of attitudes and motivation.

Behavioural change

The prevention and control of the two major dental diseases, inflammatory periodontal dis-

ease and dental caries, depend to a large extent on a change in the behaviour of the patient.

Table 22.3 Changing behaviour

The following are the steps which must be followed to establish behavioural changes

- Factual education.
- Practical demonstration.
- Motivation.
- Reinforcement.

Each of the steps listed in Table 23.3 plays a part in determining people's behaviour. One individual may be highly motivated towards preserving his or her dentition but may lack the knowledge of what is required. Another may possess both the motivation and knowledge but may lack the effective skills for brushing or interdental cleansing. However, the commonest situation is that people have both the knowledge and the practical ability to clean the teeth, but lack the will to allocate the time and effort needed to do so. In the long run, everyone requires periodic reinforcement and encouragement to continue with a newly acquired pattern of behaviour.

Factual education

Information is a necessary, but not on its own sufficient, condition for changing behaviour. The information supplied should be accurate and comprehensible to lay-people. Part of this information should include realistic goals that the patient can achieve. For example, with some patients it would be preferable to concentrate solely on the improvements achievable by brushing before progressing to interdental cleansing.

The amount of education should be appropriate to the patient. There may be a problem of retaining the advice or skill, with some patients less able to remember information. It must not be assumed that there is a standard 'education package' that can be applied to all patients without considering their age, gender, race, cultural and socioeconomic background.

Practical training

The teaching of the physical skills involved in

dental health includes disclosing, brushing, interdental cleansing and the cleaning of dentures and appliances. As a general rule the educator should use a 'tell-show-do' approach. The action should first be explained, then demonstrated to the patient, possibly at first on models, then in the mouth. Finally, the patient should carry out the procedure with the instructor supervising, correcting and giving encouragement. Care should be taken not to overload the patient. As with teaching theory, it is better to teach a little at a time.

Motivation

The Oxford dictionary defines motivation as 'that which induces a person to act'. In the field of dentistry, the phrase 'patient motivation' is often misused, implying that one can cause a third person to co-operate, comply or perform in some desired manner. This would be a very useful ability, but, unfortunately, it is simply not possible. Motivation must come from within an individual (Table 23.4).

Table 23.4 The essentials for motivation

In order to become motivated to alter a behavioural pattern an individual must be able to identify the following

- A problem exists which affects the individual personally; for example the existence of periodontal disease in the mouth.
- The problem will have an unwanted personal outcome; such as the premature loss of teeth.
- There is a practical solution; such as adequate plaque control.
- The problem is serious enough to justify the inconvenience of the solution.

In relation to dental health education, as with all other areas of education, people may be divided into three broad groups:

- those who are already motivated,
- those with latent motivation,
- those lacking the necessary motivation to change their behaviour.

The motivated have their own drive and simply require guidance and reinforcement from time to time. Latent motivation is possessed by a majority of patients. This is indicated by studies which show that approximately 60% of patients attend a dentist at least every second year, usually for a preventive check-up. This latent motivation requires a trigger to activate or release it.

Patients without the desired motivation are an intractable problem. Various forms of threat, sanction or coercion may produce an improved short-term behavioural change, but no long-term alteration. However, even these patients may not be lost for ever, as research suggests that the priority of motives may change with time and circumstances, even in adults, and this will give rise to behavioural changes.

There are a number of ways in which the dental health educator may awaken motivation in patients. Interest and enthusiasm on the part of the educator are known to increase the likelihood of achieving motivation; belief in one's product is a basic rule for any sales person. Showing the relevance of an activity to the patient's dental health, before beginning the instruction, will increase the level of motivation. Allowing patients to participate in their treatment has also been shown to increase motivation.

Fear has been used as a motivator, but studies have shown results so achieved to be generally poor. A low level of anxiety has, however, been shown to increase motivation, but it would appear that once the situation becomes too threatening the patient will tend to 'switch off' and reject the information. A further danger is that the threatened patient will reject not only the threatening information but also the educator, as the originator of the anxiety-arousing situation.

The ultimate motivator is the patient's own disease. It acts primarily as the trigger to preventive action, and its control will induce a sense of achievement which increases motivation. A hand mirror and the patient's own mouth are amongst the most useful tools of the dental health educator. Patients are thereby able to recognize that they can control their own disease and this, coupled with appropriate praise from the educator, increases motivation greatly.

Reinforcement

There is ample evidence that without frequent encouragement, correction and assistance many patients will be unable to continue with their new standards of oral home care. In terms of the control of inflammatory periodontal disease this is paralleled by the need for frequent professional prophylaxis and, if necessary, root planing. Once the progression of the disease has been controlled, then most patients require a regular (possibly three monthly) maintenance programme of visits. This can be coupled with reinforcement of the oral hygiene regimen.

The frequency of reinforcement will vary from person to person and will depend to a large extent on their attitudes and the type of problem present.

Domains of learning

- **Cognitive domain**: theoretical knowledge.
- **Skills domain**: practical ability.
- **Affective domain**: attitudes and motivation.
- **Behavioural change**: the role of
  theoretical teaching
  practical training
  motivation
  reinforcement.

Table 23.5 Session planning

Any teaching session must be carefully planned, going through these stages

- Obtain background information.
- Choose aims and objectives.
- Select appropriate teaching method.
- Prepare effective visual aids.
- Plan evaluation.
- Rehearse sufficiently.
- Deliver effectively.

The organization of teaching sessions

No successful teaching session can take place without careful organization and management and the commonest mistake made by the amateur is underestimating this. Time is a valuable commodity and there can be no excuse for wasting the time of those receiving instruction. When invited to give a dental health education session, there are certain basic steps to be taken in the preparation. Following them will help to avoid the embarrassment and unprofessionalism of having to apologize for inadequate visual aids, poor time keeping, etc. (Table 23.5).

Background information

It is important to find out various details in relation to the location, the group to be taught and the time allocated.

The location

It is senseless to arrive at the location with a slide projector and 35 mm slides only to find that there is no screen, or no black-out, or that the electricity supply is inadequate. If at all possible, the location should be visited in advance to check the various items, such as those listed below.

Seating
Is there sufficient seating for the numbers expected to attend? Can it be arranged in a formal or informal manner, depending on what is required? Will everyone be able to see the visual aids?

Electricity
Is there a suitable power point within reach of any apparatus to be used? If not, an extension cable will be required. Does the socket match the plug on any projector being taken?

Visual aids
What aids are available at the location: whiteboard, overhead projector, etc.?

Windows
Where are they situated? It is undesirable to have the teacher standing in front of a window with the students looking towards it. Is there any black-out? Can the windows be opened for ventilation?

Any other features
Obviously it is impossible to list every detail which may influence the lesson preparation, but items such as sinks are important if disclosing agents are to be used or toothbrushing taught and there might be a need to ensure wheelchair access.

The group

The content and format of a lesson will be influenced by the group to be taught in a number of ways, including the following.

Age

The design and content of the visual aids will depend on the age of the group, both in relation to what might motivate them and their reading age. The topics covered by the lesson will also vary with age of the group. Caries is likely to be more relevant to children, whereas periodontal disease tends to be more relevant to older groups. Since young children can concentrate for a much shorter time than adults the age of the group will also influence the amount of content in the lesson.

Ability

Obviously, a teaching session must take into account the ability and knowledge of the group. This is particularly important when dealing with those with handicaps. In this respect, any previous instruction which they may have had will need to be considered.

Number

The size of the group affects the teaching method selected and the content of the lesson. For example, it is impossible to teach a practical skill such as toothbrushing to a large group. A large group may also be harder to control.

Curriculum needs

Why has the dental health education been requested? Is it part of an overall health education programme? It is obvious that a lesson aimed at pregnant women would be quite unsuited to a group of army recruits!

Time

It takes experience and training to estimate accurately how much can be put into a given period of teaching, but even the experienced must rehearse the session or sessions to ensure that the allocated time is being fully used, but not overextended. If more than one session has been allotted, the content of each must be decided from the outset. When the teaching session forms part of an overall programme of lectures or is part of a school timetable, there is no room for extension beyond the allocated time.

Aims and objectives

An aim is defined as being a general statement of what the teacher intends to teach. Although it is a general statement, it should not be vague. Aims are essentially teacher-orientated; that is, they are what the teacher wishes to do. Although this may seem somewhat theoretical, it would be wrong and foolish to underestimate the importance of deciding on very clear appropriate aims, based on the information already acquired.

An example of aims chosen for a forty five minute lesson to be given to a small group of 10-year-old children might be:

- to teach the basic cause of tooth decay,
- to demonstrate and practise efficient toothbrushing,
- to give examples of sensible and damaging foodstuffs.

The aims selected for another group or for a different period of time would quite naturally be different.

Objectives are much more detailed than the aims and should be a full and precise statement of what is hoped to be achieved in the group being taught. They should relate to the three domains of education discussed above and include:

- the theory they will have learned,
- the practical skills they will have acquired,
- the attitudes they will have developed.

Once again, it would be quite wrong to dismiss these ideas as being of only theoretical importance. They have important practical implications and it is the failure to recognize these three distinct domains of learning that leads to so much waste of opportunity in dental health education. The person who sees no practical significance in this information is likely to be the one who fails to see the deficiencies in his or her teaching. As has been pointed out before, it is important to judge whether a patient needs more teaching about plaque, or further demonstrations of brushing, or encouragement to become more motivated to following the instructions given. The careful planning of detailed objectives will ensure that the correct message is being given to the group and that the correct quantity of information has been included in each session.

Teaching methods

There is no single teaching method which is best suited to all situations. The dental hygienist should be aware of the wide range of teaching methods available and be prepared to select that method of delivery which best suits the lesson content, the location, the group and the time allocated. There is no excuse for becoming stereotyped in this respect.

Lectures

The lecture is the most formal teaching method of all, with the minimum participation by the group being instructed. Lectures are of value in presenting a good deal of information to a large number of people in a short time, but the lack of participation by those being taught may cause them to lose interest and allow their concentration to wander. Also there is limited feedback from the group to the lecturer, which makes it difficult to judge whether or not the content of the lecture has been correctly pitched. Whereas a formal lecture may be appropriate as part of a large conference, it has obvious drawbacks in relation to a small group of young children.

Tutorials or seminars

These are less formal teaching situations and are probably the most popular methods used by dental hygienists. The temptation must be avoided, however, to use this format on all occasions. A tutorial or seminar is suited to smaller numbers than a lecture and the degree of informality means that the students feel relatively free to ask questions to clarify any points raised. However, the informality does not imply that there is less need for preparation. Quite the reverse. If questions are to be fielded, the hygienist must know the subject all the more thoroughly and, despite interruptions, she must be able to follow the original lesson plan and keep to the planned time schedule. Obviously, time must be allowed when planning the lesson for such interruptions.

Discussion

A discussion is a teaching method centred more on the group than on the teacher, but it cannot achieve its aims if it is allowed to run completely free. Judicious chairmanship by the person responsible for the instruction is required. How strict the chairmanship must be will vary with the situation.

Discussions are particularly useful for modifying attitudes, rather than teaching facts, and a possible dental topic for a discussion group might be the desirability of adding fluoride to drinking water. This example clearly illustrates the need for the person chairing the discussion to be thoroughly versed in the topic. If an argument was put forward against fluoride which went unanswered and undefended, the discussion would have the opposite effect from that desired. That is, the group might become convinced that water fluoridation was undesirable.

Demonstrations

Demonstrations are used to teach practical aspects of a subject. The dental hygienist is heavily involved in teaching the practical aspects of preventing dental disease to both individuals and groups, but there is a limit to the size of a group for which practical demonstrations are suitable. Ideally, such teaching should be restricted to individuals or very small groups. It is important to ensure that everyone in the group can see and that any models or other equipment being used are large enough to be visible to all. Furthermore, the instruction should, wherever possible, be related to the individuals in the group: their dental problems, manual dexterity, motivation, etc. Ideally a toothbrushing demonstration should be followed by the individuals brushing their own teeth, with any faults being corrected. It is impossible to learn to drive a car solely using a simulated dashboard; the only effective way to teach someone to drive is to take the learner out on the road in a car. Similarly, efficient plaque control cannot be taught solely with models of the teeth.

Role-playing

This is a very informal teaching method particularly suited to young children, who tend to be less inhibited in this respect than older children or adults. It might, for example, be used by the dental hygienist to overcome fear of the dental surgery and to change the attitude of children to dentistry. Either in a real surgery or in a simulated surgery, the children could play the part of the dentist, hygienist, dental nurse, receptionist, patient and parent. Role-playing must be well controlled by the educator if its full benefit is to be gained. It is better suited to creating changes of attitude than to factual teaching, although the opportunities which present themselves to include factual information (such as the basic shape and complexity of the dentition) should not be missed.

Project work

This is another informal teaching method which is centred largely on the group being taught and needs careful direction by the teacher. Groups of adolescents and children will often find this type of work stimulating and, in the process of discovering facts for themselves, they may be encouraged to formulate favourable ideas and attitudes towards a wide range of dental topics. Projects related to the teeth can often be run in conjunction with school-teachers as part of a term's work for a class.

Table 23.6 Visual aids

Visual aids have the following advantages

- They make it easier for those being taught to understand and remember certain points.
- They make a lesson more interesting and aid the concentration of those being taught.
- They can illustrate things which cannot readily be described in words; e.g. the appearance of healthy and inflamed gingivae.

With practice it should become apparent to the student that each of these teaching methods has its place. Some are better suited to larger or smaller groups and others to older or younger groups. The most important aspect to remember is that they vary in their suitability for achieving the three types of objectives which might have been set. Lectures are well suited to conveying factual information, but are not

suited to teaching practical skills or to motivating people. Practical skills can only be taught by demonstration and repetition on a one-to-one basis or in a very small group. The changing of attitudes might be more effectively achieved by discussion or role-playing.

Teaching methods

- **Lectures**: formal, little feedback, minimal participation, but suited to large groups and a good deal of information.
- **Tutorials/seminars**: less formal, better feedback and participation, more suited to smaller groups, but requiring careful preparation.
- **Discussions**: informal and particularly useful for changing attitudes, but require careful preparation and chairmanship.
- **Demonstrations**: important for teaching practical skills, but suited to small groups or individuals only.
- **Role playing**: ideal for children, very informal, useful for influencing attitudes, but requires careful preparation and management to be of value.
- **Projects**: useful for encouraging self-learning and developing interests, fit in well with school curriculum, but need careful planning management to be of value.

Visual aids

We learn by using all our senses: sight, hearing, smell, taste and touch; not by hearing alone. In fact, it is often the case that in learning one of the other senses is more important than hearing. It is easier to appreciate the difference between an apple and an orange by touching the two, than by listening to a description and a combination of touch, sight, hearing and taste and smell will make the difference clearer still. In other words, a combination of senses should be used whenever possible and this is the reason for using visual aids (Table 23.6).

However, visual aids must always be a *help* to teaching and must not be allowed to become a *distraction*. They must be chosen so that they are appropriate to the group being taught, the location of the lesson and the objectives chosen (Table 23.7).

Table 23.7 Selection of visual aids

When selecting a visual aid the following points should be considered

- Is it simple?.
- Is it interesting?.
- Is it relevant?.
- Does it help?.
- Is it in the most suitable form?

It is important that the use of visual aids should be well rehearsed to avoid the distraction and embarrassment of the aid being upside down or in the wrong order, etc. (Fig. 23.1). The visual aid should not be displayed until the relevant time. It should then be checked to ensure that everyone can see it and be fully explained, taking sufficient time for everyone to assimilate its message. It should then be removed to avoid it becoming a distraction (Fig. 23.2).

Black/whiteboard

A blackboard with chalk is the most traditional of all teaching aids. It has the advantage of being cheap to use, adaptable and requires no preparation before the lesson. Unfortunately, the inexperienced have difficulty in writing and drawing well enough in front of a class and they ought to prepare their aids beforehand. Diagrams drawn on a blackboard cannot be kept for future sessions and, in some situations, having to write with one's back to the class may cause disciplinary problems. Of course, black/whiteboards are not always available and are not easily transportable. There are some locations where the use of chalk is contraindicated by the dust it produces (e.g. in a dental surgery), but a whiteboard with felt pens may be well suited to such locations. Such boards have the advantage that any unexpected points which arise in discussion can be explained and illustrated.

Overhead projector

Overhead projectors are popular in situations such as colleges. They are designed to project the contents of a transparent sheet, called a viewfoil, which is placed on the flat surface of the projector, on to a large screen. Viewfoils can be produced by writing or drawing on them with suitable felt-tipped pens of various colours, or by using most photocopiers to reproduce existing documents or diagrams. As noted below, they can also be produced by computer. They can be prepared before the lesson or can be written on while the instruction is being given, with the advantages that even the inexperienced can write legibly with felt pens using letters only slightly larger than normal and the teacher can face the class whilst writing. Unlike 35 mm projectors, the overhead projector does not require the room to be blacked out.

By adding one transparency to another, more complicated diagrams, tables or lists can gradually be built up as the lesson progresses. The outline of objects such as toothbrushes of various designs can be projected by laying them on the surface of the projector.

Although most overhead projectors are large and heavy and are designed to remain *in situ,* smaller, more portable types are available, although somewhat expensive. A disadvantage of the overhead projector is that a degree of funding is required for the purchase of viewfoils, pens, etc. which are required to go with them.

35 mm slides

The value of coloured slides to the dental hygienist who is describing periodontal disease or plaque is obvious and it would be to any hygienist's advantage to build up a collection of slides on dental diseases, oral hygiene, preventive dentistry and other similar topics. Unfortunately, this is an expensive and sometimes difficult task.

A disadvantage of slides is that their use requires a projector, which may have to be taken to the location, and a darkened room and black-out is not always available. Furthermore a darkened room may require the hygienist to control discipline more carefully in certain groups!

Computerized programmes

Computer programmes, such as Microsoft PowerPoint, can be used to produce effective,

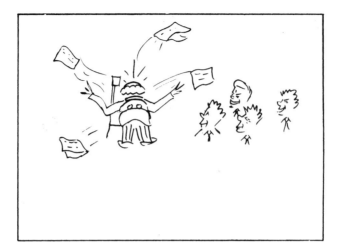

Fig. 23.1 Visual aids should be well rehearsed.

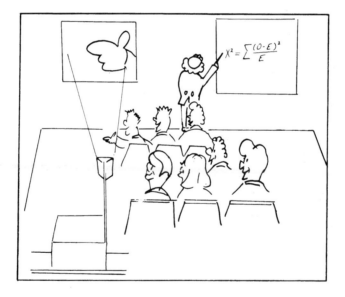

Fig. 23.2 Visual aids should not become a distraction.

colourful and professional looking viewfoils for the overhead projector. Furthermore an entire presentation can be built up and delivered using this system which, provided the equipment is available, can greatly improve the professionalism and quality of the presentation. 35 mm slides can be added into the presentation and it is an added advantage that it might only be necessary to carry a floppy disc to the session. Unfortunately the equipment needed is not yet widely available.

Videos

Sometimes suitable videos can be obtained for showing to different types of groups, but the use of videos alone should be avoided. The personal contact of the hygienist with the group can achieve many things which a video cannot. At the very least, the video should be introduced by the hygienist and then followed up in some way afterwards.

The dental hygienist should realize from the

outset that not all dental videos are well made. They are expensive to produce and it is difficult to find one that conveys the correct message and aimed at the correct group. Too often one hears apologies for the use of a video which is either out of date or directed at the wrong audience. This is totally unacceptable.

Models

Every hygienist should have, as part of the teaching armamentarium, models of the upper and lower dental arches, which can be used for explaining the structure of the dentition and the ways of caring for it. Full upper and lower dentures can serve the purpose when dealing with individuals, especially if a friendly dental technician can be persuaded to mount them on acrylic bases, but it has to be remembered that few patients have a complete dentition, regularly arranged. Such dentures often fail to reflect the true problems of plaque control and it may be better to acquire models with such common abnormalities as imbricated lower incisors or mesially inclined lower molars.

Posters

Posters are visual aids that are not really designed to enhance a teaching session, but to convey a simple message to a person in a place such as a waiting room. They might be used to lend atmosphere in a room where dental health education is to be given, but care should be taken to make certain that they are not simply a distraction.

Posters can be obtained from a variety of bodies concerned with dental health: such as the British Dental Health Foundation, or numerous commercial firms. Unfortunately, it is often difficult to find a poster that conveys the exact message needed for the intended type of person who will view the poster. There is little to be gained from putting up totally irrelevant posters on to a wall simply as a form of decoration, and too often no thought is given to the message presented in the waiting area. Many commercially produced posters are designed to advertise a product and may even contain messages which are not strictly accurate. With a little effort and imagination,

posters can be self-made, but the difficulties of producing an effective poster should not be underestimated. They should be eye-catching and have a simple, relevant message presented in a striking way. They should also be replaced at regular intervals to prevent them from becoming untidy and simply part of the wall-paper.

Flash cards

These are hand-held cards containing pictures and information which are ideally suited to teaching small groups up to four or five in number. For such groups the overhead projector or 35 mm slides might seem over-formal. Flash cards can be simply produced by the hygienist and with a little care and attention can be made to look very professional. They are easily carried and can be stored for future use.

Hand-outs

Hand-outs are duplicated notes given to the group to reinforce or expand on any particular points. They are usually given out at the end of the lesson because if they are given out sooner, they may distract the group's attention from the lesson. They may take the form of a summary of the whole lesson or they may merely illustrate a certain point of the teaching. It is often necessary to distribute a hand-out which gives important factual information which would not easily be remembered, and to which members of the group might want to refer at a later date. An example of this might be the various dosages of fluoride supplements to be given to young children.

Hand-outs can be used to involve the group, especially if they are children. For example, blank spaces could be left which have to be filled in during the lesson. However, there is a very real possibility that any hand-out given to a group may simply be thrown away straight after the lesson. Think of all the glossy leaflets picked up at dental exhibitions which are never read! It might be useful to devise a scheme whereby they must be brought back to a subsequent lesson (e.g. with a painting done by the child).

Visual aids

The value of visual aids: improve understanding, add interest, illustrate things which it is difficult to describe.

- **Criteria for selection**: simple, interesting, relevant, helpful and in a suitable form.
- **Blackboard/whiteboard**: cheap, often available, useful for impromptu illustrations, but cannot be prepared in advance, nor stored for future use.
- **Overhead projector**: adaptable, relatively cheap and simple to use, easy storage of transparencies and no blackout required.
- **35 mm slides**: well suited for use during a lecture and for illustrating clinical conditions, but require blackout, can be expensive and are less appropriate in informal situations.
- **Computerized programmes**: produce professional, imaginative and high quality visuals, provided the equipment is available.
- **Videos**: usually commercially produced and may not always be entirely relevant to or suitable for the group being taught. Because of their cost, may not be replaced when becoming dated.
- **Models**: useful for practical teaching sessions, but must be of suitable size for and relevance to the teaching situation.
- **Posters**: may be either commercially or personally produced. Best suited for locations such as waiting room walls. If commercially produced, may not always be relevant, accurate and up to date. If personally produced, may tend to appear amateurish.
- **Flash cards**: cheap and easily produced, easy to store and carry, but not suited for larger groups.
- **Hand-outs**: used to reinforce or expand on the lesson content, but should not be allowed to be a distraction and may well be discarded unread after the session.

Rehearsal

Having prepared a health education session, the next stage is to practise it. Initially this can be done in a quiet room away from any audience. If the session involves facing an audience, concentrate on the timing and talking, not reading from the notes. Note and change any areas where the talk does not flow logically into the next area. Once you are reasonably happy, grasp the nettle and ask a colleague, friend or relative to listen to and comment on the performance. Repeat the practices on a regular basis up to the time of the lesson to help you remember the main points.

Delivery

Most people find talking in public stressful and may, until they gain experience, suffer agonies of nerves and crises of confidence. The important thing to remember is that this reaction is a normal and necessary one to a situation where we must be on our toes. The release of adrenaline into the blood stream, which causes the feelings of apprehension, also provides the speaker with extra energy and more rapid reactions to the situation. It prevents us from becoming stale and boring and this communicates itself to the audience. Confidence will grow with a combination of careful preparation, knowledge of the subject and experience.

In practice, although the preparation may be very precise and thorough, the lesson inevitably will not flow exactly as planned; ideas, inspirations and interruptions will result in modifications being made. These diversions will often add interest to the lesson, but should not be allowed to distract the teacher from the planned objectives. It is a matter of getting the correct balance between the two (Table 23.8).

Many inexperienced speakers worry unduly about the style of their delivery. Although this does matter, variations in style, dialect and mannerisms make a lesson interesting. It is important to pay attention to personal appearance as this not only creates an immediate impact, but may also be a source of additional self-confidence. It is important to feel good in order to be good.

Evaluation

Having completed these basic preparations, it is sensible to consider how the value and degree of success of the lesson might be judged. A true

Table 23.8 Improving lessons

A lesson can be improved and problems avoided by giving attention to the following points

- Position yourself where you can be seen by and can see the whole group.
- Look at the audience; avoiding the temptation to stare at the visual aids.
- Spread your attention throughout the whole group, avoiding focusing too much on any one individual.
- Address comments or even questions to various individuals where appropriate.
- Attempt to 'be yourself'; being natural in your delivery will add interest.
- Speak clearly and at a reasonable pace which should be varied from time to time.
- Use a variety of tone and pitch in your voice.
- Use a range of gestures and facial expression to emphasize your points.
- Use relevant humour to lighten your talk. There can be few situations which would not benefit from an appropriate amusing story.
- Stop before the audience gets restless!

professional appreciates the importance of auditing all aspects of our working life. A novice might make the mistake of assuming that everything which is taught will be assimilated in its entirety by those on the receiving end of the instruction, but this is obviously not so. It is important to evaluate any teaching programme and, on the basis of the information gleaned, to make any modifications necessary.

Evaluation of dental health education might take a variety of forms. One method might be simply to ask questions of the group either during or after the teaching session. The answers to such questions, especially those during the lesson, can be used to make on-the-spot adjustments to the content and delivery, where this had been misjudged during preparation. A more formal method might be to construct a written questionnaire, using objective questions, to test the knowledge of the group. Obviously, such a questionnaire given to the group before and again after the instruction will give an indication of the knowledge acquired during the session or sessions. However, the difficulty of composing a relevant, unambiguous questionnaire should not be underestimated, and the inexperienced would be wise to seek the help and guidance of experienced educators if such a questionnaire is to have maximum value.

Another method of evaluating the teaching might be to assess the plaque control before and after the instruction and to note the (hoped-for) improvement. Naturally, this would only be relevant if plaque control had been included in the teaching, but this is a method of testing not only the factual knowledge gained by the students, but also their motivation. It is important to realize that such information would only be of real value if the plaque control is assessed using a reliable index of plaque levels and not mere subjective impressions. It would be of even greater value if recorded by a person other than the instructor.

Where an OHE session is delivered in a school setting, it might be valuable to invite the class teacher to provide a constructive appraisal of the lesson. However, to be of any value, it must be made clear that both negative and positive comments are invited and the request must be phrased in a way which will encourage the person doing the assessing to be honest. Whatever methods are used, evaluation is essential. It is not sufficient to simply go by an overall personal 'feeling' about the session.

- **Rehearsal of session**: careful rehearsal, using visual aids is essential.
- **Delivery**: careful attention to details such as voice, gestures, dress, eye contact, questions, variety, humour and duration.
- **Evaluation**: importance and methods, including questionnaires and independent assessment.

Sources of visual aids

A very comprehensive list of visual aids, leaflets and useful addresses has been published under the title: *Catalogue of Dental Health Resources for England, Wales and Northern Ireland* by A. S. Blinkhorn, P. J. Holloway and Y. M. Wainwright-Stringer. The hygienist should also be aware of the various dental manufacturing companies which will provide samples and literature concerning their products.

Further reading

Blinkhorn A. S., Holloway P. J., Wainwright-Stringer Y. M. (1996*) Catalogue of Dental Health Resources for England, Wales and Northern Ireland.* (2nd edition) Lancashire: Eden Bianchi Press.

Blinkhorn A. S., Kay E. J. (editors) (1996) *Notes on oral Health.* (4th edition) Lancashire: Eden Bianchi Press.

Levine R. S. (editor) (1996) *Scientific Basis of Dental Health Education.* (4th edition). London: Health Education Authority.

Schou L., Blinkhorn A. S. (editors) (1993) *Oral Health Promotion.* Oxford University Press.

Index

References in *italics* indicate figures, references in **bold** type indicate tables; there may also be textual references on these pages

Abrasion, *169*
Acidogenic hypothesis of dental caries, 124
Acids, and dental caries, 125
Acidulated phosphate fluoride, *233*–4
Acquired immunity, 101, **102**
Actinobacillus actinomycetemcomitans, 142
Actinomyces naeslundii, **113**
Actinomyces viscosus, **113**
Acute necrotizing ulcerative gingivitis (ANUG) *see* Gingivitis
Adipose tissue, 17–18
Adrenal glands, 36
Age:
　and dental caries, 155–6
　and periodontal disease, 154–5
Air scalers, 206, **207**
Airway, **27**
Aldehyde compounds, 94
Alimentary canal, 30, *31*–3
　large intestine, 32
　oral cavity, 30–1
　pharynx and oesophagus, 31
　small intestine, *32*
　stomach, 31, **32**
Alveolar bone, 80–1
Alveolar crest, 80
Alveolar ridges, *48*–9
Amelodentinal junction, 73
Amelogenesis, 69, *70*
Amine fluoride dentifrice, 224
Analgesia:
　local, 252
　　contraindications, 256, **258**
　　drugs, **254**
　　equipment, 254
　　injection techniques, 254, *255, 256*
　　unwanted effects, 256, **257**
　pre-injection topical, 253–4
　training, 5
　see also Analgesics
Analgesics, 257–8
　aspirin, 257–8
　codeine compound, 258
　moderate-strength, 258
　non-steroidal anti-inflammatory compounds, 258
　paracetamol, 258
　strong, 258
Anatomy, 38–58
　lymphatic drainage, *57*–8
　muscles of facial expression, 52–3
　muscles of mastication, **51, 52**
　oral cavity, 44–50
　　alveolar ridges and gingiva, *48*–9
　　blood supply, *55*, 56–7
　　cheeks, 45
　　floor of mouth, **45**

　　lips, 44–5
　　nerve supply, 53, *54*, **55**–6
　　palate, 49–50
　　tongue, *46*, **47**–8
　osteology, 38–44
　　cranium, 38–9, **40**
　　facial skeleton, 40, **41**
　　mandible, *42*–3
　　maxilla, *41*–2
　　skull, **38, 39**
　　temporomandibular joint, 43, **44**
　salivary glands, *50*–1
Anodontia, 170
Antibodies, 103
Antimicrobials, 258–60
　chlorhexidine, 260
　inflammatory periodontal disease, 146–9
　　mouthrinses, 146–7
　　pulsed oral irrigation, 148
　　subgingival, 147–8
　　subgingival antimicrobials, 148–9
　metronidazole, 260
　penicillin, **259**
　tetracycline, 259–60
　see also Disinfectants
Aphthous ulcers, **159**
Areolar tissue, *17*
Arteries, **23**, *55*, 56–7
　facial, 56
　inferior alveolar, 56–7
　lingual, 56
　maxillary, 56
　palatine, 57
　superior alveolar, 57
Articular capsule, 43
Aspirin, 257–8
Attrition, 168, *169*
Autoimmunity, 104–5
Autonomic nervous system, 34, **35**

Bacteria, **90**, *91*
　and dental caries, 124–5
Basic periodontal examination, 152, *153*–4
Behavioural science, 7
Bitewing films, *241*–2
Bleeding, control of, 260–1
Bleeding disorders, 164–5
Bleeding gums, 132
Bleeding index, 152
Blood, **24, 25, 26**
　clotting, 26, *27*
　plasma, **24, 25**
　platelets, 25
　red cells, *25*
　white cells, *25*, **26**

Blood vessels, 22, **23**
Bone, 18, *19*
Bone cells, 80
Borrelia vincenti, 136
Bridgework, *190, 191*
British Dental Hygienists' Association, **10**
Brushing *see* Toothbrushing
Bruxism, 168, *169*
Bullous conditions, 160

Calculus, 113, **115**–17
  attachment, 116–17
  composition, **115**
  formation, **115**, *116*, **117**
  significance, 117
Calculus index, 150
Cancer, *161*
Canines:
  lower, *63*
  permanent, *63*
  upper, *63*
Capillaries, 23
Carbohydrates, 30
Carcinogens, 110
Cardiac arrest, **179**–80
Cardiopulmonary resuscitation, **179**–80
Cardiovascular system, 21–7
  blood, **24, 25, 26**
  blood clotting, 26, *27*
  blood vessels, 22, **23**
  circulation, *23*–4
  heart, *22*
Caries *see* Dental caries
Cartilage, 18
Cell biology, 4
Cells, *11*, **12**, **13**, 16
  activity, **12**
  fibroblasts, 16
  function, **13**
  histiocytes, 16
  mast cells, 16
  plasma cells, 16
  renewal, 13
Cellular immune response, 102
Cementocytes, 76
Cementum, 75, *76*–7
  chemical composition, 76
  continued deposition, 76
  formation, 71
  functional changes, 76–7
  resorption, 76
  structure, 76
Central nervous system, *33, 34*
Cetylpyridinium chloride, 147
Cheeks, 45
  mastication, 86
Chemical trauma, 135
Chlorhexidine, 93, 94, 95, 147, 148, 228–9, *230*, 260
Chlorinated solutions, 93–4
Circulation, **23**–4
Clinical training, 8
Codeine, 258
Cognitive disability, 186, **187**–8
Collagen, 16, *17*
Complement, 103

Complex restorative dentistry, 190
Concrescence, 170–1
Connective tissue, 16
  white fibrous tissue, 18
Coronary thrombosis, 180–1
Cortical plates, 80
Cranium, 38–9, **40**
Cross-infection, 95–101
  hepatitis viruses, 95, **96**, **97**
  human immunodeficiency viruses, 97, **98**
  minimization of risk, 98, **99**, *100*
  working practices, 100–1
Curette, 206, *207, 208*
  sharpening, *202*
Curve of Spee, 246
Cytokines, 103

Dead tracts, *75*
Debridement, 137–8
Debris index, 150–1
Demonstrations, 267
Dental caries, 5, 119–28
  aetiology, 124–6
    acidogenic hypothesis, 124
    acids and dental caries, *125*
    bacteria and dental caries, 124–5
    proteolysisischelation hypothesis, 124
    proteolytic hypothesis, 124
    sugars and dental caries, 125
  classification, 119–21
    pit-and-fissure caries, 119, *120*, **121**
    root surface caries, 120–1
    smooth-surface caries, 120
  epidemiology, 155–7
    age, 155–6
    distribution within mouth, 156, **157**
    gender, 156
    geographical distribution, 156
  histopathology, **122**, **123**
  pain with, 121
  prevention, 128
  radiographic appearance, 121, *122*
  radiography, *247*
  reactions of dentine and pulp to, 123–4
  secondary factors, 126–8
    diet, 126
    iatrogenic factors, 127–8
    poor oral hygiene, 126
    pregnancy, 128
    saliva, 126, *127*
    teeth, 127
  treatment, 128
Dental lamina, 68, *69*
Dental plaque *see* Plaque
Dentifrices, **176**–7, 223–4
  desensitizing, 224
  fluoride, 22, 176, 234
  ingredients, 223–4
Dentinal tubules, *74*
Dentine, 73–5
  age changes in, 74, *75*
  caries, **123**
    reaction to, 123–4
  chemical composition, 73–4
  formation, 69, *70*

Dentine (*cont.*)
  hypoplasia, 171–2
  interglobular, 74
  nerve endings, 74
  reactionary, 124
  sensitivity, 173–7
    aetiology, 174–5
    clinical features, 173, **174**
    treatment, 175–7
  structure, *74*
  translucent, 75
Dentinogenesis, 69, *70*
Dentures:
  complete, *192*
  partial, 192, *193*
Denture stomatitis, *194*, *195*
Development of dental tissues, 68, *69*–72
  bell stage, 68–9
  cap stage, 68
  cementum formation, 71
  dental lamina, 68
  dentine formation, 69–70
  enamel formation, 69, *70*
  enamel organs, 68
  periodontal ligament, 71
  permanent teeth, *71*
  pulp formation, 70
  reduced enamel epithelium, 71
  root formation, *70*
Diabetic crises, **182**
Diabetic patients, 189–90
Diet, 236–7
  and caries, 126, 236
  and plaque formation, 237
Dietary fibre, 30
Digestive system, 28–33
  alimentary canal, 30, *31*–3
    large intestine, 32
    oral cavity, 30–1
    pharynx and oesophagus, 31
    small intestine, *32*
    stomach, 31–2
  food, 28–30
    carbohydrates, 30
    dietary fibre, 30
    fats, 30
    minerals, 29
    proteins, 30
    vitamins, 29
    water, 29
Dilaceration, 170
Disclosing agents, *217*, **218**
  erythrocin, 218
  fluorescent agents, 218
  iodine, 218
  two-tone agents, 218
Discussion, 267
Disinfectants, 92–5
  aldehyde compounds, 94
  chlorhexidine, 93
  chlorinated solutions, 93–4
  hand disinfectants, 94–5
  instrument and material disinfection, 95
  iodophor compounds, 94
  phenolics, 94
  quaternary ammonium compounds, 93

  surface disinfection, 95
  see also Antimicrobials
Drugs, 256–61
  analgesics, 257–8
    aspirin, 257–8
    codeine compound, 258
    non-steroidal anti-inflammatory compounds, 258
    paracetamol, 258
  antimicrobials, 258–60
    chlorhexidine, 260
    control of bleeding, 260–1
    metronidazole, 260
    penicillin, **259**
    tetracycline, 259–60

Elastic fibres, *17*
  yellow elastic tissue, 18
Elderly patients, 188
Emergencies, 178–84
  management, 178–82
    cardiac arrest, **179**–80
    coronary thrombosis, 180–1
    diabetic crises, **182**
    epileptic fit, 181, **182**
    fainting, 178–9
    instrument breakage, 181
  responsibilities of dental hygienist, 178
  temporary dressings, 183, **184**
Enamel, 72–3
  caries, **122**, *123*
  chemical composition, 72
  formation, 69, *70*
  function, 73
  hypoplasia, *171*–2
  structure, 72, *73*
Enamel lamellae, 72, *73*
Enamel organs, 68
Enamel prisms, 72
Enamel tufts, 72–3
Endocardial disease, 188, **189**
Endocrine system, **35**–6
  adrenals, 36
  gonads, 36
  pancreas, 36
  parathyroids, 35–6
  pituitary, 35
  thyroid, 35
Enrolment, **9**
Epidemiology, 6, 150–7
  dental caries, 155–7
    age, 155–6
    distribution within mouth, 156, **157**
    gender, 156
    geographical distribution, 156
  factors influencing chronic periodontal disease, 154–5
    age, 154–5
    ethnic group, 155
    gender, 155
    systemic disease, 155
  gingival indices, 151–2
    bleeding index, 152
    gingival index, 151–2
    PMA index, 151
  periodontal indices, 152–4
    basic periodontal examination, 152, *153*

Epidemiology (*cont.*)
  mobility index, 153–4
  periodontal index, 152
  periodontal probing, 154
  plaque indices, 150–1
    modified plaque index, 151
    oral hygiene index, 150–1
    plaque index, 151
    simplified oral hygiene index, 151
Epilepsy, 181–2
Epithelium, *14*–16
  ciliated columnar, 14
  simple columnar, 14
  simple squamous (pavement), 14
  stratified or compound squamous, 14, *15*–16
Erosion, 167, *168*
Erythrocin, 218
Ethnicity, and periodontal disease, 155
External oblique line, 246

Facial skeleton, 40, **41**
Fainting, 178–9
Fats, 30
Fibres, 16, *17*
Fibroblasts, 16
Final examination, 8, **9**
Fissure caries, 122, *123*
Fissure sealants, 234, **235**–6
  effectiveness, 235–6
  types of, 235
Floor of mouth, **45**
Flossing, *225, 226, 227*
Fluid exudate, 107
Fluorescent disclosing agents, 218
Fluoridated milk, 232
Fluoridated salt, 232
Fluoride, 229–34
  history of use, 229–31
  systemic, 231
  topical, 232–3
Fluoride dentifrices, 176, 234
Fluoride drops, 231, **232**
Fluoride mouthrinses, 234
Fluoride tablets, 231, **232**
Fluoride varnishes, 175, 234
Fluorosis, 172
Food, 28–30
  carbohydrates, 30
  dietary fibre, 30
  fats, 30
  minerals, 29
  proteins, 30
  vitamins, 29
  water, 29
Formalin dentifrices, 176–7
Foundation course, 4
Fungi, 90
Fusion, 170

Gemination, 170
Gender:
  and dental caries, 156
  and periodontal disease, 155
Genial tubercles, 246

Gingiva, *48*–9, *81*–3
  attached, 81
  bleeding, 132
  changes with inflammation, 82–3
  conditions affecting, *162*–3
  drug induced changes, *163*
  free, 81
  gingival physiology, *83*
  hyperplasia, *163*
  interdental papilla, 81
  structure, 81, **82**
  see also Gingival; Gingivitis
Gingival bleeding index, 152
Gingival crevice, 81, *82*
Gingival indices, 151–2
  bleeding index, 152
  gingival index, 151–2
  PMA index, 151
Gingivitis, 131
  acute allergic, *138, 139*
  acute necrotizing ulcerative, 135, *136*–9
    aetiology, 136
    clinical features, 135–6
    follow-up treatment, 138–9
    localized treatment, 137–8
    local stagnation areas, 137
    mental and physical stress, 136
    smoking, 137
    systemic disease, 136
    systemic effects, 136
    systemic treatment, 137
  acute non-specific, 134
  acute traumatic, 134–5
    chemical trauma, 135
    gingivitis artefacta, *135*
    thermal trauma, 135
    toothbrush damage, 134
  aetiology, 132
  clinical features, 131–2
    bleeding, 132
    colour, 132
    consistency, 132
    form, *132*
    halitosis, 132
    texture, 132
  HIV-associated, 139–40
  management, 133, *134*
  see also Periodontal disease
Gingivitis artefacta, *135*
Glass ionomer cements/resins, 175–6
Gonads, 36
Gums *see* Gingiva

Haemostasis, 26, *27*
Halitosis, 132
Hand disinfectants, 94–5
Heart, *22*
Hepatitis viruses, 95–6, **97**
  hepatitis B vaccines, 97
  hepatitis B virus, 96
  risk groups, 96
  risk of infection, 96
  risk to hygienist, 165
Histiocytes, 16
Histology, 11–20, 68

Histology (*cont.*)
  adipose tissue, 17–18
  areolar tissue, *17*
  body tissues, 14–17
    cells, 16
    connective tissues, 16
    epithelium, *14*, *15*–16
    fibres, 16, *17*
  bone, 18, *19*
  cartilage, 18
  cell, *11*, **12**, **13**
  cell renewal, 13
  microscope, 11
  muscle, 19–20
  nerve, *20*
  training, 4
  white fibrous tissue, 18
  yellow elastic tissue, 18
Histopathology, caries, **122**, *123*
Human immunodeficiency virus, 97, **98**
  and gingivitis, 139–40
  and periodontitis, 146
  risk to hygienist, 165
Humoral immune response, 102
Hydrodynamic theory, 174–75
Hydrogen peroxide, 147
Hypersensitivity, 104
Hypochlorite, 95
Hypodontia, 170

Immune response, *100*, 101, **102**
  abnormalities of, 104–5
  cellular, 102
  components of, 102–3
  humoral, 102
  role in periodontal disease, 104
  see also Immune system
Immune system, 101–5
  acquired immunity, 101, **102**
  immune response *see* Immune response
  innate immunity, 101
  pathogenicity of organisms, 103–4
Immunocompromised patients, 189
Impressions, disinfection, 95
Incisive foramen, 246
Incisors:
  lower central, 62
  lower lateral, 62, *63*
  permanent, *62*, *63*
  upper central, *62*
  upper lateral, *62*
Incremental lines:
  cementum, 76
  dentine, *74*
  enamel, *71*, 72
Inflammation:
  acute, **106**–7
    causes, **106**
    results, 107
    stages, 106–7
  chronic, 107–8
Innate immunity, 101
Instruments, 5
  air/sonic scalers, 206, **207**
  breakage, 181

  care of, **199**, *200*
  disinfection, 95, 99–100
  hand, 203–6
    dental curette, 206, *207*, *208*
    periodontal file, *205*
    periodontal hoe, *205*
    push scaler, 205
    sickle scaler, *204*
  scaling, 203, *204*
  sharpening, *200*, **201**
    techniques, *201*, *202*
  storage, 202–3
  ultrasonic scalers, 206, **207**, *208*, **209**
Interdental brushes, 227
Interdental cleaning, 224–8
  dental floss/tape, *225*, *226*, 227
  interdental/interspace brushes, 227
  interdental woodsticks, 226–7, *228*
  water irrigation units, 227–8
Interdental papilla, 81
Interdental woodsticks, 226–7, *228*
International Dental Federation Classification, **60**
Interspace brushes, 227
Iodine, 95, 218
Iodophor compounds, 94

Keratosis, *160*–1

Lactobacillus acidophilus, 125
Lamina dura, 80, *245*, 246
Large intestine, 32
Lectures, 267
Lichen planus, *161*–2
Lips, 44–5
  mastication, 86
Listerine, 147
Local anaesthesia *see* Analgesia, local
Local analgesia *see* Analgesia
Lungs, 27, *28*
Lymphatic system, 36, *37*
Lymph glands, *57*–8
Lymph nodes, *37*, *57*–8

Macrodontia, 170
Mandible, *42*–3
Mandibular canal, *245*, 246
Mast cells, 16
Mastication, 86, **87**
Maxilla, **41**–2
Maxillary sinus, *245*, 246
Mental foramen, 246
Mesiodens, 170, *171*
Metronidazole, 137, 148, 260
Microbiology, 90–5
  bacteria, **90**, *91*
  disinfectants, 92–5
    aldehyde compounds, 94
    chlorhexidine, 93
    chlorinated solutions, 93–4
    hand disinfectants, 94–5
    instrument and material disinfection, 95
    iodophor compounds, 94
    phenolics, 94

Microbiology (*cont.*)
  quaternary ammonium compounds, 93
  surface disinfection, 95
  fungi, 90
  sterilization, 91, *92*
  training, 5
  viruses, 91
Microdontia, 170
Microscope, 11
Minerals, 29
Minocycline, 148
Mobility index, 153–4
Modified plaque index, 151
Molars:
  lower first, 65, *66*
  lower second, 65, *66*
  lower third, 66
  permanent, 64, *65, 66*
  primary, 56
  upper first, *65*
  upper second, *65*
  upper third, *65*
Motor disabilities, 185, **186**
Mouthrinses, 146–7
Muscles, 19–20
  cardiac, 19–20
  of facial expression, 52–3
  involuntary, 19
  lateral pterygoid, 51, *52*
  masseter, 51, *52*
  of mastication, **51, 52**
  medial pterygoid, 51, *52*
  temporalis, 51, *52*
  of tongue, **47**–8
  voluntary, 19

Nasal cavity, 246
Neoplasia, 108–10
  causes of malignancy, 110
  classification, 108, **109**
  precancerous state, 109–10
Nerves, *20*, 53, *54*, **55**–6
  alveolar branches, *54*
  buccal, **55**, 56
  infraorbital, *54*
  lingual, 56
  mandibular, *54*
  maxillary, *54*
  muscular branches, 56
  palatal, *54*–5
  periodontal ligament, 79
  taste, 86
Nervous system, 33–5
  autonomic nervous system, *34*, **35**
  central nervous system, *33, 34*
  peripheral nervous system, **34**
Neural transmission, *20*
Nifedipine, and gingival hyperplasia, *163*
Non-steroidal anti-inflammatory drugs, 258

Occlusal films, *241*, 242
Odontomes, 171
Odontoblasts, 174, 176
Oesophagus, 31

Oral cavity, 30–1, 44–50
  alveolar ridges and gingiva, *48*–9
  blood supply, *55*, 56–7
  cheeks, 45
  floor of mouth, **45**
  lips, 44–5
  nerve supply, 53, *54*, **55**–6
  palate, 49–50
  tongue, *46*, **47**–8
Oral health education, 7, 262–74
  background, **262**–3
  behavioural change, **263**–5
    factual education, 263
    motivation, **264**
    practical training, 263–4
    reinforcement, 264–5
  delivery, 272
  domains of learning, **263**
  evaluation, 272, **273**
  organization of teaching sessions, **265**–7
    aims and objectives, 266–7
    group, 266
    location, 265–6
    time, 266
  rehearsal, 272
  teaching methods, 267–8
    demonstrations, 267
    discussion, 267
    lectures, 267
    project work, 268
    role-playing, 267–8
    tutorials and seminars, 267
  visual aids, **268**, **269**, *270*–2
    black/whiteboard, 269
    computerized programmes, 269–70
    flash cards, 271
    hand-outs, 271–2
    35 mm slides, 269
    models, 271
    overhead projector, 269
    posters, 271
    sources of, 273–4
    videos, 270–1
Oral hygiene:
  acute necrotizing ulcerative gingivitis, 138
  and caries, 126
  and periodontitis, 144
Oral hygiene index, 150–1
  calculus index, 150
  debris index, 150–1
Oral medicine, 158–66
  bleeding disorders, 164–5
  conditions affecting gingiva, *162*–3
  conditions influencing hygienist treatment, 163–4
    pregnancy, 164
    rheumatic fever, 163–4
  conditions putting hygienist's health at risk, 165, **166**
  drug induced gingival changes, *163*
  lichen planus, *161*–2
  medical history, **158**
  oral ulceration, 158–60
    bullous conditions affecting oral mucosa, 160
    recurrent aphthous ulceration, **159**
    traumatic ulceration, 159
    viral ulceration, 159, *160*
  premalignant and malignant conditions, *161*

Oral medicine (*cont.*)
  systemic conditions, 162
  white patches, *160–1*
Oral physiology, 83
Oral surgery, 195–6
Orthodontics, 196–7
  appliance fitment, 196
  assessment appointment, 196
  completion of active treatment, 196
  recall visits, 196
  review, 196, **197**
Orthopaedic prostheses, 188–9
Osseointegrated implants, 191, *192*
Osteology, 38–44
  cranium, 38–9, **40**
  facial skeleton, 40, **41**
  mandible, *42–3*
  maxilla, *41–2*
  skull, **38**, **39**
  temporomandibular joint, *43*, *44*
Overdentures, 193, *194*

Pain, with carious lesions, 121
Palate, 49–50
  mastication, 87
Pancreas, 36
Panoramic radiographs, *242*
Paracetamol, 258
Parathyroid glands, 35–6
Parotid gland, *50*
Pathogenicity of organisms, 103–4
Pathology, 106–10
  acute inflammation, **106**–7
  chronic inflammation, 107–8
  inflammatory periodontal disease, 129, *130*, *131*
  neoplasia, 108–10
Penicillin, 137, **259**
Periapical films, 240, *241*
  techniques, 243–4
    angulation, 244
    bisecting angle, *243*
    paralleling technique, *244*
Periodontal disease, 5–6, 129–49
  antimicrobials in management of, 146–9
    mouthrinses, 146–7
    subgingival antimicrobials, 147–9
  factors influencing, 154–5
    age, 154–5
    ethnic group, 155
    gender, 155
    systemic disease, 155
  gingivitis, 131
    aetiology, 132
    chronic, 131, *132*
    management, 133, *134*
    types of, 133–4, *135*, *136*–7, *138*, *139*–40
  pathology, 129–31
    advanced lesion, 130, *131*
    early lesion, *130*
    established lesion, 130, *131*
    initial lesion, 129, *130*
  periodontitis, *140*–6
    adult, 142, *143*, *144*
    HIV-associated, 146
    juvenile, *141*, *142*

    prepubertal, *141*
    rapidly progressive, *142*
    refractory, *144*, *145*–6
  prevention of *see* Prevention of dental disease
Periodontal file, *205*
Periodontal hoe, 205
Periodontal indices, 152–4
  basic periodontal examination, 152, *153*–4
  mobility index, 153–4
  periodontal index, 152
Periodontal ligament, 77–80
  blood vessels, 79
  cells, 78, *79*
  development, 71
  fibres, *78*, *79*
  lymphatics, 79, **80**
  nerves, 79
  structure, 77, **78**, *79*, **80**
Periodontal probing, 154
Periodontal screening, 216–17
Periodontitis, *140*–6
  adult, 142, *143*, *144*
  HIV-associated, 146
  juvenile, *141*, *142*
  prepubertal, *141*
  rapidly progressive, *142*
  refractory, *144*–6
    inadequate host response, 145
    inadequate oral hygiene, 144
    management, 145–6
    root surface defects, 144, *145*
    root surface deposits, 144, *145*
    unidentified systemic factors, 145
Peripheral nervous system, **34**
  physiology, **252**, *253*
Permanent teeth, 59, 59–60, 66–7, 89
  canines, *63*
  development, *71*
  eruption, 88
  incisors, *62*, *63*
  molars, 64, *65*, *66*
Personal protection, 99
Phagocytosis, *13*
Pharmacology, training, 5
Pharynx, 31
Phenolics, 94
Phenytoin, and gingival hyperplasia, *163*
Pit-and-fissure caries, 119, *120*, **121**
Pituitary gland, 35
Plaque, 5, 111–13
  composition, *112*, **113**, **114**
  control, 217–23
    brushing frequency, 223
    chemical, 228–9, *230*
    disclosing agents, *217*, **218**
    special brushes, 219, *220*–1
    toothbrush design, 218, *219*
    toothbrushing, 218, 221, *222*–3
  and diet, 237
  formation, *111*, *112*
Plaque indices, 150–1
  modified plaque index, 151
  oral hygiene index, 150–1
  plaque index, 151
  simplified oral hygiene index, 151
Plasma, **24**, **25**

Plasma cells, 16
PMA index, 151
Potassium dentifrices, 176
Pre-clinical training, 7–8
Pregnancy, 164
  and caries, 128
  epulis, *162*
Premolars, *63*, *64*
Prevention of dental disease, 215, *216*–38
  dentifrices, 223–4
  diet, 236–7
  fissure sealants, 234, **235**–6
  fluoride, 229–34
    fluoridated milk and salt, 232
    fluoride dentifrices, 234
    fluoride mouthrinses, 234
    fluoride tablets and drops, 231, **232**
    fluoride varnishes, 234
    history of use, 229–31
    stannous fluoride solutions, 233–4
    systemic fluorides, 231, *235*
    topical fluorides, 232, *233*
  interdental cleaning, 224–8
    dental floss, *225*, *226*, 227
    interdental/interspace brushes, 227
    interdental woodsticks, 226–7, *228*
    water irrigation units, 227–8
  periodontal screening and monitoring, 216–17
  plaque control, *217*–23
    chemical, 228–9, *230*
    disclosing agents, *217*, 218
    special brushes, 219, *220*–1
    toothbrush design, 218, *219*
    toothbrushing, 211, 218, *222*–3
    brushing frequency, 223
Primary teeth, 59, 89
  eruption, *87*–8
  shedding, 88
Professional indemnity, 9, **10**
Project work, 268
Prophyromonas gingivalis, 142
Proteins, 30
Proteolysischelation hypothesis of dental caries, 124
Proteolytic hypothesis of dental caries, 124
Pulp, 61, **77**, 246
  anatomy, **77**
  cells, **77**
  fibres, 77
  formation, 70
  reaction to caries, 123–4
Pulsed oral irrigation, 148
Push scaler, 205
  sharpening, *202*

Quaternary ammonium compounds, 93

Radiography, 6–7, 239–51
  anatomical landmarks, *245*, 246–7
    curve of Spee, 246
    external oblique line, 246
    genial tubercles, 246
    incisive foramen, 246
    lamina dura, *245*, 246
    mandibular canal, *245*, 246

    maxillary sinus, *245*, 246
    mental foramen, 246
    nasal cavity, 246
    orientation of film, 246–7
    pulp, 246
    roots, 246
    zygomatic arch, 246
  caries, 121, *122*
  dental films, 240, *241*–5
    bitewing, *241*, *242*
    density of image, *243*
    exposure of film, 243
    occlusal, *241*, *242*
    panoramic, 242
    periapical, 240, *241*, *243*, *244*
    processing, 244–5
  diagnosing faults, 248–9
  pathology, 247
  production of X-rays, 239, *240*
  regulations, 249–51
  restorations, *247*–8
Red cells, *25*
Removable dental prostheses, 191–4
  complete dentures, *192*
  overdentures, 193, *194*
  partial dentures, 192, *193*
Respiration, 28
Respiratory system, **27**, *28*
  air passages, **27**
  lungs, 27, *28*
  respiration, 28
Restorations, *247*–8
Reticular fibres, 17
Rheumatic fever, 163–4
Role-playing, 267–8
Root planing, 203, *204*
Roots, 61, 246
  formation, *70*
  resorption, 88
Root surface caries, 120–1
Root surface defects, 144, *145*
Root surface deposits, 144, *145*
Rubber dam, 210–14
  application, *212*, *213*, *214*
  equipment, 210, *211*–12
  purpose of, 210

Saliva, **84**, **85**, **86**
  and caries, 126–7
Salivary glands, *50*–1
Salivary pellicle, 111
Sanguinaria, 147
Scalers:
  air/sonic, 206, **207**
  push, 205
  sickle, *204*
Scaling, 203, *204*
Seminars, 267
Sharpey's fibres, 76
Sickle scaler, *204*
  sharpening, *201*, *202*
Siloxane esters, 175
Simplified oral hygiene index, 151
Skull, **38**, **39**
Small intestine, *32*

Smoking, and acute necrotizing ulcerative gingivitis, 137
Smooth-surface caries, 120
Snacking, dangers of, 236
Sodium fluoride dentifrice, 224
Sodium monofluorophosphate dentifrice, 224
Sonic scalers, 206, **207**
Special needs, 185–98
  cleft palate, 197
  cognitive disability, **172**–3, 186
  complex restorative dentistry, 190
  dental bridgework, *190, 191*
  denture stomatitis, *194, 195*
  diabetic patients, 189–90
  endocardial disease and orthopaedic prostheses, 188, **189**
  immunocompromised patients, 189
  motor disabilities, 185, **186**
  older patients, 188
  oral surgery, 195–6
  orthodontic patients, 196, **197**
  osseointegrated implants, 191, *192*
  post-surgical maintenance, 195
  removable dental prostheses, 191–4
    complete dentures, *192*
    overdentures, 193, *194*
    partial dentures, 192, *193*
Sphenomandibular ligament, 43
Stains, 117, **118**
Stannous fluoride, 147, 233–4
  applicators, *233*
  dentifrice, 224
Sterilization, 91–2
  boiling water, 92
  gamma radiation, 92
  heat, 91, *92*
Stomach, 31, **32**
Stratum corneum, 16
Stratum germinativum, 15
Stratum granulosum, 16
Stratum spinosum, 15–16
Streptococcus mitior, **113**
Streptococcus mutans, **113**, 125, 217
Streptococcus salivarius, **113**, 125
Streptococcus sanguis, **113**, 125
Stylomandibular ligament, 43
Sublingual gland, *50*–1
Submandibular gland, *50*
Sugar:
  added, 237
  and caries, 125, 236
  hidden, 236
  substitutes, 237
Suppuration, 107
Surface barriers, 175–6
Surface disinfection, 95

Taste, 85, **86**
Teeth, 59–67
  caries *see* Dental caries
  crown, 60, **61**
  dentine *see* Dentine
  developmental abnormalities, 170–2
    tooth number, 170, *171*
    tooth shape, 170–1
    tooth size, 170
    tooth structure, *171*–2

  eruption and shedding, *87*, **88**, **89**
  identification, **59**
  International Dental Federation Classification, **60**
  permanent, 59
  permanent canines, *63*
  permanent incisors, *62, 63*
  permanent molars, *64, 65, 66*
  premolars, *63, 64*
  primary, 59–60, 66–7
  pulp *see* Pulp
  roots *see* Roots
  structure, *60*–1
  surface wear, 167–70
    abrasion, *169*, **170**
    attrition, 168, *169*
    erosion, 167, *168*
    management of, 169–70
Temporary dressings, 183, **184**
Temporomandibular joint, *43, 44*
Temporomandibular ligament, 43
Tetracycline, 148, 259–60
Thermal trauma, 135
Thyroid gland, 35
Tongue, *46*, **47**–8
  functions, 48
  mastication, 87
  muscles, **47**–8
  surfaces, *46*, **47**
  taste, 85, **86**
Toothbrushes
  design, 218, *219*
  special brushes, 219, *220*–1
Toothbrushing, 218
damage, 134, *169*
  frequency, 223
  techniques, 221–3
    Bass technique, 222
    Charter's technique, 222
    horizontal, 221
    roll technique, 221, *222*
    scrub-brush technique, 222–3
    vertical, 221
Toothpaste, allergic reaction to, *138, 139*
Training, 1–10
  British Dental Hygienists' Association, **10**
  course content, 4–7
  employment, **9**
  enrolment, **9**
  final examination, 8, **9**
  history, 1, **2**
  practical, 7–8
  preparation for employment, 8
  professional indemnity, 9, **10**
  scope of work, 2, **3**
Translucent zone, 124
Traumatic ulceration, 159
Treponema vincenti, 136
Triclosan, 147
Tubular sclerosis, 124
Tutorials, 267
Two-tone disclosing agents, 218

Ulceration, 158–60
  recurrent aphthous ulceration, **159**
  traumatic ulceration, 159

Ulceration (*cont.*)
   viral ulceration, 159, *160*
Ultrasonic scalers, 206, **207**, *208*, **209**

Veins, 23
Venous drainage, 57
Viral ulceration, 159, *160*
Viruses, 91
   hepatitis, 95–7
   human immunodeficiency virus, 97, **98**
Visual aids, **268**, **269**, *270*–2
   black/whiteboard, 269
   computerized programmes, 269–70
   flash cards, 271
   hand-outs, 271
   35 mm slides, 269
   models, 271
   overhead projector, 269

   posters, 271
   sources of, 273–4
   videos, 270–1
Vitamins, 29

Water, 29
Water irrigation units, 227–8
White cells, *25*, **26**
White fibrous tissue, 18
White patches, *160*–1
Working practices, 100–1

Yellow elastic tissue, 18

Zygomatic arch, 246